Pain Management

Pain Management

Edited by Kieron Gillen

hayle medical

New York

Hayle Medical,
750 Third Avenue, 9th Floor,
New York, NY 10017, USA

Visit us on the World Wide Web at:
www.haylemedical.com

ISBN: 978-1-63241-511-0

Printed in China.

Cataloging-in-Publication Data

Pain management / edited by Kieron Gillen.
p. cm.
Includes bibliographical references and index.
ISBN 978-1-63241-511-0
1. Pain--Treatment. 2. Pain medicine. I. Gillen, Kieron.
RB127 .P35 2018
616.047 2--dc23

Table of Contents

Preface

As a branch of medicine science, pain management refers to the practice and study of improving the quality of life for people suffering from chronic pain. The primary treatment of pain includes drugs such as analgesics, anticonvulsants, etc. Other common treatment methods include physical therapy and rehabilitation such as acupuncture, transcutaneous electrical nerve simulation, etc. This book elucidates the concepts and innovative models around prospective developments with respect to pain management. It discusses in detail all the theories and concepts used under this area. It is a valuable compilation of topics, ranging from the basic to the most complex theories and principles in the field of pain management.

A detailed account of the significant topics covered in this book is provided below:

Chapter 1- The branch of medicine concerned with decreasing the pain of a patient and improving their quality of life is known as pain management. It mostly includes pharmacists, physiotherapists, occupational therapists, nurse practitioners and clinical nurse specialists. The chapter on pain management offers an insightful focus, keeping in mind the complex subject matter.

Chapter 2- Pain is a feeling of discomfort or of distress. The different types of pain are back pain, chronic pain, neuropathic pain, psychogenic pain, phantom pain, etc. The topics discussed in the chapter are of great importance to broaden the existing knowledge on pain.

Chapter 3- Pain scale is the measurement of pain that a patient is suffering. The measurement can be done by observing the patient, self-report or physiological data. Schmidt sting pain index, pain tolerance, pain assessment, pain ladder, etc. are some of the other indicators of pain and its management. The aspects elucidated in this chapter are of vital importance, and provide a better understanding of pain scale and assessment.

Chapter 4- Analgesics or painkillers, are drugs given to patients to reduce their pain. These medicines are prescribed to the patient on the bases of the type of pain. Analgesics mainly include morphine, opioid drugs and nonsteroidal anti-inflammatory drugs. This chapter will provide an integrated understanding of analgesic.

Chapter 5- Anesthesia is given to a patient to temporarily make them unconscious. It can be of various types like general anesthesia, local anesthesia and spinal anesthesia. This chapter is an overview of the subject matter incorporating all the major aspects of anesthesia.

It gives me an immense pleasure to thank our entire team for their efforts. Finally in the end, I would like to thank my family and colleagues who have been a great source of inspiration and support.

Editor

1

An Introduction to Pain Management

The branch of medicine concerned with decreasing the pain of a patient and improving their quality of life is known as pain management. It mostly includes pharmacists, physiotherapists, occupational therapists, nurse practitioners and clinical nurse specialists. The chapter on pain management offers an insightful focus, keeping in mind the complex subject matter.

Pain Management

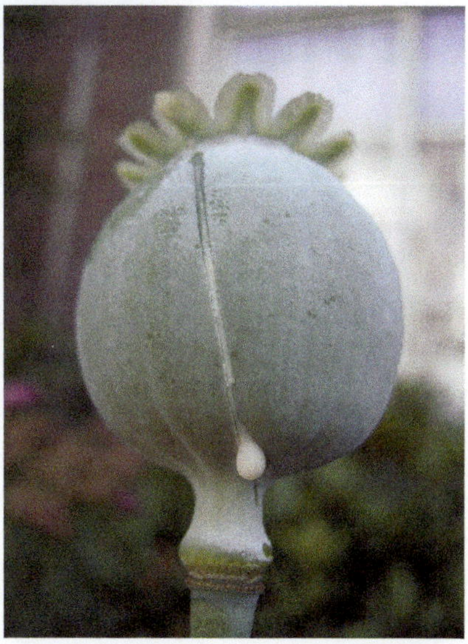

Opium poppies such as this one provide ingredients for the class of analgesics called opiates

Pain management, pain medicine, pain control or algiatry, is a branch of medicine employing an interdisciplinary approach for easing the suffering and improving the quality of life of those living with chronic pain The typical pain management team includes medical practitioners, pharmacists, clinical psychologists, physiotherapists, occupational therapists, physician assistants, nurse practitioners, and clinical nurse specialists. The team may also include other mental health specialists and massage therapists. Pain sometimes resolves promptly once the underlying trauma or pathology has healed, and is treated by one practitioner, with drugs such as analgesics and (occasionally) anxiolytics. Effective management of chronic (long-term) pain, however, frequently requires the coordinated efforts of the management team.

Medicine treats injury and pathology to support and speed healing; and treats distressing symptoms such as pain to relieve suffering during treatment and healing. When a painful injury or pathology is resistant to treatment and persists, when pain persists after the injury or pathology has healed, and when medical science cannot identify the cause of pain, the task of medicine is to relieve suffering. Treatment approaches to chronic pain include pharmacological measures, such as analgesics, antidepressants and anticonvulsants, interventional procedures, physical therapy, physical exercise, application of ice and/or heat, and psychological measures, such as biofeedback and cognitive behavioral therapy.

Uses

Pain can have many causes and there are many possible treatments for it. In the nursing profession, one common definition of pain is any problem that is "whatever the experiencing person says it is, existing whenever the experiencing person says it does". Different sorts of pain management address different sorts of pain.

Pain management includes patient communication about the pain problem. To define the pain problem, a health care provider will likely ask questions such as these:

- How intense is the pain?
- How does the pain feel?
- Where is the pain?
- What, if anything, makes the pain lessen?
- When did the pain start?

After asking questions such as these, the health care provider will have a description of the pain. Pain management will then be used to address that pain.

Adverse Effects

There are many types of pain management, and each of them have their own benefits, drawbacks, and limits.

A common difficulty in pain management is communication. People experiencing pain may have difficulty recognizing or describing what they feel and how intense it is. Health care providers and patients may have difficulty communicating with each other about how pain responds to treatments. There is a continuing risk in many types of pain management for the patient to take treatment which is less effective than needed or which causes other difficulty and side effects. Some treatments for pain can be harmful if overused. A goal of pain management for the patient and their health care provider to identify the amount of treatment which addresses the pain but which is not too much treatment.

Another problem with pain management is that pain is the body's natural way of communicating a problem. Pain is supposed to resolve as the body heals itself with time and pain management. Sometimes pain management covers a problem, and the patient might be less aware that they need treatment for a deeper problem.

Physical Approach

Physical Medicine and Rehabilitation

Physical medicine and rehabilitation employs diverse physical techniques such as thermal agents and electrotherapy, as well as therapeutic exercise and behavioral therapy, alone or in tandem with interventional techniques and conventional pharmacotherapy to treat pain, usually as part of an interdisciplinary or multidisciplinary program.

TENS

Transcutaneous electrical nerve stimulation has been found to be ineffective for lower back pain, however, it might help with diabetic neuropathy. Although there has not been adequate evidence based research on acute sensory TENS, chronic conditions are efficacious in relieving pain. TENS is indicated for any chronic musculoskeletal condition under the gate control theory of pain. Essentially, the gate control theory states that sensory fibers carry their signal faster than pain fibers, and thus make their way to the dorsal root ganglion of the spine (the gate) much faster. This in turn causes the pain signal to be blocked by the sensory TENS signal. This theory explains why rubbing a stubbed toe relieves pain. A study conducted by Oncel M and team compared the efficacy of TENS with a non-steroidal anti-inflammatory drug (NSAID, Naproxen sodium) in patients who had patients with uncomplicated minor rib fractures. The researchers found that TENS therapy given twice a day for 3 days resulted in significant pain reduction and was found to be more effective than NSAID or placebo.

Acupuncture

Acupuncture involves the insertion and manipulation of needles into specific points on the body to relieve pain or for therapeutic purposes. An analysis of the 13 highest quality studies of pain treatment with acupuncture, published in January 2009 in the *British Medical Journal*, was unable to quantify the difference in the effect on pain of real, sham and no acupuncture.

Acupuncture is believed by its followers to restore the energy balance in the body through stimulation of energy channels called the meridians. It is believed acupuncture therapy reduces pain signals through production of endorphins that are known to be the natural painkillers. Clinical studies suggest that acupuncture can reduce joint pain and so the therapy can be effective in reducing pain caused by knee osteoarthritis.

Light Therapy

Research has not found evidence that light therapy such as low level laser therapy is an effective therapy for relieving low back pain.

Interventional Procedures

Interventional procedures - typically used for chronic back pain - include epidural steroid injections, facet joint injections, neurolytic blocks, spinal cord stimulators and intrathecal drug delivery system implants.

Pulsed radiofrequency, neuromodulation, direct introduction of medication and nerve ablation may be used to target either the tissue structures and organ/systems responsible for persistent nociception or the nociceptors from the structures implicated as the source of chronic pain.

An intrathecal pump used to deliver very small quantities of medications directly to the spinal fluid. This is similar to epidural infusions used in labour and postoperatively. The major differences are that it is much more common for the drug to be delivered into the spinal fluid (intrathecal) rather than epidurally, and the pump can be fully implanted under the skin. Interestingly, it is suggested this approach allows a smaller dose of the drug to be delivered directly to the site of action, with fewer systemic side effects, which is thus therapeutically questionable due to the fact that the three main opioid receptors; chiefly the [μ-,κ-,and δ (Mu-,Kappa-, and Delta- respectively] are limited in their anatomical locations. The 3 main receptors are found dominantly within the brain, CNS and Digestive tract.

A spinal cord stimulator is an implantable medical device that creates electric impulses and applies them near the dorsal surface of the spinal cord provides a paresthesia ("tingling") sensation that alters the perception of pain by the patient.

A small number of patients, especially those with severe pain from untreatable cancer, may benefit surgical treatment such as cordotomy.

Psychological Approach

Cognitive Behavioral Therapy

Cognitive behavioral therapy (CBT) for pain helps patients with pain to understand the relationship between one's physiology (e.g., pain and muscle tension), thoughts, emotions, and behaviors. A main goal in treatment is cognitive restructuring to encourage helpful thought patterns, targeting a behavioral activation of healthy activities such as regular exercise and pacing. Lifestyle changes are also trained to improve sleep patterns and to develop better coping skills for pain and other stressors using various techniques (e.g., relaxation, diaphragmatic breathing, and even biofeedback).

Studies have demonstrated the usefulness of cognitive behavioral therapy in the management of chronic low back pain, producing significant decreases in physical and psychosocial disability. A study published in the January 2012 issue of the *Archives of Internal Medicine* found CBT is significantly more effective than standard care in treatment of people with body-wide pain, like fibromyalgia. Evidence for the usefulness of CBT in the management of adult chronic pain is generally poorly understood, due partly to the proliferation of techniques of doubtful quality, and the poor quality of reporting in clinical trials. The crucial content of individual interventions has not been isolated and the important contextual elements, such as therapist training and development of treatment manuals, have not been determined. The widely varying nature of the resulting data makes useful systematic review and meta-analysis within the field very difficult.

In 2012, a systematic review of randomized controlled trials (RCTs) evaluated the clinical effectiveness of psychological therapies for the management of adult chronic pain (excluding headaches). There is no evidence that behaviour therapy (BT) is effective for reducing this type of pain, however BT may be useful for improving a persons mood immediately after treatment. This improvement appears to be small, and is short term in duration. CBT may have a small positive short-term effect on pain immediately following treatment. CBT may also have a small effect on reducing disability and potential catastrophizing that may be associated with adult chronic pain. These benefits do not appear to last very long following the therapy. CBT may contribute towards improving the mood of an adult who experiences chronic pain, and there is a possibility that this benefit may be maintained for longer periods of time.

For children and adolescents, a review of RCTs evaluating the effectiveness of psychological therapy for the management of chronic and recurrent pain found that psychological treatments are effective in reducing pain when people under 18 years old have headaches. This beneficial effect may be maintained for at least three months following the therapy. Psychological treatments may also improve pain control for children or adolescents who experience pain not related to headaches. It is not known if psychological therapy improves a child or adolescents mood and the potential for disability related to their chronic pain.

Hypnosis

A 2007 review of 13 studies found evidence for the efficacy of hypnosis in the reduction of pain in some conditions, though the number of patients enrolled in the studies was small, bringing up issues of power to detect group differences, and most lacked credible controls for placebo and/or expectation. The authors concluded that "although the findings provide support for the general applicability of hypnosis in the treatment of chronic pain, considerably more research will be needed to fully determine the effects of hypnosis for different chronic-pain conditions."

Hypnosis has reduced the pain of some noxious medical procedures in children and adolescents, and in clinical trials addressing other patient groups it has significantly reduced pain compared to no treatment or some other non-hypnotic interventions. However, no studies have compared hypnosis to a convincing placebo, so the pain reduction may be due to patient expectation (the "placebo effect"). The effects of self hypnosis on chronic pain are roughly comparable to those of progressive muscle relaxation.

Mindfulness Meditation

A meta-analysis of studies that used techniques centered around the concept of mindfulness, concluded, "Findings suggest that MBIs decrease the intensity of pain for chronic pain patients."

Medications

The World Health Organization (WHO) recommends a *pain ladder* for managing analgesia. It was first described for use in cancer pain, but it can be used by medical professionals as a general principle when dealing with analgesia for any type of pain. In the treatment of chronic pain, whether due to malignant or benign processes, the three-step WHO Analgesic Ladder provides guidelines for selecting the kind and stepping up the amount of analgesia. The exact medications recommended will vary with the country and the individual treatment center, but the following gives an example of the WHO approach to treating chronic pain with medications. If, at any point, treatment fails to provide adequate pain relief, then the doctor and patient move onto the next step.

Common types of pain and typical drug management		
Pain type	**typical initial drug treatment**	**comments**
headache	paracetamol /acetaminophen, NSAIDs	doctor consultation is appropriate if headaches are severe, persistent, accompanied by fever, vomiting, or speech or balance problems; self-medication should be limited to two weeks
migraine	paracetamol, NSAIDs	triptans are used when the others do not work, or when migraines are frequent or severe
menstrual cramps	NSAIDs	some NSAIDs are marketed for cramps, but any NSAID would work
minor trauma, such as a bruise, abrasions, sprain	paracetamol, NSAIDs	opioids not recommended
severe trauma, such as a wound, burn, bone fracture, or severe sprain	opioids	more than two weeks of pain requiring opioid treatment is unusual
strain or pulled muscle	NSAIDs, muscle relaxants	if inflammation is involved, NSAIDs may work better; short-term use only

Common types of pain and typical drug management		
Pain type	**typical initial drug treatment**	**comments**
minor pain after surgery	paracetamol, NSAIDs	opioids rarely needed
severe pain after surgery	opioids	combinations of opioids may be prescribed if pain is severe
muscle ache	paracetamol, NSAIDs	if inflammation involved, NSAIDs may work better.
toothache or pain from dental procedures	paracetamol, NSAIDs	this should be short term use; opioids may be necessary for severe pain
kidney stone pain	paracetamol, NSAIDs, opioids	opioids usually needed if pain is severe.
pain due to heartburn or gastroesophageal reflux disease	antacid, H2 antagonist, proton-pump inhibitor	heartburn lasting more than a week requires medical attention; aspirin and NSAIDs should be avoided
chronic back pain	paracetamol, NSAIDs	opioids may be necessary if other drugs do not control pain and pain is persistent
osteoarthritis pain	paracetamol, NSAIDs	medical attention is recommended if pain persists.
fibromyalgia	antidepressant, anticonvulsant	evidence suggests that opioids are not effective in treating fibromyalgia

Mild Pain

Paracetamol (acetaminophen), or a non-steroidal anti-inflammatory drug (NSAID) such as ibuprofen.

Mild to Moderate Pain

Paracetamol, an NSAID and/or paracetamol in a combination product with a weak opioid such as tramadol, may provide greater relief than their separate use. Also a combination of opioid with acetaminophen can be frequently used such as Percocet, Vicodin, or Norco.

Moderate to Severe Pain

When treating moderate to severe pain, the type of the pain, acute or chronic, needs to be considered. The type of pain can result in different medications being prescribed. Certain medications may work better for acute pain, others for chronic pain, and some may work equally well on both. Acute pain medication is for rapid onset of pain such as from an inflicted trauma or to treat post-operative pain. Chronic pain medication is for alleviating long-lasting, ongoing pain.

Morphine is the gold standard to which all narcotics are compared. Semi-synthetic derivatives of morphine such as hydromorphone (Dilaudid), oxymorphone (Numorphan, Opana), nicomorphine (Vilan), hydromorphinol and others vary in such ways as duration of action, side effect profile and milligramme potency. Fentanyl has the benefit of less histamine release and thus fewer side effects. It can also be administered via transdermal patch which is convenient for chronic pain management. In addition to the intrathecal patch and injectable Sublimaze, the FDA has approved various immediate release fentanyl products for breakthrough cancer pain (Actiq/OTFC/Fentora/Onsolis/Subsys/Lazanda/Abstral). Oxycodone is used across the Americas and Europe for relief of serious chronic pain; its main slow-release formula is known as OxyContin, and short-acting tablets, capsules, syrups and ampules are available making it suitable for acute intractable pain or breakthrough pain. Diamorphine, methadone and buprenorphine are used less frequently. Pethidine, known in North America as meperidine, is not recommended for pain management due to its low potency, short duration of action, and toxicity associated with repeated use. Pentazocine, dextromoramide and dipipanone are also not recommended in new patients except for acute pain where other analgesics are not tolerated or are inappropriate, for pharmacological and misuse-related reasons. In some countries potent synthetics such as piritramide and ketobemidone are used for severe pain, and tapentadol is a newer agent introduced in the last decade.

For moderate pain, tramadol, codeine, dihydrocodeine, and hydrocodone are used, with nicocodeine, ethylmorphine and propoxyphene and dextropropoxyphene less commonly.

Drugs of other types can be used to help opioids combat certain types of pain, for example, amitriptyline is prescribed for chronic muscular pain in the arms, legs, neck and lower back with an opiate, or sometimes without it and/or with an NSAID.

While opiates are often used in the management of chronic pain, high doses are associated with an increased risk of opioid overdose.

Opioids

From the Food and Drug Administration's website: "According to the National Institutes of Health, studies have shown that properly managed medical use of opioid analgesic compounds (taken exactly as prescribed) is safe, can manage pain effectively, and rarely causes addiction."

Opioid medications can provide short, intermediate or long acting analgesia depending upon the specific properties of the medication and whether it is formulated as an extended release drug. Opioid medications may be administered orally, by injection, via nasal mucosa or oral mucosa, rectally, transdermally, intravenously, epidurally and intrathecally. In chronic pain conditions that are opioid responsive a combination of a long-acting (OxyContin, MS Contin, Opana ER, Exalgo and Methadone) or extended release medication is often prescribed in conjunction with a shorter-acting medication (oxycodone, morphine or hydromorphone) for breakthrough pain, or exacerbations.

Most opioid treatment used by patients outside of healthcare settings is oral (tablet, capsule or liquid), but suppositories and skin patches can be prescribed. An opioid injection is rarely needed for patients with chronic pain.

Although opioids are strong analgesics, they do not provide complete analgesia regardless of whether the pain is acute or chronic in origin. Opioids are efficacious analgesics in chronic malignant pain and modestly effective in nonmalignant pain management. However, there are associated adverse effects, especially during the commencement or change in dose. When opioids are used for prolonged periods drug tolerance, chemical dependency, diversion and addiction may occur.

Clinical guidelines for prescribing opioids for chronic pain have been issued by the American Pain Society and the American Academy of Pain Medicine. Included in these guidelines is the importance of assessing the patient for the risk of substance abuse, misuse, or addiction; a personal or family history of substance abuse is the strongest predictor of aberrant drug-taking behavior. Physicians who prescribe opioids should integrate this treatment with any psychotherapeutic intervention the patient may be receiving. The guidelines also recommend monitoring not only the pain but also the level of functioning and the achievement of therapeutic goals. The prescribing physician should be suspicious of abuse when a patient reports a reduction in pain but has no accompanying improvement in function or progress in achieving identified goals.

Commonly-used long-acting opioids and their parent compound:

- OxyContin (oxycodone)
- Hydromorph Contin (hydromorphone)
- MS Contin (morphine)
- M-Eslon (morphine)
- Exalgo (hydromorphone)
- Opana ER (oxymorphone)
- Duragesic (fentanyl)
- Nucynta ER (tapentadol)
- Metadol/Methadose (methadone)*
- Hysingla ER (hydrocodone bitartrate)
- Zohydro ER (hydrocodone bicarbonate)

*Methadone can be used for either treatment of opioid addiction/detoxification when taken once daily or as a pain medication usually administered on an every 12-hour or 8-hour dosing interval.

Non-steroidal anti-inflammatory Drugs

The other major group of analgesics are non-steroidal anti-inflammatory drugs (NSAID). Acetaminophen/paracetamol is not always included in this class of medications. However, acetaminophen may be administered as a single medication or in combination with other analgesics (both NSAIDs and opioids). The alternatively prescribed NSAIDs such as ketoprofen and piroxicam have limited benefit in chronic pain disorders and with long-term use are associated with significant adverse effects. The use of selective NSAIDs designated as selective COX-2 inhibitors have significant cardiovascular and cerebrovascular risks which have limited their utilization.

Antidepressants and Antiepileptic Drugs

Some antidepressant and antiepileptic drugs are used in chronic pain management and act primarily within the pain pathways of the central nervous system, though peripheral mechanisms have been attributed as well. These mechanisms vary and in general are more effective in neuropathic pain disorders as well as complex regional pain syndrome. Drugs such as gabapentin have been widely prescribed for the off-label use of pain control. The list of side effects for these classes of drugs are typically much longer than opiate or NSAID treatments for chronic pain, and many antiepileptics cannot be suddenly stopped without the risk of seizure.

Cannabinoids

Chronic pain is one of the most commonly cited reasons for the use of medical marijuana. A 2012 Canadian survey of participants in their medical marijuana program found that 84% of respondents reported using medical marijuana for the management of pain.

Evidence of medical marijuana's pain mitigating effects is generally conclusive. Detailed in a 1999 report by the Institute of Medicine, "the available evidence from animal and human studies indicates that cannabinoids can have a substantial analgesic effect". In a 2013 review study published in *Fundamental & Clinical Pharmacology*, various studies were cited in demonstrating that cannabinoids exhibit comparable effectiveness to opioids in models of acute pain and even greater effectiveness in models of chronic pain.

Other Analgesics

Other drugs are often used to help analgesics combat various types of pain, and parts of the overall pain experience, and are hence called adjuvant medications. Gabapentin—an anti-epileptic—not only exerts effects alone on neuropathic pain, but can potentiate opiates. While perhaps not prescribed as such, other drugs such as Tagamet (cimetidine) and even simple grapefruit juice may also potentiate opiates, by inhibiting

CYP450 enzymes in the liver, thereby slowing metabolism of the drug. In addition, orphenadrine, cyclobenzaprine, trazodone and other drugs with anticholinergic properties are useful in conjunction with opioids for neuropathic pain. Orphenadrine and cyclobenzaprine are also muscle relaxants, and therefore particularly useful in painful musculoskeletal conditions. Clonidine has found use as an analgesic for this same purpose, and all of the mentioned drugs potentiate the effects of opioids overall.

Society and Culture

Undertreatment

Undertreatment of pain is the absence of pain management therapy for a person in pain when treatment is indicated.

Consensus in evidence-based medicine and the recommendations of medical specialty organizations establish the guidelines which determine the treatment for pain which health care providers ought to offer. For various social reasons, persons in pain may not seek or may not be able to access treatment for their pain. At the same time, health care providers may not provide the treatment which authorities recommend.

In Children

Acute pain is common in children and adolescents as a result of injury, illness, or necessary medical procedures. Chronic pain is present in approximately 15–25% of children and adolescents, and may be caused by an underlying disease, such as sickle cell anemia, cystic fibrosis, rheumatoid arthritis, or cancer or by functional disorders such as migraines, fibromyalgia, or complex regional pain.

Assessment

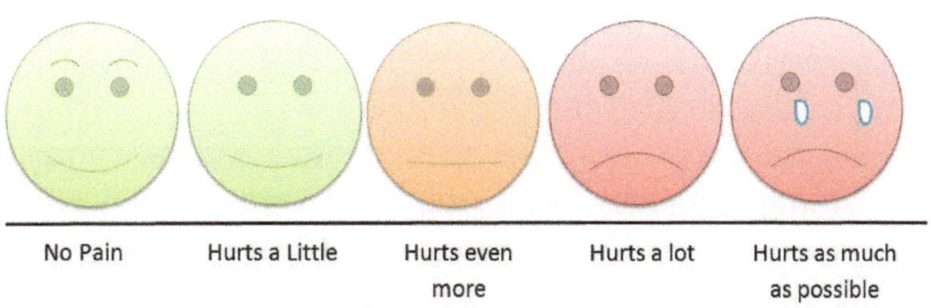

Young children can indicate their level of pain by pointing to the appropriate face on a children's pain scale.

Pain assessment in children is often challenging due to limitations in developmental level, cognitive ability, or their previous pain experiences. Clinicians must observe physiological and behavioral cues exhibited by the child to make an assessment. Self-report, if possible, is the most accurate measure of pain; self-report pain scales developed for young children involve matching their pain intensity to photographs of other children's faces, such as the Oucher Scale, pointing to schematics of faces showing different pain levels, or pointing out the location of pain on a body outline. Questionnaires for older children and adolescents include the Varni-Thompson Pediatric Pain Questionnaire (PPQ) and the Children's Comprehensive Pain Questionnaire, which are often utilized for individuals with chronic or persistent pain.

Nonpharmacologic

Caregivers may provide nonpharmacological treatment for children and adolescents because it carries minimal risk and is cost effective compared to pharmacological treatment. Nonpharmacologic interventions vary by age and developmental factors. Physical interventions to ease pain in infants include swaddling, rocking, or sucrose via a pacifier, whereas those for children and adolescents include hot or cold application, massage, or acupuncture. Cognitive behavioral therapy (CBT) aims to reduce the emotional distress and improve the daily functioning of school-aged children and adolescents with pain through focus on changing the relationship between their thoughts and emotions in addition to teaching them adaptive coping strategies. Integrated interventions in CBT include relaxation technique, mindfulness, biofeedback, and acceptance (in the case of chronic pain). Many therapists will hold sessions for caregivers to provide them with effective management strategies.

Pharmacologic

Acetaminophen, nonsteroidal anti-inflammatory agents, and opioid analgesics are commonly used to treat acute or chronic pain symptoms in children and adolescents, but a pediatrician should be consulted before administering any medication.

Professional Certification

Pain management practitioners come from all fields of medicine. In addition to medical practitioners, a pain management team may often benefit from the input of pharmacists, physiotherapists, clinical psychologists and occupational therapists, among others. Together the multidisciplinary team can help create a package of care suitable to the patient.

Pain physicians are often fellowship-trained board-certified anesthesiologists, neurologists, physiatrists or psychiatrists. Palliative care doctors are also specialists in pain management. The American Board of Anesthesiology, the American Osteopathic Board of Anesthesiology (recognized by the AOABOS), the American Board of Physical Medicine and Rehabilitation, and the American Board of Psychiatry and Neurology each provide certification for a subspecialty in pain management following fellowship training which is recognized by the American Board of Medical Specialties (ABMS) or the American Osteopathic Association Bureau of Osteopathic Specialists (AOABOS). As the field of pain medicine has grown rapidly, many practitioners have entered the field, some non-ACGME board-certified.

Interventional Pain Management

Interventional pain management or interventional pain medicine is a medical subspecialty which treats pain with invasive interventions such as facet joint injections, nerve blocks (interrupting the flow of pain signals along specific nervous system pathways), neuroaugmentation (including spinal cord stimulation and peripheral nerve stimulation), vertebroplasty, kyphoplasty, nucleoplasty, endoscopic discectomy and implantable drug delivery systems.

History

Early efforts at interventional pain management date back to the origins of regional analgesia and neural blockade, and gradually evolved into a distinct specialty. Tuffer described the first therapeutic nerve block for pain management in 1899. Von Gaza developed diagnostic blockade in pain management, using procaine for determining the pain's pathways. Modern day contributors include Bonica, Winnie, Raj, Racz, Bogduk, and others. The term "interventional pain management" was first used by pain management specialist Steven D. Waldman in 1996 to define the emerging specialty. The subspecialty of interventional pain management has received a specific specialty designation by the United States National Uniform Billing Committeeto allow its practitioners to bill Federal healthcare programs including Medicare and Medicaid. Physicians who practice interventional pain management are represented by a variety of pain management organizations including the Society For Pain Practice Management and the American Society of Interventional Pain Physicians.

Radiation

Radiotherapy is used when drug treatment is failing to control the pain of a growing tumor, such as in bone metastisis (most commonly), penetration of soft tissue, or compression of sensory nerves. Often, low doses are adequate to produce analgesia, thought to be due to reduction in pressure or, possibly, interference with the tumor's production of pain-promoting chemicals. Radiopharmaceuticals that target specific tumors have been used to treat the pain of metastatic illnesses. Relief may occur within a week of treatment and may last from two to four months.

Neurolytic Block

A neurolytic block is the deliberate injury of a nerve by the application of chemicals (in which case the procedure is called "neurolysis") or physical agents such as freezing or heating ("neurotomy"). These interventions cause degeneration of the nerve's fibers and temporary interference with the transmission of pain signals. In these procedures, the thin protective layer around the nerve fiber, the basal lamina, is preserved so that, as a damaged fiber regrows, it travels within its basal lamina tube and connects with the correct loose end, and function may be restored. Surgically cutting a nerve severs these basal lamina tubes, and without them to channel the regrowing fibers to their lost connections, a painful neuroma or deafferentation pain pain may develop. This is why the neurolytic is preferred over the surgical block.

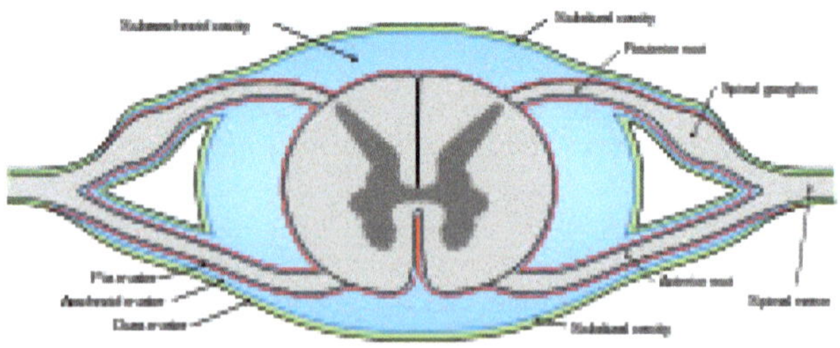

Cross section of the spinal cord showing the subarachnoid cavity, and spinal nerve roots including the dorsal root ganglion

Cutting or Destruction of Nervous Tissue

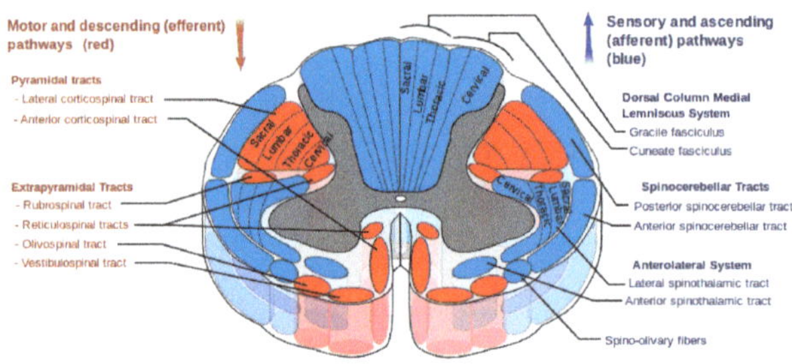

Cross-section of the spinal cord showing the dorsal column and the anterolateral spinothalamic tracts

Surgical cutting or destruction of peripheral or central nervous tissue is now rarely used in the treatment of pain. Procedures include neurectomy, cordotomy, dorsal root entry zone lesioning, and cingulotomy.

Neurectomy involves cutting a nerve, and is (rarely) used in patients with short life expectancy who are unsuitable for drug therapy due to ineffectiveness or intolerance. The dorsal root or dorsal root ganglion (that carry mostly sensory signals) may be usefully targeted (called rhizotomy); with the dorsal root ganglion possibly the more effective target because some sensory fibers enter the spinal cord from the dorsal root ganglion via the *ventral* (motor) root, and these would not be interrupted by dorsal root neurectomy. Because nerves often carry both sensory and motor fibers, motor impairment is a possible side effect of neurectomy. A common result of this procedure is "deafferentation pain" where, 6–9 months after surgery, pain returns at greater intensity.

Cordotomy involves cutting into the spinothalamic tracts, which run up the front/side (anterolateral) quadrant of the spinal cord, carrying heat and pain signals to the brain.

Pancoast tumor pain has been effectively treated with dorsal root entry zone (DREZ) lesioning – damaging a region of the spinal cord where peripheral pain signals cross to spinal cord fibers. This is major surgery, carrying the risk of significant neurological side effects.

Cingulotomy involves cutting the fibers that carry signals directly from the cingulate gyrus to the entorhinal cortex in the brain. It reduces the unpleasantness of pain (without affecting its intensity), but may have cognitive side effects.

Intrathecal Infusion

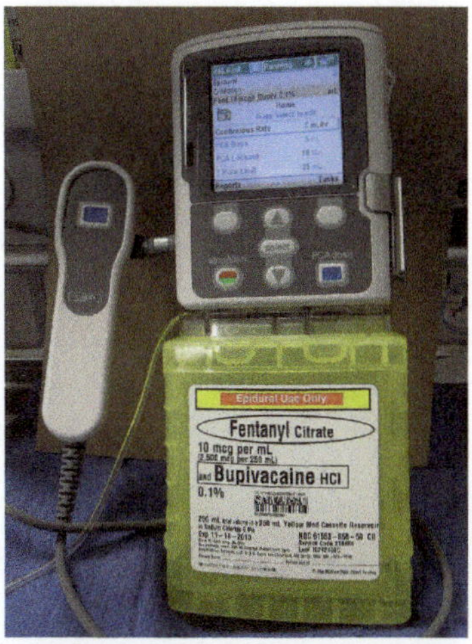

A patient-controlled analgesia infusion pump, configured for epidural administration of fentanyl and bupivacaine

Delivery of an opioid such as morphine, hydromorphone, fentanyl, sufentanyl or meperidine directly into the subarachnoid cavity (the space between the spinal cord's inner, waterproof sheath and its outer protective sheaths) provides enhanced analgesia with reduced systemic side effects, and has reduced the level of pain in otherwise intractable cases. The anxiolytic clonidine, or the nonopioid analgesic ziconotide, and local anesthetics such as bupivacaine, ropivacaine or tetracaine may also be infused along with the opioid.

Epidural Infusion

The outermost, protective sheath surrounding the spinal cord is called the dura mater. Between this and the surrounding vertebrae is the epidural space, filled with connective tissue, fat and blood vessels, and crossed by the spinal nerve roots. A catheter may be inserted into this space for three to six months, to deliver anesthetics or analgesics. The line carrying the drug may be threaded under the skin to emerge at the front of the patient, a process called tunneling. This is recommended with long term use so as to reduce the chance of any infection at the exit site reaching the epidural space.

Spinal Cord Stimulation

Electrical stimulation of the dorsal columns of the spinal cord can produce analgesia. First, the leads are implanted, guided by the patient's report and fluoroscopy, and the generator is worn externally for several days to assess efficacy. If pain is reduced by more than half, the therapy is deemed to be suitable. A small pocket is cut into the tissue beneath the skin of the upper buttocks, chest wall or abdomen and the leads are threaded under the skin from the stimulation site to the pocket, where they are attached to the snugly-fitting generator. It seems to be more helpful with neuropathic and ischemic pain than nociceptive pain, and is not often used in the treatment of cancer pain.

Deep Brain Stimulation

Ongoing electrical stimulation of structures deep within the brain – the periaqueductal gray and periventricular gray for nociceptive pain, and the internal capsule, ventral posterolateral nucleus and ventral posteromedial nucleus for neuropathic pain – has produced impressive results with some patients but results vary and appropriate patient selection is important. One study of seventeen patients with intractable cancer pain found that thirteen were virtually painless and only four required opioid analgesics on release from hospital after the intervention. Most ultimately did resort to opioids, usually in the last few weeks of life.

Hypophysectomy

Hypophysectomy is the destruction of the pituitary gland, and has been used successfully on metastatic breast and prostate cancer pain.

Undertreatment of Pain

Undertreatment of pain is the absence of pain management therapy for a person in pain when treatment is indicated.

Consensus in evidence-based medicine and the recommendations of medical specialty organizations establish the guidelines which determine the treatment for pain which health care providers ought to offer. For various social reasons, persons in pain may not seek or may not be able to access treatment for their pain. At the same time, health care providers may not provide the treatment which authorities recommend.

Classification

When pain is a symptom of a disease, then treatment may focus on addressing the cause of the disease. Because of the hope that treatment which ends the disease would eliminate the pain, sometimes pain management is not recognized as a priority in favor of efforts to address an underlying cause of the pain.

In other cases, the pain itself might need its own treatment plan. Palliative care could be used to address the pain as its own priority. Palliative care might be used either with or alongside any treatment for an underlying condition.

Signs

Some organizations advise that health care providers treat pain whenever it is present. The perspective is that when a person complains of serious pain, then that person is in need of treatment.

Various publications offer guidance on recognizing pain and advising when a person with pain needs additional treatment.

Causes

Reasons for deficiencies in pain management include cultural, societal, religious, and political attitudes. Moreover, the biomedical model of disease, focused on pathophysiology rather than quality of life, reinforces entrenched attitudes that marginalize pain management as a priority. Other reasons may have to do with inadequate training, personal biases or fear of prescription drug abuse.

Prevention and Screening

Current strategies for improvement in pain management include framing it as an ethical issue; promoting pain management as a legal right; providing constitutional guarantees and statutory regulations that span negligence law, criminal law, and elder abuse; defining pain management as a fundamental human right; categorizing failure to provide pain management as professional misconduct, and issuing guidelines and standards of practice by professional bodies.

Epidemiology

Undertreatment of pain is common, and is experienced by all age groups from neonates to the elderly.

Global Incidence

In September 2008, the World Health Organization (WHO) estimated that approximately 80 percent of the world population has either no or insufficient access to treatment for moderate to severe pain. Every year tens of millions of people around the world, including around four million cancer patients and 0.8 million HIV/AIDS patients at the end of their lives suffer from such pain without treatment. Yet the medications to treat pain are cheap, safe, effective, generally straightforward to administer, and international law obliges countries to make adequate pain medications available.

United States

In the United States, women and Hispanic and African Americans are more likely to be undertreated.

History

In 1961 the Single Convention on Narcotic Drugs established that certain drugs are "indispensible for the relief of pain and suffering" and that states should make them available to people who need them.

In 2009, a World Health Organization report noted that accessing treatment for pain was difficult for many people in many places in the world for a range of reasons.

In 2010 the Commission on Narcotic Drugs and adopted a resolution on access to pain treatments. Also in 2010 the United Nations Office on Drugs and Crime published a feature explaining the problem of lack of access to pain treatment and expressing interest in the topic. In 2011 the International Narcotics Control Board published a supplement to its annual report which highlighted the issue as a concern to be addressed.

Society and Culture

There is a complicated history of politics which influences practice in the treatment of pain.

Undertreatment may be due to physicians' fear of being accused of over-prescribing, despite the relative rarity of prosecutions, or physicians' poor understanding of the health risks attached to opioid prescription As a result of two recent cases in California though, where physicians who failed to provide adequate pain relief were successfully sued for elder abuse, the North American medical and health care communities appear to be undergoing a shift in perspective. The California Medical Board publicly reprimanded the physician in the second case; the federal Center for Medicare and Medicaid Services has declared a willingness to charge with fraud health care providers who accept payment for providing adequate pain relief while failing to do so; and clinical practice guidelines and standards are evolving into clear, unambiguous statements on acceptable pain management, so health care providers, in California at least, can no longer avoid culpability by claiming that poor or no pain relief meets community standards.

Special Populations

Undertreatment in the elderly can be due to a variety of reasons including the misconception that pain is a normal part of aging, therefore it is unrealistic to expect older adults to be pain free. Other misconceptions surrounding pain and older adults are that older adults have decreased pain sensitivity, especially if they have a cognitive dysfunction such as dementia and that opioids should not be administered to older adults as they are too dangerous. However, with appropriate assessment and careful administration and monitoring older adults can have to same level of pain management as any other population of care.

References

- King, Nicholas B.; Fraser, Veronique (2013). "Untreated Pain, Narcotics Regulation, and Global Health Ideologies". PLoS Medicine. 10 (4): e1001411. doi:10.1371/journal.pmed.1001411. ISSN 1549-1676
- Hoskin PJ. Radiotherapy. In: Sykes N, Bennett MI & Yuan C-S. Clinical pain management: Cancer pain. 2nd ed. London: Hodder Arnold; 2008. ISBN 978-0-340-94007-5. p. 251–55
- Young RF & Brechner T. Electrical stimulation of the brain for relief of intractable pain due to cancer. Cancer. 1986;57:1266–72. doi:10.1002/1097-0142(19860315)57:6<1266::aid-cn-cr2820570634>3.0.co;2-q. PMID 3484665
- Human Rights Watch (2 June 2011), Global State of Pain Treatment: Access to Medicines and Palliative Care, Human Rights Watch, retrieved 28 July 2016
- Lipman, Arthur G. (17 August 2009). "Pain as a Human Right". Journal of Pain & Palliative Care Pharmacotherapy. 19 (3): 85–100. doi:10.1080/j354v19n03_16
- Atallah JN. Management of cancer pain. In: Vadivelu N, Urman RD, Hines RL. Essentials of pain management. New York: Springer; 2011. doi:10.1007/978-0-387-87579-8. ISBN 978-0-387-87578-1. p. 597–628
- Fishman, Scott M. (July 2007). "Recognizing Pain Management as a Human Right: A First Step". Anesthesia & Analgesia. 105 (1): 8–9. doi:10.1213/01.ane.0000267526.37663.41
- Cleeland, CS (1998). "Undertreatment of cancer pain in elderly patients". Journal of the American Medical Association. 279 (23): 1914–5. doi:10.1001/jama.279.23.1914. PMID 9634265
- Scott Fishman; Jane Ballantyne; James P. Rathmell (January 2010). Bonica's Management of Pain. Lippincott Williams & Wilkins. p. 1458. ISBN 978-0-7817-6827-6. Retrieved 15 August 2013
- Lohman, Diederik; Schleifer, Rebecca; Amon, Joseph J (20 January 2010). "Access to pain treatment as a human right". BMC Medicine. 8 (1): 8. doi:10.1186/1741-7015-8-8. PMC 2823656. PMID 20089155
- Hoffmann, DE; Tarzian, AJ (2001). "The Girl Who Cried Pain: A Bias Against Women in the Treatment of Pain" (PDF). Journal of law, medicine & ethics. 29 (1): 13–27. PMID 11521267
- Williams JE. Nerve blocks: Chemical and physical neurolytic agents. In: Sykes N, Bennett MI & Yuan C-S. Clinical pain management: Cancer pain. 2nd ed. London: Hodder Arnold; 2008. ISBN 978-0-340-94007-5. p. 225–35
- Bonham, VL (2001). "Race, ethnicity, and pain treatment: Striving to understand the causes and solutions to the disparities in pain treatment" (PDF). Journal of law, medicine & ethics. 29: 52–68
- Blomqvist, K (2003). "Older people in persistent pain: Nursing and paramedical staff perceptions and pain management". Journal of Advanced Nursing. 4 (6): 575–584. doi:10.1046/j.1365-2648.2003.02569.x

2

Pain and its Types

Pain is a feeling of discomfort or of distress. The different types of pain are back pain, chronic pain, neuropathic pain, psychogenic pain, phantom pain, etc. The topics discussed in the chapter are of great importance to broaden the existing knowledge on pain.

Pain

Pain is a distressing feeling often caused by intense or damaging stimuli, such as stubbing a toe, burning a finger, putting alcohol on a cut, or bumping the "funny bone". Because it is a complex, subjective phenomenon, defining pain has been a challenge. The International Association for the Study of Pain's widely used definition states: "Pain is an unpleasant sensory and emotional experience associated with actual or potential tissue damage, or described in terms of such damage." In medical diagnosis, pain is regarded as a symptom of an underlying condition.

Pain motivates the individual to withdraw from damaging situations, to protect a damaged body part while it heals, and to avoid similar experiences in the future. Most pain resolves once the noxious stimulus is removed and the body has healed, but it may persist despite removal of the stimulus and apparent healing of the body. Sometimes pain arises in the absence of any detectable stimulus, damage or disease.

Pain is the most common reason for physician consultation in most developed countries. It is a major symptom in many medical conditions, and can interfere with a person's quality of life and general functioning. Simple pain medications are useful in 20% to 70% of cases. Psychological factors such as social support, hypnotic suggestion, excitement, or distraction can significantly affect pain's intensity or unpleasantness. In some arguments put forth in physician-assisted suicide or euthanasia debates, pain has been used as an argument to permit people who are terminally ill to end their lives.

One judgment on the value of pain is given by German philosopher, Friedrich Nietzsche, who wrote: "Only great pain is the ultimate liberator of the spirit... I doubt that such pain makes us 'better'; but I know that it makes us more profound". Nietzsche and philosophers influenced by him thus oppose the entirely negative valuation of pain, instead holding that 'What does not destroy me, makes me stronger".

Classification

In 1994, responding to the need for a more useful system for describing chronic pain, the International Association for the Study of Pain (IASP) classified pain according to specific characteristics:

1. region of the body involved (e.g. abdomen, lower limbs),
2. system whose dysfunction may be causing the pain (e.g., nervous, gastrointestinal),
3. duration and pattern of occurrence,
4. intensity and time since onset, and
5. cause

However, this system has been criticized by Clifford J. Woolf and others as inadequate for guiding research and treatment. Woolf suggests three classes of pain:

1. nociceptive pain,
2. inflammatory pain which is associated with tissue damage and the infiltration of immune cells, and
3. pathological pain which is a disease state caused by damage to the nervous system or by its abnormal function (e.g. fibromyalgia, peripheral neuropathy, tension type headache, etc.).

Duration

Pain is usually transitory, lasting only until the noxious stimulus is removed or the underlying damage or pathology has healed, but some painful conditions, such as rheumatoid arthritis, peripheral neuropathy, cancer and idiopathic pain, may persist for years. Pain that lasts a long time is called *chronic* or persistent, and pain that resolves quickly is called *acute*. Traditionally, the distinction between *acute* and *chronic* pain has relied upon an arbitrary interval of time from onset; the two most commonly used markers being 3 months and 6 months since the onset of pain, though some theorists and researchers have placed the transition from acute to chronic pain at 12 months. Others apply *acute* to pain that lasts less than 30 days, *chronic* to pain of more than six months' duration, and *subacute* to pain that lasts from one to six months. A popular alternative definition of *chronic pain*, involving no arbitrarily fixed durations, is "pain that extends beyond the expected period of healing". Chronic pain may be classified as cancer pain or else as benign.

Nociceptive

Nociceptive pain is caused by stimulation of sensory nerve fibers that respond to stimuli approaching or exceeding harmful intensity (nociceptors), and may be classified according to the mode of noxious stimulation. The most common categories are "thermal" (e.g. heat or cold), "mechanical" (e.g. crushing, tearing, shearing, etc.) and "chemical" (e.g. iodine in a cut or chemicals released during inflammation). Some nociceptors respond to more than one of these modalities and are consequently designated polymodal.

Nociceptive pain may also be divided into "visceral", "deep somatic" and "superficial somatic" pain. Visceral structures are highly sensitive to stretch, ischemia and inflammation, but relatively insensitive to other stimuli that normally evoke pain in other structures, such as burning and cutting. *Visceral pain* is diffuse, difficult to locate and often referred to a distant, usually superficial, structure. It may be accompanied by nausea and vomiting and may be described as sickening, deep, squeezing, and dull. *Deep somatic* pain is initiated by stimulation of nociceptors in ligaments, tendons, bones, blood vessels, fasciae and muscles, and is dull, aching, poorly-localized pain. Examples include sprains and broken bones. *Superficial* pain is initiated by activation of nociceptors in the skin or other superficial tissue, and is sharp, well-defined and clearly located. Examples of injuries that produce superficial somatic pain include minor wounds and minor (first degree) burns.

Neuropathic

Neuropathic pain is caused by damage or disease affecting any part of the nervous system involved in bodily feelings (the somatosensory system). Peripheral neuropathic pain is often described as "burning", "tingling", "electrical", "stabbing", or "pins and needles". Bumping the "funny bone" elicits acute peripheral neuropathic pain.

Phantom

Phantom pain is pain felt in a part of the body that has been lost or from which the brain no longer receives signals. It is a type of neuropathic pain. Phantom limb pain is a common experience of amputees.

The prevalence of phantom pain in upper limb amputees is nearly 82%, and in lower limb amputees is 54%. One study found that eight days after amputation, 72% of patients had phantom limb pain, and six months later, 67% reported it. Some amputees experience continuous pain that varies in intensity or quality; others experience several bouts a day, or it may occur only once every week or two. It is often described as shooting, crushing, burning or cramping. If the pain is continuous for a long period, parts of the intact body may become sensitized, so that touching them evokes pain in the phantom limb. Phantom limb pain may accompany urination or defecation.

Local anesthetic injections into the nerves or sensitive areas of the stump may relieve pain for days, weeks, or sometimes permanently, despite the drug wearing off in a matter of hours; and small injections of hypertonic saline into the soft tissue between vertebrae produces local pain that radiates into the phantom limb for ten minutes or so and may be followed by hours, weeks or even longer of partial or total relief from phantom pain. Vigorous vibration or electrical stimulation of the stump, or current from electrodes surgically implanted onto the spinal cord, all produce relief in some patients.

Mirror box therapy produces the illusion of movement and touch in a phantom limb which in turn may cause a reduction in pain.

Paraplegia, the loss of sensation and voluntary motor control after serious spinal cord damage, may be accompanied by girdle pain at the level of the spinal cord damage, visceral pain evoked by a filling bladder or bowel, or, in five to ten per cent of paraplegics, phantom body pain in areas of complete sensory loss. This phantom body pain is initially described as burning or tingling but may evolve into severe crushing or pinching pain, or the sensation of fire running down the legs or of a knife twisting in the flesh. Onset may be immediate or may not occur until years after the disabling injury. Surgical treatment rarely provides lasting relief.

Psychogenic

Psychogenic pain, also called *psychalgia* or *somatoform pain*, is pain caused, increased, or prolonged by mental, emotional, or behavioral factors. Headache, back pain, and stomach pain are sometimes diagnosed as psychogenic. Sufferers are often stigmatized, because both medical professionals and the general public tend to think that pain from a psychological source is not “real”. However, specialists consider that it is no less actual or hurtful than pain from any other source.

People with long-term pain frequently display psychological disturbance, with elevated scores on the Minnesota Multiphasic Personality Inventory scales of hysteria, depression and hypochondriasis (the “neurotic triad”). Some investigators have argued that it is this neuroticism that causes acute pain to turn chronic, but clinical evidence points the other way, to chronic pain causing neuroticism. When long-term pain is relieved by therapeutic intervention, scores on the neurotic triad and anxiety fall, often to normal levels. Self-esteem, often low in chronic pain patients, also shows improvement once pain has resolved.

The term ‘psychogenic’ assumes that medical diagnosis is so perfect that all organic causes of pain can be detected; regrettably, we are far from such infallibility... All too often, the diagnosis of neurosis as the cause of pain hides our ignorance of many aspects of pain medicine.

—*Ronald Melzack, 1996.*

Breakthrough Pain

Breakthrough pain is transitory acute pain that comes on suddenly and is not alleviated by the patient’s regular pain management. It is common in cancer patients who often have background pain that is generally well-controlled by medications, but who also sometimes experience bouts of severe pain that from time to time "breaks through" the medication. The characteristics of breakthrough cancer pain vary from person to person and according to the cause. Management of breakthrough pain can entail intensive use of opioids, including fentanyl.

Incident Pain

Incident pain is pain that arises as a result of activity, such as movement of an arthritic joint, stretching a wound, etc.

Pain Asymbolia and Insensitivity

The ability to experience pain is essential for protection from injury, and recognition of the presence of injury. Episodic analgesia may occur under special circumstances, such as in the excitement of sport or war: a soldier on the battlefield may feel no pain for many hours from a traumatic amputation or other severe injury.

Although unpleasantness is an essential part of the IASP definition of pain, it is possible to induce a state described as intense pain devoid of unpleasantness in some patients, with morphine injection or psychosurgery. Such patients report that they have pain but are not bothered by it; they recognize the sensation of pain but suffer little, or not at all. Indifference to pain can also rarely be present from birth; these people have normal nerves on medical investigations, and find pain unpleasant, but do not avoid repetition of the pain stimulus.

Insensitivity to pain may also result from abnormalities in the nervous system. This is usually the result of acquired damage to the nerves, such as spinal cord injury, diabetes mellitus (diabetic neuropathy), or leprosy in countries where that disease is prevalent. These individuals are at risk of tissue damage and infection due to undiscovered injuries. People with diabetes-related nerve damage, for instance, sustain poorly-healing foot ulcers as a result of decreased sensation.

A much smaller number of people are insensitive to pain due to an inborn abnormality of the nervous system, known as "congenital insensitivity to pain". Children with this condition incur carelessly-repeated damage to their tongues, eyes, joints, skin, and muscles. Some die before adulthood, and others have a reduced life expectancy. Most people with congenital insensitivity to pain have one of five hereditary sensory and autonomic neuropathies (which includes familial dysautonomia and congenital insensitivity to pain with anhidrosis). These conditions feature decreased sensitivity to pain together with other neurological abnormalities, particularly of the autonomic nervous system. A very rare syndrome with isolated congenital insensitivity to pain has been linked with mutations in the *SCN9A* gene, which codes for a sodium channel ($Na_v1.7$) necessary in conducting pain nerve stimuli.

Effect on Functioning

Experimental subjects challenged by acute pain and patients in chronic pain experience impairments in attention control, working memory, mental flexibility, problem solving, and information processing speed. Acute and chronic pain are also associated with increased depression, anxiety, fear, and anger.

If I have matters right, the consequences of pain will include direct physical distress, unemployment, financial difficulties, marital disharmony, and difficulties in concentration and attention...

—Harold Merskey 2000

Theory

Historical Theories

Before the relatively recent discovery of neurons and their role in pain, various different body functions were proposed to account for pain. There were several competing early theories of pain among the ancient Greeks: Hippocrates believed that it was due to an imbalance in vital fluids. In the 11th century, Avicenna theorized that there were a number of feeling senses including touch, pain and titillation.

In 1644, René Descartes theorized that pain was a disturbance that passed down along nerve fibers until the disturbance reached the brain, a development that transformed the perception of pain from a spiritual, mystical experience to a physical, mechanical sensation. Descartes's work, along with Avicenna's, prefigured the 19th-century development of specificity theory. Specificity theory saw pain as "a specific sensation, with its own sensory apparatus independent of touch and other senses". Another theory that came to prominence in the 18th and 19th centuries was intensive theory, which conceived of pain not as a unique sensory modality, but an emotional state produced by stronger than normal stimuli such as intense light, pressure or temperature. By the mid-1890s, specificity was backed mostly by physiologists and physicians, and the intensive theory was mostly backed by psychologists. However, after a series of clinical observations by Henry Head and experiments by Max von Frey, the psychologists migrated to specificity almost en masse, and by century's end, most textbooks on physiology and psychology were presenting pain specificity as fact.

In 1955, DC Sinclair and G Weddell developed peripheral pattern theory, based on a 1934 suggestion by John Paul Nafe. They proposed that all skin fiber endings (with the exception of those innervating hair cells) are identical, and that pain is produced by intense stimulation of these fibers. Another 20th-century theory was gate control theory, introduced by Ronald Melzack and Patrick Wall in the 1965 *Science* article "Pain Mechanisms: A New Theory". The authors proposed that both thin (pain) and large diameter (touch, pressure, vibration) nerve fibers carry information from the site of injury to two destinations in the dorsal horn of the spinal cord, and that the more large fiber activity relative to thin fiber activity at the inhibitory cell, the less pain is felt.

Three Dimensions of Pain

In 1968 Ronald Melzack and Kenneth Casey described pain in terms of its three dimensions: "sensory-discriminative" (sense of the intensity, location, quality and duration of the pain), "affective-motivational" (unpleasantness and urge to escape the unpleasantness), and "cognitive-evaluative" (cognitions such as appraisal, cultural values, distraction and hypnotic suggestion). They theorized that pain intensity (the sensory discriminative dimension) and unpleasantness (the affective-motivational dimension) are not simply determined by the magnitude of the painful stimulus, but "higher" cognitive activities can influence perceived intensity and unpleasantness. Cognitive activities "may affect both sensory and affective experience or they may modify primarily the affective-motivational dimension. Thus, excitement in games or war appears to block both dimensions of pain, while suggestion and placebos may modulate the affective-motivational dimension and leave the sensory-discriminative dimension relatively undisturbed." (p. 432) The paper ends with a call to action: "Pain can be treated not only by trying to cut down the sensory input by anesthetic block, surgical intervention and the like, but also by influencing the motivational-affective and cognitive factors as well." (p. 435)

Theory Today

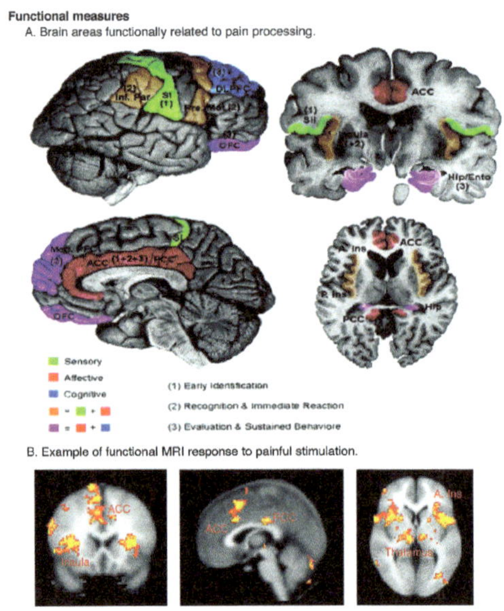

Regions of the cerebral cortex associated with pain.

Wilhelm Erb's (1874) "intensive" theory, that a pain signal can be generated by intense enough stimulation of *any* sensory receptor, has been soundly disproved. Some sensory fibers do not differentiate between noxious and non-noxious stimuli, while others, nociceptors, respond only to noxious, high intensity stimuli. At the peripheral end of the nociceptor, noxious stimuli generate currents that, above a given threshold, send signals along the nerve fiber to the spinal cord. The "specificity" (whether it responds to thermal, chemical or mechanical features of its environment) of a nociceptor is determined by which ion channels it expresses at its peripheral end. Dozens of different types of nociceptor ion channels have so far been identified, and their exact functions are still being determined.

The pain signal travels from the periphery to the spinal cord along an A-delta or C fiber. Because the A-delta fiber is thicker than the C fiber, and is thinly sheathed in an electrically insulating material (myelin), it carries its signal faster (5–30 m/s) than the unmyelinated C fiber (0.5–2 m/s). Pain evoked by the A-delta fibers is described as sharp and is felt first. This is followed by a duller pain, often described as burning, carried by the C fibers. These "first order" neurons enter the spinal cord via Lissauer's tract.

These A-delta and C fibers connect with "second order" nerve fibers in the central gelatinous substance of the spinal cord (laminae II and III of the dorsal horns). The second order fibers then cross the cord via the anterior white commissure and ascend in the spinothalamic tract. Before reaching the brain, the spinothalamic tract splits into the lateral, neospinothalamic tract and the medial, paleospinothalamic tract.

Second order neospinothalamic tract neurons carry information from A-delta fibers and terminate at the ventral posterolateral nucleus of the thalamus, where they connect with third order neurons of the somatosensory cortex. Paleospinothalamic neurons carry information from C fibers and terminate throughout the brain stem, a tenth of them in the thalamus and the rest in the medulla, pons and periaqueductal gray matter.

Second order, spinal cord fibers dedicated to carrying A-delta fiber pain signals, and others that carry both A-delta and C fiber pain signals to the thalamus have been identified. Other spinal cord fibers, known as wide dynamic range neurons, respond to A-delta and C fibers, but also to the large A-beta fibers that carry touch, pressure and vibration signals. Pain-related activity in the thalamus spreads to the insular cortex (thought to embody, among other things, the feeling that distinguishes pain from other homeostatic emotions such as itch and nausea) and anterior cingulate cortex (thought to embody, among other things, the affective/motivational element, the unpleasantness of pain). Pain that is distinctly located also activates primary and secondary somatosensory cortex.

Evolutionary and Behavioral Role

Pain is part of the body's defense system, producing a reflexive retraction from the painful stimulus, and tendencies to protect the affected body part while it heals, and avoid that harmful situation in the future. It is an important part of animal life, vital to healthy survival. People with congenital insensitivity to pain have reduced life expectancy.

In his book, *The Greatest Show on Earth: The Evidence for Evolution*, biologist Richard Dawkins grapples with the question of why pain has to be so very painful. He describes the alternative as a simple, mental raising of a "red flag". To argue why that red flag might be insufficient, Dawkins explains that drives must compete with each other within living beings. The most fit creature would be the one whose pains are well balanced. Those pains which mean certain death when ignored will become the most powerfully felt. The relative intensities of pain, then, may resemble the relative importance of that risk to our ancestors (lack of food, too much cold, or serious injuries are felt as agony, whereas minor damage is felt as mere discomfort). This resemblance will not be perfect, however, because natural selection can be a poor designer. The result is often glitches in animals, including supernormal stimuli. Such glitches help explain pains which are not, or at least no longer directly adaptive (e.g. perhaps some forms of toothache, or injury to fingernails).

Idiopathic pain (pain that persists after the trauma or pathology has healed, or that arises without any apparent cause), may be an exception to the idea that pain is helpful to survival, although some psychodynamic psychologists argue that such pain is psychogenic, enlisted as a protective distraction to keep dangerous emotions unconscious.

Thresholds

In pain science, thresholds are measured by gradually increasing the intensity of a stimulus such as electric current or heat applied to the body. The pain perception threshold is the point at which the stimulus begins to hurt, and the pain tolerance threshold is reached when the subject acts to stop the pain.

Differences in pain perception and tolerance thresholds are associated with, among other factors, ethnicity, genetics, and sex. People of Mediterranean origin report as painful some radiant heat intensities that northern Europeans describe as nonpainful. And Italian women tolerate less intense electric shock than Jewish or Native American women. Some individuals in all cultures have significantly higher than normal pain perception and tolerance thresholds. For instance, patients who experience painless heart attacks have higher pain thresholds for electric shock, muscle cramp and heat.

Assessment

A person's self-report is the most reliable measure of pain. Some health care professionals may underestimate pain severity. A definition of pain widely employed in nursing, emphasizing its subjective nature and the importance of believing patient reports, was introduced by Margo McCaffery in 1968: "Pain is whatever the experiencing person says it is, existing whenever he says it does". To assess intensity, the patient may be asked to locate their pain on a scale of 0 to 10, with 0 being no pain at all, and 10 the worst pain they have ever felt. Quality can be established by having the patient complete the McGill Pain Questionnaire indicating which words best describe their pain.

Multidimensional Pain Inventory

The Multidimensional Pain Inventory (MPI) is a questionnaire designed to assess the psychosocial state of a person with chronic pain. Analysis of MPI results by Turk and Rudy (1988) found three classes of chronic pain patient: "(a) dysfunctional, people who perceived the severity of their pain to be high, reported that pain interfered with much of their lives, reported a higher degree of psychological distress caused by pain, and reported low levels of activity; (b) interpersonally distressed, people with a common perception that significant others were not very supportive of their pain problems; and (c) adaptive copers, patients who reported high levels of social support, relatively low levels of pain and perceived interference, and relatively high levels of activity." Combining the MPI characterization of the person with their IASP five-category pain profile is recommended for deriving the most useful case description.

People who are Non-verbal

When a person is non-verbal and cannot self-report pain, observation becomes critical, and specific behaviors can be monitored as pain indicators. Behaviors such as facial grimacing and guarding indicate pain, as well as an increase or decrease in vocalizations, changes in routine behavior patterns and mental status changes. Patients experiencing pain may exhibit withdrawn social behavior and possibly experience a decreased appetite and decreased nutritional intake. A change in condition that deviates from baseline such as moaning with movement or when manipulating a body part, and limited range of motion are also potential pain indicators. In patients who possess language but are incapable of expressing themselves effectively, such as those with dementia, an increase in confusion or display of aggressive behaviors or agitation may signal that discomfort exists, and further assessment is necessary.

Infants feel pain but they lack the language needed to report it, so communicate distress by crying. A non-verbal pain assessment should be conducted involving the parents, who will notice changes in the infant not obvious to the health care provider. Preterm babies are more sensitive to painful stimuli than full term babies.

Other Barriers to Reporting

The experience of pain has many cultural dimensions. For instance, the way in which one experiences and responds to pain is related to sociocultural characteristics, such as gender, ethnicity, and age. An aging adult may not respond to pain in the way that a younger person would. Their ability to recognize pain may be blunted by illness or the use of multiple prescription drugs. Depression may also keep the older adult from reporting they are in pain. The older adult may also stop doing activities they love because it hurts too much. Decline in self-care activities (dressing, grooming, walking, etc.) may also be indicators that the older adult is experiencing pain. The older adult may refrain from reporting pain because they are afraid they will have to have surgery or will be put on a drug they might become addicted to. They may not want others to see them as weak, or may feel there is something impolite or shameful in complaining about pain, or they may feel the pain is deserved punishment for past transgressions.

Cultural barriers can also keep a person from telling someone they are in pain. Religious beliefs may prevent the individual from seeking help. They may feel certain pain treatment is against their religion. They may not report pain because they feel it is a sign that death is near. Many people fear the stigma of addiction and avoid pain treatment so as not to be prescribed potentially addicting drugs. Many Asians do not want to lose respect in society by admitting they are in pain and need help, believing the pain should be borne in silence, while other cultures feel they should report pain right away and get immediate relief. Gender can also be a factor in reporting pain. Sexual differences can be the result of social and cultural expectations, with women expected to be emotional and show pain and men stoic, keeping pain to themselves.

As an aid to Diagnosis

Pain is a symptom of many medical conditions. Knowing the time of onset, location, intensity, pattern of occurrence (continuous, intermittent, etc.), exacerbating and relieving factors, and quality (burning, sharp, etc.) of the pain will help the examining physician to accurately diagnose the problem. For example, chest pain described as extreme heaviness may indicate myocardial infarction, while chest pain described as tearing may indicate aortic dissection.

Physiological Measurement of Pain

fMRI brain scanning has been used to measure pain, giving good correlations with self-reported pain.

Hedonic Adaptation

Hedonic adaptation means that actual long-term suffering due to physical illness is often much lower than expected.

Legal Awards for Pain and Suffering

One area where assessments of pain are effectively required to be made is in legal awards for pain and suffering. In the Western world these are typically discretionary awards made by juries and are regarded as difficult to predict, variable and subjective, for instance in the US, UK, Australia and New Zealand.

Management

Inadequate treatment of pain is widespread throughout surgical wards, intensive care units, accident and emergency departments, in general practice, in the management of all forms of chronic pain including cancer pain, and in end of life care. This neglect is extended to all ages, from neonates to the frail elderly. African and Hispanic Americans are more likely than others to suffer needlessly in the hands of a physician; and women's pain is more likely to be undertreated than men's.

The International Association for the Study of Pain advocates that the relief of pain should be recognized as a human right, that chronic pain should be considered a disease in its own right, and that pain medicine should have the full status of a specialty. It is a specialty only in China and Australia at this time. Elsewhere, pain medicine is a subspecialty under disciplines such as anesthesiology, physiatry, neurology, palliative medicine and psychiatry. In 2011, Human Rights Watch alerted that tens of millions of people worldwide are still denied access to inexpensive medications for severe pain.

Breastfeeding may decrease pain when babies are immunized.

Medication

Acute pain is usually managed with medications such as analgesics and anesthetics. Caffeine, when added to pain medications such as ibuprofen, may provide some additional benefit. Management of chronic pain, however, is much more difficult and may require the coordinated efforts of a pain management team, which typically includes medical practitioners, clinical pharmacists, clinical psychologists, physiotherapists, occupational therapists, physician assistants, and nurse practitioners.

Sugar (sucrose) when taken by mouth reduces pain in newborn babies undergoing some medical procedures (a single lancing of the heel, venipuncture, and intramuscular injections). Sugar does not remove pain from circumcision, and it is unknown if sugar reduces pain for other procedures. Sugar did not affect pain-related electrical activity in the brains of newborns one second after the heel lance procedure. Sweet liquid by mouth moderately reduces the rate and duration of crying caused by immunization injection in children between one and twelve months of age.

Psychological

Individuals with more social support experience less cancer pain, take less pain medication, report less labor pain and are less likely to use epidural anesthesia during childbirth or suffer from chest pain after coronary artery bypass surgery.

Suggestion can significantly affect pain intensity. About 35% of people report marked relief after receiving a saline injection they believe to have been morphine. This "placebo" effect is more pronounced in people who are prone to anxiety, so anxiety reduction may account for some of the effect, but it does not account for all of it. Placebos are more effective in intense pain than mild pain; and they produce progressively weaker effects with repeated administration.

It is possible for many people with chronic pain to become so absorbed in an activity or entertainment that the pain is no longer felt, or is greatly diminished.

Cognitive behavioral therapy (CBT) has been shown effective for improving quality of life in those with chronic pain but the reduction in suffering is quite modest, and the CBT method employed seems to have no effect on outcome. Acceptance and Commitment Therapy (ACT) is likely also effective in the treatment of chronic pain.

A number of meta-analyses have found clinical hypnosis to be effective in controlling pain associated with diagnostic and surgical procedures in both adults and children, as well as pain associated with cancer and childbirth. A 2007 review of 13 studies found evidence for the efficacy of hypnosis in the reduction of chronic pain in some conditions, though the number of patients enrolled in the studies was low, bringing up issues of power to detect group differences, and most lacked credible controls for placebo and/or expectation. The authors concluded that "although the findings provide support for the general applicability of hypnosis in the treatment of chronic pain, considerably more research will be needed to fully determine the effects of hypnosis for different chronic-pain conditions."

Alternative Medicine

Pain is the most common reason for people to use complementary and alternative medicine. An analysis of the 13 highest quality studies of pain treatment with acupuncture, published in January 2009, concluded there is little difference in the effect of real, sham and no acupuncture. However other reviews have found benefit. Additionally, there is tentative evidence for a few herbal medicines. There is interest in the relationship between vitamin D and pain, but the evidence so far from controlled trials for such a relationship, other than in osteomalacia, is unconvincing.

A 2003 meta-analysis of randomized clinical trials found that spinal manipulation was "more effective than sham therapy but was no more or less effective than general practitioner care, analgesics, physical therapy, exercise, or back school" in the treatment of low back pain.

Epidemiology

Pain is the main reason for visiting the emergency department in more than 50% of cases and is present in 30% of family practice visits. Several epidemiological studies from different countries have reported widely varying prevalence rates for chronic pain, ranging from 12 to 80% of the population. It becomes more common as people approach death. A study of 4,703 patients found that 26% had pain in the last two years of life, increasing to 46% in the last month.

A survey of 6,636 children (0–18 years of age) found that, of the 5,424 respondents, 54% had experienced pain in the preceding three months. A quarter reported having experienced recurrent or continuous pain for three months or more, and a third of these reported frequent and intense pain. The intensity of chronic pain was higher for girls, and girls' reports of chronic pain increased markedly between ages 12 and 14.

Society and Culture

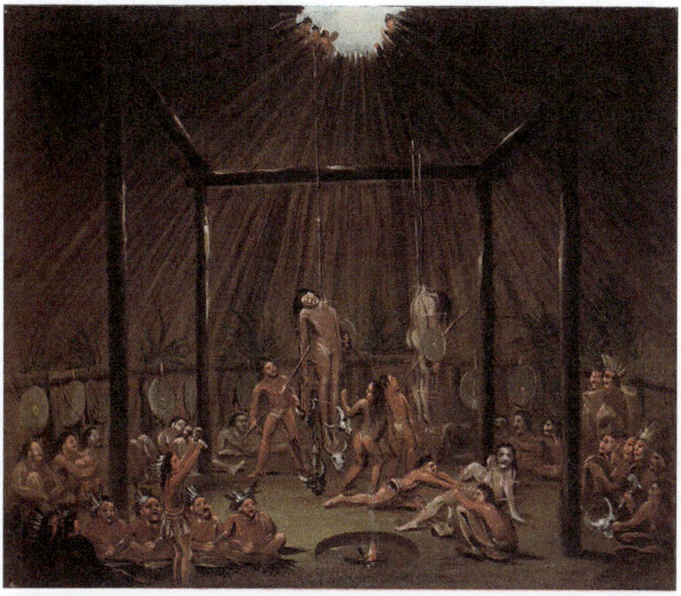

The okipa ceremony as witnessed by George Catlin, circa 1835.

The nature or meaning of physical pain has been diversely understood by religious or secular traditions from antiquity to modern times.

Physical pain is an important political topic in relation to various issues, including pain management policy, drug control, animal rights or animal welfare, torture, and pain compliance. In various contexts, the deliberate infliction of pain in the form of corporal punishment is used as retribution for an offence, or for the purpose of disciplining or reforming a wrongdoer, or to deter attitudes or behaviour deemed unacceptable. The slow slicing, or death by a thousand cuts, was a form of execution in China reserved for crimes viewed as especially severe, such as high treason or patricide. In some cultures, extreme practices such as mortification of the flesh or painful rites of passage are highly regarded. For example, the Sateré-Mawé people of Brazil use intentional bullet ant stings as part of their initiation rites to become warriors.

Philosophy of pain is a branch of philosophy of mind that deals essentially with physical pain, especially in connection with such views as dualism, identity theory, and functionalism.

More generally, it is often as a part of pain in the broad sense, i.e. suffering, that physical pain is dealt with in culture, religion, philosophy, or society.

Other Animals

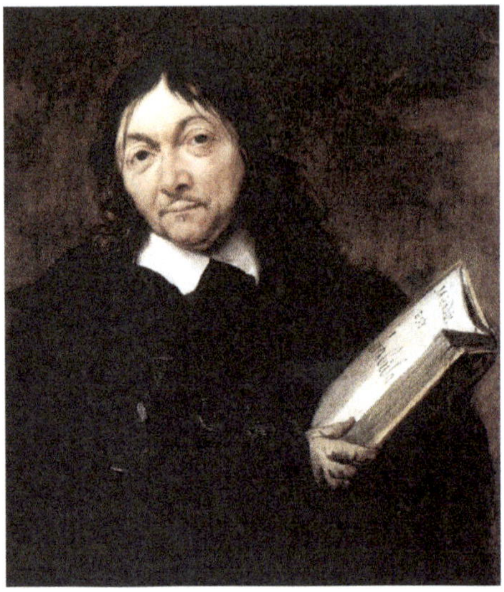

Portrait of René Descartes by Jan Baptist Weenix 1647-1649

The most reliable method for assessing pain in most humans is by asking a question: a person may report pain that cannot be detected by any known physiological measure. However, like infants, animals cannot answer questions about whether they feel pain; thus the defining criterion for pain in humans cannot be applied to them. Philosophers and scientists have responded to this difficulty in a variety of ways. René Descartes for example argued that animals lack consciousness and therefore do not experience pain and suffering in the way that humans do. Bernard Rollin of Colorado State University, the principal author of two U.S. federal laws regulating pain relief for animals, writes that researchers remained unsure into the 1980s as to whether animals experience pain, and that veterinarians trained in the U.S. before 1989 were simply taught to ignore animal pain. In his interactions with scientists and other veterinarians, he was regularly asked to "prove" that animals are conscious, and to provide "scientifically acceptable" grounds for claiming that they feel pain. Carbone writes that the view that animals feel pain differently is now a minority view. Academic reviews of the topic are more equivocal, noting that although the argument that animals have at least simple conscious thoughts and feelings has strong support, some critics continue to question how reliably animal mental states can be determined. The ability of invertebrate species of animals, such as insects, to feel pain and suffering is also unclear.

The presence of pain in an animal cannot be known for certain, but it can be inferred through physical and behavioral reactions. Specialists currently believe that all vertebrates can feel pain, and that certain invertebrates, like the octopus, might too. As for other animals, plants, or other entities, their ability to feel physical pain is at present a question beyond scientific reach, since no mechanism is known by which they could have such a feeling. In particular, there are no known nociceptors in groups such as plants, fungi, and most insects, except for instance in fruit flies.

In vertebrates, endogenous opioids are neuromodulators that moderate pain by interacting with opioid receptors. Opioids and opioid receptors occur naturally in crustaceans and, although at present no certain conclusion can be drawn, their presence indicates that lobsters may be able to experience pain. Opioids may mediate their pain in the same way as in vertebrates. Veterinary medicine uses, for actual or potential animal pain, the same analgesics and anesthetics as used in humans.

Etymology

First attested in English in 1297, the word *peyn* comes from the Old French *peine*, in turn from Latin *poena* meaning "punishment, penalty" (in L.L. also meaning "torment, hardship, suffering") and that from Greek (*poine*), generally meaning "price paid, penalty, punishment".

Chronic Pain

Chronic pain is pain that lasts a long time. In medicine, the distinction between acute and chronic pain is sometimes determined by an arbitrary interval of time since onset; the two most commonly used markers being 3 months and 6 months since onset, though some theorists and researchers have placed the transition from acute to chronic pain at 12 months. Others apply *acute* to pain that lasts less than 30 days, *chronic* to pain of more than six months duration, and *subacute* to pain that lasts from one to six months. A popular alternative definition of *chronic pain*, involving no arbitrarily fixed duration, is "pain that extends beyond the expected period of healing". Epidemiological studies have found that 10.1% to 55.2% of people in various countries have chronic pain.

Chronic pain may originate in the body, or in the brain or spinal cord. It is often difficult to treat. Various nonopioid medicines are recommended initially, depending on whether the pain originates from tissue damage or is neuropathic. Psychological treatments including cognitive behavioral therapy and acceptance and commitment therapy may be effective for improving quality of life in those with chronic pain. Some people with chronic pain may benefit from opioid treatment while others are harmed. A trial of opioids is only recommended in those with non cancer pain who have no history of either mental illness or substance use disorder and should be stopped if not effective.

Severe chronic pain is associated with increased 10 year mortality, particularly from heart disease and respiratory disease. People with chronic pain tend to have higher rates of depression, anxiety, and sleep disturbances; these are correlations and it is often not clear which factor causes another. Chronic pain may contribute to decreased physical activity due to fear of exacerbating pain, often resulting in weight gain. Pain intensity, pain control, and resiliency to pain are influenced by different levels and types of social support that a person with chronic pain receives.

Classification

The International Association for the study of pain defines chronic pain as pain with no biological value, that persists past normal tissue healing. The DSM-5 recognizes one chronic pain disorder, somatic symptom disorders, a reduction from the three previously recognized pain disorders. The criteria include it lasting for greater than six month.

The suggested ICD-11 chronic pain classification suggests 7 categories for chronic pain.

1. Chronic primary pain: defined by 3 months of persistent pain in one or more anatomical regions that is unexplainable by another pain condition.
2. Chronic cancer pain: defined as cancer or treatment related visceral, musculoskeletal, or bony pain.
3. Chronic posttraumatic pain: pain lasting 3 months post trauma or surgery, excluding infectious or preexisting conditions.
4. Chronic neuropathic pain: pain caused by damage to the somatosensory nervous system damage.
5. Chronic headache and orofacial pain: pain that originates in the head or face, and occurs for 50% or more days over a 3 months period.
6. Chronic visceral pain: pain originating in an internal organ.
7. Chronic musculoskeletal pain: pain originating in the bones, muscles, joints or connective tissue.

Chronic pain may be divided into "nociceptive" (caused by inflamed or damaged tissue activating specialised pain sensors called nociceptors), and "neuropathic" (caused by damage to or malfunction of the nervous system).

Nociceptive pain may be divided into "superficial" and "deep", and deep pain into "deep somatic" and "visceral". *Superficial* pain is initiated by activation of nociceptors in the skin or superficial tissues. *Deep somatic* pain is initiated by stimulation of nociceptors in ligaments, tendons, bones, blood vessels, fasciae and muscles, and is dull, aching, poorly-localized pain. *Visceral* pain originates in the viscera (organs). Visceral pain may be well-localized, but often it is extremely difficult to locate, and several visceral regions produce "referred" pain when damaged or inflamed, where the sensation is located in an area distant from the site of pathology or injury.

Neuropathic pain is divided into "peripheral" (originating in the peripheral nervous system) and "central" (originating in the brain or spinal cord). Peripheral neuropathic pain is often described as "burning", "tingling", "electrical", "stabbing", or "pins and needles".

Pathophysiology

Under persistent activation nociceptive transmission to the dorsal horn may induce a pain wind-up phenomenon. This induces pathological changes that lower the threshold for pain signals to be transmitted. In addition it may generate nonnociceptive nerve fibers to respond to pain signals. Nonnociceptive nerve fibers may also be able to generate and transmit pain signals. The type of nerve fibers that are believed to propagate the pain signals are the C-fibers, since they have a slow conductivity and give rise to a painful sensation that persists over a long time. In chronic pain this process is difficult to reverse or eradicate once established. In some cases, chronic pain can be caused by genetic factors which interfere with neuronal differentiation, leading to a permanent reduction in the threshold for pain.

Chronic pain of different etiologies has been characterized as a disease affecting brain structure and function. Magnetic resonance imaging studies have shown abnormal anatomical and functional connectivity, even during rest involving areas related to the processing of pain. Also, persistent pain has been shown to cause grey matter loss, reversible once the pain has resolved.

These structural changes can be explained by the phenomenon known as neuroplasticity. In the case of chronic pain, the somatotopic representation of the body is inappropriately reorganized following peripheral and central sensitization. This maladaptive change results in the experience of allodynia or hyperalgesia. Brain activity in individuals with chronic pain, measured via electroencephalogram (EEG), has been demonstrated to be altered, suggesting pain-induced neuroplastic changes. More specifically, the relative beta activity (compared to the rest of the brain) is increased, the relative alpha activity is decreased, and the theta activity both absolutely and relatively is diminished.

Dopaminergic dysfunction has been hypothesized to act as a shared mechanism between chronic pain, insomnia and major depressive disorder. Increased tonic dopamine activity and a compensatory decrease in phasic dopamine activity, which is important in inhibiting pain. This is supported by the implication of COMT in fibromyalgia and temporomandibular joint syndrome. Astrocytes, microglia, and Satellite glial cells have been found to be dysfunctional in chronic pain. Increased activity of microglia, alterations of microglial networks as well as increased production of chemokines and cytokines by microglia are proposed to act to potentiate pain. Astrocytes have been observed to lose their ability to regulate the excitability of neurons, increasing spontaneous neural activity in pain circuits.

Management

Pain management is the branch of medicine employing an interdisciplinary approach to the relief of pain and improvement in the quality of life of those living with pain. The typical pain management team includes medical practitioners (particularly anesthesiologists), clinical psychologists, physiotherapists, occupational therapists, physician assistants, and nurse practitioners. Acute pain usually resolves with the efforts of one practitioner; however, the management of chronic pain frequently requires the coordinated efforts of the treatment team. Complete and sustained remission of many types of chronic pain is rare, though some can be done to improve quality of life.

Nonopioids

Initially recommended efforts are non opioid based therapies.

Various nonopioid medicines are used, depending on whether the pain originates from tissue damage or is neuropathic. Limited evidence suggests that chronic pain from tissue inflammation or damage (as in rheumatoid arthritis and cancer pain) is best treated with opioids, while for neuropathic pain (pain caused by a damaged or dysfunctional nervous system) other drugs may be more effective, such as tricyclic antidepressants, serotonin-norepinephrine reuptake inhibitors, and anticonvulsants. Because of the weakness of the evidence, it is not clear which are the best approaches to treating many types of pain, and doctors must rely on their own clinical experience. Doctors often cannot predict who will use opioids just for pain management and who will go on to develop addiction, and cannot always distinguish between those who are and those who are not seeking opioids due primarily to an existing addiction. Withholding, interrupting or withdrawing opioid treatment in people who benefit from it can cause harm.

Interventional pain management may be appropriate, including techniques such as trigger point injections, neurolytic blocks, and radiotherapy. While there is no high quality evidence to support ultrasound, it has been found to have a small effect on improving function in non-specific chronic low back pain.

Psychological treatments, including cognitive behavioral therapy and acceptance and commitment therapy have been shown effective for improving quality of life and reducing pain interference in those with chronic pain.

While exercise has been offered as a method to lessen chronic pain and there is some evidence of benefit, this evidence is tentative. Side effects from exercise are few in this population.

Opioids

In those who have not benefited from other measures and have no history of either mental illness or substance use disorder treatment with opioids may be tried. If significant benefit does not occur it is recommended that they be stopped.

Some people with chronic pain benefit from opioid treatment and others do not; some are harmed by the treatment. Possible harms include reduced sex hormone production, hypogonadism, infertility, impaired immune system, falls and fractures in older adults, neonatal abstinence syndrome, heart problems, sleep-disordered breathing, opioid-induced hyperalgesia, physical dependence, addiction, and overdose.

Alternative Medicine

Hypnosis, including self-hypnosis, has tentative evidence. Evidence does not support hypnosis for chronic pain due to a spinal cord injury. Preliminary studies have found medical marijuana to be beneficial in treating chronic pain, but further research is needed.

Tai Chi has been shown to improve pain, stiffness, and quality of life in chronic conditions such as osteoarthritis, low back pain, and osteoporosis. Acupuncture has also been found to be an effective and safe treatment in reducing pain and improving quality of life for chronic pelvic pain syndrome specifically.

Transcranial magnetic stimulation for reduction of chronic pain is not currently supported by high quality evidence, and the demonstrated effects are small and short-term.

Epidemiology

A systematic literature review of chronic pain found that the prevalence of chronic pain varied studies in various countries from 10.1% to 55.2% of the population, affected women at a higher rate than men, and that chronic pain consumes a large amount of healthcare resources around the globe.

A large-scale telephone survey of 15 European countries and Israel, 19% of respondents over 18 years of age had suffered pain for more than 6 months, including the last month, and more than twice in the last week, with pain intensity of 5 or more for the last episode, on a scale of 1 (no pain) to 10 (worst imaginable). 4839 of these respondents with chronic pain were interviewed in depth. Sixty six percent scored their pain intensity at moderate (5–7), and 34% at severe (8–10); 46% had constant pain, 56% intermittent; 49% had suffered pain for 2–15 years; and 21% had been diagnosed with depression due to the pain. Sixty one percent were unable or less able to work outside the home, 19% had lost a job, and 13% had changed jobs due to their pain. Forty percent had inadequate pain management and less than 2% were seeing a pain management specialist.

In the United States, the prevalence of chronic pain has been estimated to be approximately 35%, with approximately 50 million Americans experiencing partial or total disability as a consequence. According to the Institute of Medicine, there are about 116 million Americans living with chronic pain, which suggests that approximately half of American adults have some chronic pain condition. The Mayday Fund estimate of 70 million Americans with chronic pain is slightly more conservative. In an internet study, the prevalence of chronic pain in the United States was calculated to be 30.7% of the population: 34.3% for women and 26.7% for men.

Outcomes

Chronic pain is associated with higher rates of depression and anxiety. Sleep disturbance, and insomnia due to medication and illness symptoms are often experienced by those with chronic pain. Chronic pain may contribute to decreased physical activity due to fear of exacerbating pain, often resulting in weight gain. Such comorbid disorders can be very difficult to treat due to the high potential of medication interactions, especially when the conditions are treated by different doctors.

Severe chronic pain is associated with increased 10 year mortality, particularly from heart disease and respiratory disease. Several mechanisms have been proposed for the increased mortality, e.g. abnormal endocrine stress response. Additionally, chronic stress seems to affect cardiovascular risk by acceleration of the atherosclerotic process. However, further research is needed to elucidate the relationship between severe chronic pain, stress and cardiovascular health.

Psychology

Personality

Two of the most frequent personality profiles found in people with chronic pain by the Minnesota Multiphasic Personality Inventory (MMPI) are the *conversion V* and the *neurotic triad*. The conversion V personality, so called because the higher scores on MMPI scales 1 and 3, relative to scale 2, form a "V" shape on the graph, expresses exaggerated concern over body feelings, develops bodily symptoms in response to stress, and often fails to recognize their own emotional state, including depression. The neurotic triad personality, scoring high on scales 1, 2 and 3, also expresses exaggerated concern over body feelings and develops bodily symptoms in response to stress, but is demanding and complaining.

Some investigators have argued that it is this neuroticism that causes acute pain to turn chronic, but clinical evidence points the other way, to chronic pain causing neuroticism. When long term pain is relieved by therapeutic intervention, scores on the neurotic triad and anxiety fall, often to normal levels. Self-esteem, often low in people with chronic pain, also shows striking improvement once pain has resolved.

It has been suggested that catastrophizing may play a role in the experience of pain. *Pain catastrophizing* is the tendency to describe a pain experience in more exaggerated terms than the average person, to think a great deal more about the pain when it occurs, or to feel more helpless about the experience. People who score highly on measures of catastrophization are likely to rate a pain experience as more intense than those who score low on such measures. It is often reasoned that the tendency to catastrophize *causes* the person to experience the pain as more intense. One suggestion is that catastrophizing influences pain perception through altering attention and anticipation, and heightening emotional responses to pain. However, at least some aspects of catastrophization may be the *product* of an intense pain experience, rather than its cause. That is, the more intense the pain feels to the person, the more likely they are to have thoughts about it that fit the definition of catastrophization.

Social Support

Social support has important consequences for individuals with chronic pain. In particular, pain intensity, pain control, and resiliency to pain has been implicated as outcomes influenced by different levels and types of social support. Much of this research has focused on emotional, instrumental, tangible and informational social support. People with persistent pain conditions tend to rely on their social support as a coping mechanism and therefore have better outcomes when they are a part of larger more supportive social networks. Across a majority of studies investigated, there was a direct significant association between social activities or social support and pain. Higher levels of pain were associated with a decrease in social activities, lower levels of social support, and reduced social functioning.

Effect on Cognition

Chronic pain's impact on cognition is an under-researched area, but several tentative conclusions have been published. Most people with chronic pain complain of cognitive impairment, such as forgetfulness, difficulty with attention, and difficulty completing tasks. Objective testing has found that people in chronic pain tend to experience impairment in attention, memory, mental flexibility, verbal ability, speed of response in a cognitive task, and speed in executing structured tasks.

Childhood Chronic Pain

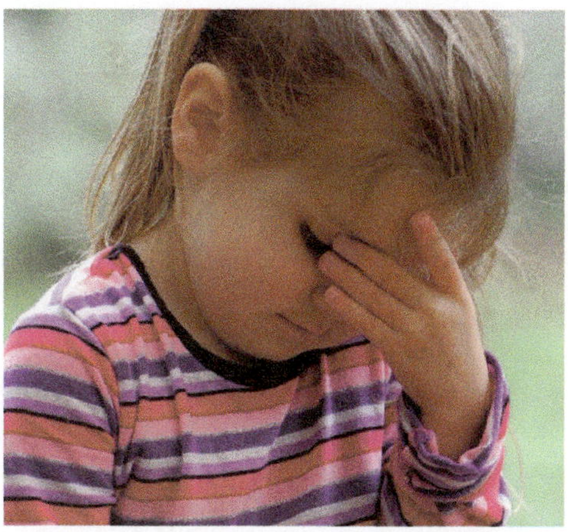

Headaches are one of the most common forms of childhood chronic pain.

Childhood chronic pain affects at least 5% of the population under the age of 18, according to conservative epidemiological studies. Rates of paediatric chronic pain have also increased in the past 20 years. While chronic pain conditions vary significantly in severity, they often affect children's mental health, academic performance, and general quality of life. The outcomes of childhood chronic pain are affected by a number of factors, including demographic factors, genetics, and school and family support.

Classification and Epidemiology

Chronic pain is defined as pain that lasts at least 3–6 months and, in the case of injury or surgery, remains present after standard recovery time has elapsed. The ICD-11 provides seven categories for diagnosing chronic pain:

- Chronic primary pain
- Chronic cancer pain
- Chronic postsurgical and posttraumatic pain
- Chronic neuropathic pain
- Chronic headache and orofacial pain
- Chronic visceral pain
- Chronic musculoskeletal pain

Childhood chronic pain can be caused by a number of conditions, including the following:

Condition	Symptoms	Known causes and risk factors	Estimated prevalence	Treatments
Chronic abdominal pain	Recurrent abdominal pain, usually without a known organic cause	Usually unknown	8.4%	Drug therapies, cognitive behavioural therapy (CBT)
Chronic headache	Recurrent headache (at least 15 days per month, 4 hours per day)	Sex (more common in females), psychological disturbances, obesity, overuse of caffeine or headache medication, other chronic pain conditions	1.5% - 3.4%	Antidepressants, beta blockers, anticonvulsants, NSAIDs, botulinum toxin, CBT
Complex regional pain syndrome	Severe burning/throbbing pain (usually in a limb), swelling, sensitivity, changes in skin colour and texture	Injury or trauma	Unknown	Pain relievers, corticosteroids, bone-loss medication, sympathetic nerve-blocking medication, intravenous ketamine, physical therapy, biofeedback, spinal cord stimulation

Juvenile fibromyalgia	Widespread muskulo-skeletal pain, headache, sleep disturbances, fatigue	Genetics, sex (more common in females), infections, trauma, rheumatic disease	1.2% - 6.2%	Antidepressants, anticonvulsants, pain relievers, CBT
Juvenile rheumatoid arthritis	Joint pain, swelling, and stiffness	Genetics, sex (more common in females)	0.4%	NSAIDs, TNF blockers, immune suppressants, corticosteroids, physical therapy

Management

Chronic pain can be treated in a number of ways, and varies depending on the type and severity of the condition. Common pain medications prescribed to children include paracetamol, ibuprofen, and acetylsalicylic acid. Researchers have also found that psychotherapies are often helpful in reducing functional disability in children with chronic pain. A meta-analysis by Christopher Eccleston and colleagues found that cognitive behavioural therapy (CBT) significantly reduced pain severity for children with chronic headaches. Additionally, biofeedback and relaxation therapy can be used in conjunction with CBT to treat chronic pain. Research thus far has typically found small effects for improving psychological wellbeing, but more robust outcomes for pain relief. Studies have also found significant pain relief effect for alternative medicine treatments, such as acupuncture and herbal medicine. Further research is needed to evaluate the efficacy of other alternative medicine techniques, such as arts therapy, homeopathy, and hypnosis.

Outcomes

Education

Chronic pain often interferes with children's ability to attend and succeed in school. Children with severe disorders are particularly likely to miss school because of debilitating pain, as well as for medical appointments. High rates of school absence are associated with poor adjustment and psychosocial wellbeing among children with chronic illnesses. For children with severe chronic pain disorders, school districts may provide a variety of services, including inpatient, homebound, and special education.

Inpatient Education

Some hospitals employ or contract tutors to assist children in inpatient care with their schoolwork. Hospital teachers are typically certified to teach a wide variety of ages and subjects. At the same time, in a study by Steinke et al., around one-third of hospital teachers reported teaching ages or subjects beyond their areas of certification. The number of hospital teachers is declining due to reduced hospitalization and shorter hospital stays.

Homebound Education

In many school districts in the United States, homebound education is offered to students who miss more than 15 days in a row. Homebound education typically consists of 45 minutes of instruction per day in the child's home. Other nations, including Australia and Belgium, have implemented programs to use technology to include chronically ill students in their regular class sessions, and these programs have generally had positive results. Many critics of homebound education believe that it is not a sufficient substitute for classroom learning. Additionally, many children with chronic pain have intermittent rather than extended absences, which makes them ineligible for homebound education services. Even when homebound education is an option, it is often difficult for students from low-income or otherwise disadvantaged backgrounds. Programs typically require a computer, Internet connection, a quiet and well-lit space, and parental supervision, demands that may burdensome for economically disadvantaged families.

Special Education Services

While children with chronic pain are typically not placed in special education classrooms, they may receive health-related accommodations. Such accommodations may include shorter school days, exemption from requirements like physical education classes, arrangements to deliver medication and other treatments, and programs to educate classmates about their disorder. These measures require extensive communication between teachers, doctors, and school nurses.

Family Impacts

Paediatric chronic pain often impacts quality of life for the families of children affected, with mothers having particularly low health-related quality of life on average. Parents of children with chronic pain conditions allocate considerable physical, financial, and emotional resources towards health care for their child. For example, a study by Ho and colleagues found that primary caregivers for chronically ill children spent an average of around $8800 and 28.5 hours on medical appointments in the past three months, causing them to miss an average of 4 days of work.

Mental Health

Childhood chronic pain often exists alongside mental health conditions like anxiety disorders, depression, and post-traumatic stress disorder (PTSD), with elevated rates of these disorders lasting into adulthood. There are a variety of theories that address this relationship. Chronic pain is emotionally stressful both to the child affected and to his or her family, which may increase their risks for mental illness. Chronic pain and PTSD can also be "mutually maintaining", with cognitive, behavioural, and affective patterns creating a cycle of worsening physical and mental symptoms. Under this model, depressive symptoms (such as reduced activity and increased physiological arousal) aggravate pain symptoms, and unhealthy coping strategies (such as catastrophic thinking) worsen mental health.

Many mental health disorders also share neurobiological mechanisms with psychological disorders, such as activating the HPA axis and increasing the production of stress hormones. Chronic pain, anxiety, depression, and PTSD are also all associated dysfunction involving serotonin and brain-derived neurotrophic factor. New research has also linked both chronic pain and mental illness to inflammation.

Quality of Life

In a study of patients at a paediatric pain clinic, researchers found that chronic pain had a significant negative impact on quality of life. Depression was also prevalent, and was correlated with functional disability. Additionally, psychosocial adjustment is a better predictor of school attendance than pain severity, which suggests that it is an important variable in examining outcomes of children with chronic pain. The psychological consequences of chronic pain may be exacerbated with the stigma associated with it. Many people do not typically associate chronic pain with children, and so may minimize or dismiss its impact.

Factors Affecting Outcomes

Demographic Factors

Chronic pain, especially chronic headache, is more common in girls, older children, and children from low socioeconomic status backgrounds. According to researchers Anna Huguet and Jordi Miró, the most common locations for paediatric chronic pain are the head and abdomen. These two locations are more likely to be sources of chronic pain for girls, whereas boys are more likely to experience lower limb pain. Girls are also more likely than boys to experience multiple sources of pain. The prevalence of chronic pain among girls increases sharply between the ages of 12 and 14, which leads some researchers to believe that it is linked to menarche and other hormonal changes during puberty.

Age also has a significant impact on children's experiences with chronic pain. Young children often cannot describe their pain in ways that adults understand, and even older children may lack the vocabulary to clearly communicate with medical professionals. Doctors, especially general practitioners, may also lack experience diagnosing or treating paediatric chronic pain disorders, and so make and so make patients and their families feel "judged, disbelieved, and labeled as difficult or dysfunctional".

Genetics and Family Factors

Chronic pain can run in families, with the risk of paediatric chronic pain increasing dramatically for offspring of adults with chronic pain. This is often attributable to genetic predispositions to certain disorders, but can also be associated with individual differences in stress response. Researchers at UCLA found that adults with the *5-HT-*

TLPR S allele had higher cortisol levels, which can contribute both to the progression of chronic pain disorders and to less positive parenting.

For chronic pain patients, family support is an important factor in promoting successful pain management and rehabilitation. While healthy family interaction has a positive impact on paediatric pain patients, overprotectiveness and unhealthy relationship demands can foster depressive symptoms.

School Support

School support is also an important factor influencing paediatric chronic pain outcomes. When children receive appropriate support from teachers and school counsellors, they are more likely to achieve attain success and psychological wellbeing. This process can often be facilitated by a paediatric nurse practitioner (PNP), who coordinates a child's education with his or her medical treatment.

Peer Education

An important component of school support for many children with chronic pain is peer education. These children often face bullying and exclusion from peers, especially when they have visible markers of disability (i.e. a wheelchair) or are unable to participate in school activities (i.e. physical education classes or recess games). Peer education programs vary based on the child's age and medical condition, but often include informative presentations, role playing, and question and answer sessions. Evaluations of the efficacy of these programs have generally shown positive effects for increasing peers' disease-related knowledge, but uncertainty remains about whether they can produce changes in attitudes and behaviours.

Teacher Education

The majority of teachers feel some degree of anxiety about having children with chronic health conditions in their classrooms. Only 40% of teachers in a study by Clay and colleagues received formal training about teaching children with chronic illnesses, and so many were concerned about providing appropriate accommodations and handling any medical emergencies. Teacher education programs have found moderate positive effects in increasing school personnel's knowledge about chronic pain and comfortableness teaching children with chronic pain disorders.

Back Pain

Back pain is pain felt in the back. Episodes of back pain may be acute, sub-acute, or chronic depending on the duration. The pain may be characterized as a dull ache, shooting or piercing pain, or a burning sensation. The pain may radiate into the arms and hands as well as the legs or feet, and may include paresthesia (tingling with no apparent cause), weakness or numbness in the legs and arms. The anatomic classification of back pain follows the segments of the spine: neck pain (cervical), middle back pain (thoracic), lower back pain (lumbar) or coccydynia (tailbone or sacral pain) with the lumbar vertebrae area most common for pain.

The pain may originate from the muscles, nerves, bones, joints or other structures in the vertebral column (spine). Internal structures such as the gallbladder and pancreas may also cause referred pain in the back.

Back pain is common with about nine out of ten adults experiencing it at some point in their life, and five out of ten working adults having it every year. However, it is rare for it to be permanently disabling, and in most cases of herniated disks and stenosis, rest, injections or surgery have similar general pain resolution outcomes on average after one year. In the United States, acute low back pain is the fifth most common reason for physician visits and causes 40% of missed days off work. Additionally, it is the single leading cause of disability worldwide.

Classification

Back pain may be classified by various methods to aid its diagnosis and management. The duration of back pain is considered in three categories, following the expected pattern of healing of connective tissue. Acute pain lasts up to 12 weeks, subacute pain refers to the second half of the acute period (6 to 12 weeks), and chronic pain is pain which persists beyond 12 weeks.

Nonspecific back pain is believed to result from soft tissues such as muscles, fascia, and ligaments. Radicular pain with or without spinal stenosis indicates involvement of nervous tissue. Secondary back pain results from a known medical diagnosis such as infection or cancer. Non specific pain indicates that the cause is not known precisely but is believed to be due from the soft tissues such as muscles, fascia, and ligaments.

Back pain has several causes. Approximately 98 percent of back pain patients are diagnosed with nonspecific acute back pain in which no serious underlying pathology is identified. Nearly 2 percent are comprised by metastatic cancers, while serious infections such as spinal osteomyelitis and epidural abscesses account for fewer than 1 percent. The most common cause of neurologic impairment including weakness or numbness results from a herniated disc. Nearly 95 percent of disc herniations occur at the lowest two lumbar intervertebral levels.

Associated Conditions

Back pain does not usually require immediate medical intervention. The vast majority of episodes of back pain are self-limiting and non-progressive. Most back pain syndromes are due to inflammation, especially in the acute phase, which typically lasts from two weeks to three months.

Back pain can be a sign of a serious medical problem, although this is not most frequently the underlying cause:

- Typical warning signs of a potentially life-threatening problem are bowel and/or bladder incontinence or progressive weakness in the legs.
- Severe back pain (such as pain that is bad enough to interrupt sleep) that occurs with other signs of severe illness (*e.g.* fever, unexplained weight loss) may also indicate a serious underlying medical condition.
- Back pain that occurs after a trauma, such as a car accident or fall, may indicate a bone fracture or other injury.
- Back pain in individuals with medical conditions that put them at high risk for a spinal fracture, such as osteoporosis or multiple myeloma, also warrants prompt medical attention.
- Back pain in individuals with a history of cancer (especially cancers known to spread to the spine like breast, lung and prostate cancer) should be evaluated to rule out metastatic disease of the spine.

A few observational studies suggest that two conditions to which back pain is often attributed, lumbar disc herniation and degenerative disc disease, may not be more prevalent among those in pain than among the general population, and that the mechanisms by which these conditions might cause pain are not known. Other studies suggest that for as many as 85% of cases, no physiological cause can be shown.

A few studies suggest that psychosocial factors such as on-the-job stress and dysfunctional family relationships may correlate more closely with back pain than structural abnormalities revealed in X-rays and other medical imaging scans.

Causes

There are several potential sources and causes of back pain. However, the diagnosis of specific tissues of the spine as the cause of pain presents problems. This is because symptoms arising from different spinal tissues can feel very similar and it is difficult to differentiate without the use of invasive diagnostic intervention procedures, such as local anesthetic blocks.

One potential source of back pain is skeletal muscle of the back. Potential causes of pain in muscle tissue include muscle strains (pulled muscles), muscle spasm, and muscle imbalances. However, imaging studies do not support the notion of muscle tissue damage in many back pain cases, and the neurophysiology of muscle spasm and muscle imbalances is not well understood.

Another potential source of lower back pain is the synovial joints of the spine (e.g. zygapophysial joints/facet joints). These have been identified as the primary source of the pain in approximately one third of people with chronic low back pain, and in most people with neck pain following whiplash. However, the cause of zygapophysial joint pain is not fully understood. Capsule tissue damage has been proposed in people with neck pain following whiplash. In people with spinal pain stemming from zygapophysial joints, one theory is that intra-articular tissue such as invaginations of their synovial membranes and fibro-adipose meniscoids (that usually act as a cushion to help the bones move over each other smoothly) may become displaced, pinched or trapped, and consequently give rise to nociception (pain).

There are several common other potential sources and causes of back pain– these include spinal disc herniation and degenerative disc disease or isthmic spondylolisthesis, osteoarthritis (degenerative joint disease) and lumbar spinal stenosis, trauma, cancer, infection, fractures, and inflammatory disease. The anterior ligaments of the intervertebral disc are extremely sensitive, and even the slightest injury can cause significant pain.

Radicular pain (sciatica) is distinguished from 'non-specific' back pain, and may be diagnosed without invasive diagnostic tests.

New attention has been focused on *non-discogenic back pain*, where patients have normal or near-normal MRI and CT scans. One of the newer investigations looks into the role of the dorsal ramus in patients that have no radiographic abnormalities (Posterior Rami Syndrome).

Another possible cause of chronic back pain in people with otherwise normal scans is central sensitization, where an initial injury or infection causes a longer-lasting state of heightened sensitivity to pain. This persistent state maintains pain even after the initial injury has healed. Treatment of sensitization typically involves low doses of anti-depressants.

Risk Factors

- Smokers are more likely to get back pain than others.

Diagnosis

In most cases of low back pain medical consensus advises not seeking an exact diagnosis but instead beginning to treat the pain. This assumes that there is no reason to expect that the person has an underlying problem. In most cases, the pain goes away naturally after a few weeks. Typically, people who do seek diagnosis through imaging are not likely to have a better outcome than those who wait for the condition to resolve.

Prevention

There is moderate quality evidence that suggests the combination of education and exercise may reduce an individual's risk of developing an episode of low back pain. Lesser quality evidence points to exercise alone as a possible deterrent to the risk of the onset of this condition.

Management

The management goals when treating back pain are to achieve maximal reduction in pain intensity as rapidly as possible, to restore the individual's ability to function in everyday activities, to help the patient cope with residual pain, to assess for side-effects of therapy, and to facilitate the patient's passage through the legal and socioeconomic impediments to recovery. For many, the goal is to keep the pain to a manageable level to progress with rehabilitation, which then can lead to long-term pain relief. Also, for some people the goal is to use non-surgical therapies to manage the pain and avoid major surgery, while for others surgery may be the quickest way to feel better.

Not all treatments work for all conditions or for all individuals with the same condition, and many find that they need to try several treatment options to determine what works best for them. The present stage of the condition (acute or chronic) is also a determining factor in the choice of treatment. Only a minority of back pain patients (most estimates are 1% - 10%) require surgery.

Pain

- Heat therapy is useful for back spasms or other conditions. A review concluded that heat therapy can reduce symptoms of acute and sub-acute low-back pain. Some patients find that moist heat works best (e.g. a hot bath or whirlpool) or continuous low-level heat (e.g. a heat wrap that stays warm for 4 to 6 hours).
- Cold compression therapy (e.g. ice or cold pack application) may be effective at relieving back pain in some cases.
- Use of medications in chronic back pain is controversial. The short term use of muscle relaxants is effective in the relief of acute back pain. Opioids have not always been shown to be better than placebo for chronic back pain when the risks and benefits are considered. Non-steroidal anti-inflammatory drugs (NSAIDs/NSAIAs) have been shown to be more effective than placebo, and are usually more effective than paracetamol (acetaminophen). There is insufficient clinical trials to determine if injection therapy, usually with corticosteroids, helps in cases of low back pain.
- "Back school" is an intervention that consists of both education and physical exercises. A 2016 Cochrane review found the evidence concerning back school to be very low quality and was not able to make generalizations as to whether back school is effective or not.

- There is limited evidence that massage may help those with lower back pain. Massage may give short-term pain relief, but not functional improvement, for those with acute lower back pain. Massage may give short-term pain relief and functional improvement for those with long-term (chronic) and sub-acute lower pack pain, but this benefit does not appear to be sustained after 6 months of treatment. There does not appear to be any serious adverse effects associated with massage.
- Exercises can be an effective approach to reducing pain, but should be done under supervision of a licensed health professional. Generally, some form of consistent stretching and exercise is believed to be an essential component of most back treatment programs. However, one study found that exercise is effective for chronic back pain, but not for acute pain. Another study found that back-mobilizing exercises in acute settings are *less effective* than continuation of ordinary activities as tolerated.
- Education and attitude adjustment to focus on psychological or emotional causes - respondent-cognitive therapy and progressive relaxation therapy can reduce chronic pain.

Procedures

For back pain with sciatica, injecting the spine with steroids into the epidural space under X-ray guidance may improve pain and reduce the need for surgery.

For sacroiliac joints radiofrequency neurotomy is of unclear benefit.

Surgery

Surgery may sometimes be appropriate for people with:

- Lumbar disc herniation or degenerative disc disease
- Lumbar spinal stenosis from lumbar disc herniation, degenerative joint disease, or spondylolisthesis
- Scoliosis
- Compression fracture

Surgery is usually the last resort in the treatment of back pain. It is usually only recommended if all other treatment options have been tried or in an emergency situation. A 2009 systematic review of back surgery studies found that, for certain diagnoses, surgery is moderately better than other common treatments, but the benefits of surgery often decline in the long term.

The main procedures used in back pain surgery are discetomies, spinal fusions, laminectomies, removal of tumors, and vertebroplasties.

There are different types of surgical procedures that are used in treating various conditions causing back pain. Nerve decompression, fusion of body segments and deformity correction surgeries are examples. The first type of surgery is primarily performed in older patients who suffer from conditions causing nerve irritation or nerve damage. Fusion of bony segments is also referred to as a spinal fusion, and it is a procedure used to fuse together two or more bony fragments with the help of metalwork. The latter type of surgery is normally performed to correct congenital deformities or those that were caused by a traumatic fracture. In some cases, correction of deformities involves removing bony fragments or providing stability provision for the spine. Another procedure to repair common intervertebral disc lesions which may offer rapid recovery (just a few days) involves the simple removal of the fibrous nucleus of the affected intervertebral disc. Various techniques, such as in the following paragraph, are described in the literature.

A discectomy is performed when the intervertebral disc have herniated or torn. It involves removing the protruding disc, either a portion of it or all of it, that is placing pressure on the nerve root. The disc material which is putting pressure on the nerve is removed through a small incision that is made over that particular disc. The recovery period after this procedure does not last longer than 6 weeks. The type of procedure in which the bony fragments are removed through an endoscope is called percutaneous disc removal. Microdiscetomies may be performed as a variation of standard discetomies in which a magnifier is used to provide the advantage of a smaller incision, thus a shorter recovery process.

Spinal fusions are performed in cases in which the patient has had the entire disc removed or when another condition has caused the vertebrae to become unstable. The procedure consists in uniting two or more vertebrae by using bone grafts and metalwork to provide more strength for the healing bone. Recovery after spinal fusion may take up to one year, depending greatly on the age of the patient, the reason why surgery has been performed and how many bony segments needed to be fused.

In cases of spinal stenosis and disc herniation, a laminectomy can be performed. During this procedure, pressure on the nerves is reduced, thereby relieving some pain. A specifically designed exercise program during recovery can increase functional status and decrease low back pain as compared to the common recommendation to “stay active”.

Back surgery can be performed to prevent the growth of benign and malignant tumors. In the first case, surgery has the goal of relieving the pressure from the nerves which is caused by a benign growth, whereas in the latter the procedure is aimed to prevent the spread of cancer to other areas of the body. Recovery depends on the type of tumor that is being removed, the health status of the patient and the size of the tumor.

Doubtful Benefit

- Cold compression therapy is advocated for a strained back or chronic back pain and is postulated to reduce pain and inflammation, especially after strenuous exercise such as golf, gardening, or lifting. However, a meta-analysis of randomized controlled trials by the Cochrane Collaboration concluded "The evidence for the application of cold treatment to low-back pain is even more limited, with only three poor quality studies located. No conclusions can be drawn about the use of cold for low-back pain".

- Bed rest is rarely recommended as it can exacerbate symptoms, and when necessary is usually limited to one or two days. Prolonged bed rest or inactivity is actually counterproductive, as the resulting stiffness leads to more pain.
- Inversion therapy is useful for temporary back relief due to the traction method or spreading of the vertebrae through (in this case) gravity. The patient hangs in an upside down position for a period of time from ankles or knees until this separation occurs. The effect can be achieved without a complete vertical hang (90 degree) and noticeable benefits can be observed at angles as low as 10 to 45 degrees.
- Ultrasound has been shown not to be beneficial and has fallen out of favor.

Chronic Back Pain

People with back pain lasting for 3 months or more are at risk of physical, psychological and social dysfunctions. Such individuals are likely to experience less pain and disability if they receive a multidisciplinary intervention. This typically involves a combination of physical, psychological and educational interventions delivered by a team of specialists with different skills. Such multidisciplinary treatment programs are often quite intensive and expensive. They are more appropriate for people with severe or complex problems.

People who have chronic back pain may have limited range of motion and/or tenderness upon touch. If the pain continues to worsen, or certain red flags that might indicate a variety of serious conditions are present further testing may be recommended. These red flags include weakness, numbness or tingling, fever, weight loss or problems with bowel and/or bladder control.

Alternative Medicine

- Studies of manipulation suggest that this approach has a benefit similar to other therapies and is superior to placebo.
- Acupuncture has some proven benefit for back painpages however, a recent randomized controlled trial suggested insignificant difference between real and sham acupuncture.
- Electrotherapy, such as a transcutaneous electrical nerve stimulation (TENS) has been proposed. Two randomized controlled trials found con-

flicting results. This has led the Cochrane Collaboration to conclude that there is inconsistent evidence to support use of TENS. In addition, spinal cord stimulation, where an electrical device is used to interrupt the pain signals being sent to the brain, has been studied for various underlying causes of back pain.

- It is unclear if low level laser therapy is useful for low back pain.
- A 2017 systematic review found tai chi and mindfulness-based stress reduction are effective interventions.

Pregnancy

About 50% of women experience low back pain during pregnancy. Back pain in pregnancy may be severe enough to cause significant pain and disability and pre-dispose patients to back pain in a following pregnancy. No significant increased risk of back pain with pregnancy has been found with respect to maternal weight gain, exercise, work satisfaction, or pregnancy outcome factors such as birth weight, birth length, and Apgar scores.

Biomechanical factors of pregnancy that are shown to be associated with low back pain of pregnancy include abdominal sagittal and transverse diameter and the depth of lumbar lordosis. Typical factors aggravating the back pain of pregnancy include standing, sitting, forward bending, lifting, and walking. Back pain in pregnancy may also be characterized by pain radiating into the thigh and buttocks, night-time pain severe enough to wake the patient, pain that is increased during the night-time, or pain that is increased during the day-time.

The avoidance of high impact, weight-bearing activities and especially those that asymmetrically load the involved structures such as extensive twisting with lifting, may help. Direct bending to the ground without bending the knee causes severe impact on the lower back in pregnancy and in normal individuals, which leads to strain, especially in the lumbo-sacral region that as a result strains the multifidus.

Economics

Back pain is regularly cited by national governments as having a major impact on productivity, through loss of workers on sick leave. Some national governments, notably Australia and the United Kingdom, have launched campaigns of public health awareness to help combat the problem, for example the Health and Safety Executive's Better Backs campaign. In the United States lower back pain's economic impact reveals that it is the number one reason for individuals under the age of 45 to limit their activity, second highest complaint seen in physician's offices, fifth most common requirement for hospitalization, and the third leading cause for surgery.

Evolutionary Perspective

An evolutionary perspective has been used to try to explain why humans have back pain. Selective pressures often resulted in our evolution as a species. At times we are able to postulate the reason for these changes, and other times we cannot seem to arrive at a logical conclusion about the possible benefits of the tradeoff. In the case of back pain, researcher Aaron G. Filler believes the evolutionary changes seen in the human skeleton occurred to ensure the survival of the species. Of special mention here is our ability to walk upright. Walking upright meant that our hands were now free to carry heavy objects and the young across great distances.

Research

A study with 80 patients found magnesium to be useful in those with chronic back pain.

Abdominal Pain

Abdominal pain, also known as stomach pain or tummy ache, is a common symptom associated with non-serious and serious causes.

Common causes of pain in the abdomen include gastroenteritis and irritable bowel syndrome. In a third of cases the exact cause is unclear. About 10% of people have a more serious underlying condition such as appendicitis, leaking or ruptured abdominal aortic aneurysm, diverticulitis, or ectopic pregnancy. Determining the cause can be difficult, because many diseases can cause this symptom.

Differential Diagnosis

The most frequent reason for abdominal pain are gastroenteritis (13%), irritable bowel syndrome (8%), urinary tract problems (5%), inflammation of the stomach (5%) and constipation (5%). In about 30% of cases, the cause is not determined. About 10% of cases have a more serious cause including gallbladder (gallstones or biliary dyskinesia) or pancreas problems (4%), diverticulitis (3%), appendicitis (2%) and cancer (1%). More common in those who are older, mesenteric ischemia and abdominal aortic aneurysms are other serious causes.

A more extensive list includes the following:

- Gastrointestinal
    - GI tract
        - Inflammatory: gastroenteritis, appendicitis, gastritis, esophagitis, diverticulitis, Crohn's disease, ulcerative colitis, microscopic colitis

        - Obstruction: hernia, intussusception, volvulus, post-surgical adhesions, tumours, severe constipation, hemorrhoids
        - Vascular: embolism, thrombosis, hemorrhage, sickle cell disease, abdominal angina, blood vessel compression (such as celiac artery compression syndrome), superior mesenteric artery syndrome, postural orthostatic tachycardia syndrome
        - Digestive: peptic ulcer, lactose intolerance, coeliac disease, food allergies
    - Glands
        - Bile system
            - Inflammatory: cholecystitis, cholangitis
            - Obstruction: cholelithiasis, tumours
        - Liver
            - Inflammatory: hepatitis, liver abscess
        - Pancreatic
            - Inflammatory: pancreatitis
- Renal and urological
    - Inflammation: pyelonephritis, bladder infection, indigestion
    - Obstruction: kidney stones, urolithiasis, urinary retention, tumours
    - Vascular: left renal vein entrapment
- Gynaecological or obstetric
    - Inflammatory: pelvic inflammatory disease
    - Mechanical: ovarian torsion
    - Endocrinological: menstruation, Mittelschmerz
    - Tumors: endometriosis, fibroids, ovarian cyst, ovarian cancer
    - Pregnancy: ruptured ectopic pregnancy, threatened abortion
- Abdominal wall
    - muscle strain or trauma
    - muscular infection

    - neurogenic pain: herpes zoster, radiculitis in Lyme disease, abdominal cutaneous nerve entrapment syndrome (ACNES), tabes dorsalis
- Referred pain
    - from the thorax: pneumonia, pulmonary embolism, ischemic heart disease, pericarditis
    - from the spine: radiculitis
    - from the genitals: testicular torsion
- Metabolic disturbance
    - uremia, diabetic ketoacidosis, porphyria, C1-esterase inhibitor deficiency, adrenal insufficiency, lead poisoning, black widow spider bite, narcotic withdrawal
- Blood vessels
    - aortic dissection, abdominal aortic aneurysm
- Immune system
    - sarcoidosis
    - vasculitis
    - familial Mediterranean fever
- Idiopathic
    - irritable bowel syndrome (affecting up to 20% of the population, IBS is the most common cause of recurrent, intermittent abdominal pain)

Acute Abdominal Pain

Acute abdomen can be defined as severe, persistent abdominal pain of sudden onset that is likely to require surgical intervention to treat its cause. The pain may frequently be associated with nausea and vomiting, abdominal distention, fever and signs of shock. One of the most common conditions associated with acute abdominal pain is acute appendicitis.

Selected Causes of Acute Abdomen

- Traumatic: blunt or perforating trauma to the stomach, bowel, spleen, liver, or kidney
- Inflammatory:

  - Infections such as appendicitis, cholecystitis, pancreatitis, pyelonephritis, pelvic inflammatory disease, hepatitis, mesenteric adenitis, or a subdiaphragmatic abscess
  - Perforation of a peptic ulcer, a diverticulum, or the caecum
  - Complications of inflammatory bowel disease such as Crohn's disease or ulcerative colitis
- Mechanical:
  - Small bowel obstruction secondary to adhesions caused by previous surgeries, intussusception, hernias, benign or malignant neoplasms
  - Large bowel obstruction caused by colorectal cancer, inflammatory bowel disease, volvulus, fecal impaction or hernia
- Vascular: occlusive intestinal ischemia, usually caused by thromboembolism of the superior mesenteric artery

By Location

Location

- Upper middle abdominal pain
  - Stomach (gastritis, stomach ulcer, stomach cancer)
  - Pancreas pain (pancreatitis or pancreatic cancer, can radiate to the left side of the waist, back, and even shoulder)
  - Duodenal ulcer, diverticulitis
  - Appendicitis (starts here, after some time moves to lower right abdomen)
- Upper right abdominal pain
  - Liver (caused by hepatomegaly due to fatty liver, hepatitis, or caused by liver cancer, abscess)
  - Gallbladder and biliary tract (gallstones, inflammation, roundworms)
  - Colon pain (below the area of liver – bowel obstruction, functional disorders, gas accumulation, spasm, inflammation, colon cancer)
- Upper left abdominal pain
  - Spleen pain (splenomegaly)
  - Pancreas

  - Colon pain (below the area of spleen – bowel obstruction, functional disorders, gas accumulation, spasm, inflammation, colon cancer)
- Middle abdominal pain (pain in the area around belly button)
  - Appendicitis (starts here)
  - Small intestine pain (inflammation, intestinal spasm, functional disorders)
- Lower abdominal pain (diarrhea, colitis and dysentery)
- Lower right abdominal pain
  - Cecum (intussusception, bowel obstruction)
  - Appendix point (Appendicitis location)
- Lower left abdominal pain
  - diverticulitis, sigmoid volvulus, obstruction or gas accumulation
- Pelvic pain
  - bladder (cystitis, may be secondary to diverticulum and bladder stone, bladder cancer)
  - pain in women (uterus, ovaries, fallopian tubes)
- Right lumbago and back pain
  - liver pain (hepatomegaly)
  - right kidney pain (its location below the area of liver pain)
- Left lumbago and back pain
  - less in spleen pain
  - left kidney pain
- Low back pain
  - kidney pain (kidney stone, kidney cancer, hydronephrosis)
  - Ureteral stone pain

Diagnostic Approach

When a health care practitioner assesses a patient to determine the etiology and subsequent treatment for abdominal pain the history of the presenting complaint and physical examination should derive a diagnosis in over 90% of cases.

Investigations that aid diagnosis include

- Blood tests including full blood count, electrolytes, urea, creatinine, liver function tests, pregnancy test, amylase and lipase.
- Urinalysis
- Imaging including erect chest X-ray and plain films of the abdomen
- An electrocardiograph to rule out a heart attack which can occasionally present as abdominal pain

If diagnosis remains unclear after history, examination and basic investigations as above then more advanced investigations may reveal a diagnosis. These as such would include

- Computed tomography of the abdomen/pelvis
- Abdominal or pelvic ultrasound
- Endoscopy and colonoscopy (not used for diagnosing acute pain)

Management

Butylscopolamine (Buscopan) is used to treat cramping abdominal pain with some success.

Epidemiology

Abdominal pain is the reason about 3% of adults see their family physician. Rates of emergency department visits in the United States for abdominal pain increased 18% from 2006 through 2011. This was the largest increase out of 20 common conditions seen in the ED. The rate of ED use for nausea and vomiting also increased 18%.

Appendicitis

Appendicitis is inflammation of the appendix. Symptoms commonly include right lower abdominal pain, nausea, vomiting, and decreased appetite. However, approximately 40% of people do not have these typical symptoms. Severe complications of a ruptured appendix include widespread, painful inflammation of the inner lining of the abdominal wall and sepsis.

Appendicitis is caused by a blockage of the hollow portion of the appendix. This is most commonly due to a calcified "stone" made of feces. Inflamed lymphoid tissue from a viral infection, parasites, gallstone, or tumors may also cause the blockage. This blockage leads to increased pressures in the appendix, decreased blood flow to the tissues of the appendix, and bacterial growth inside the appendix causing inflammation. The combination of inflammation, reduced blood flow to the appendix and distention of the appendix causes tissue injury and tissue death. If this process is left untreated, the appendix may burst, releasing bacteria into the abdominal cavity, leading to severe abdominal pain and increased complications.

The diagnosis of appendicitis is largely based on the person's signs and symptoms. In cases where the diagnosis cannot be made based on the person's history and physical exam, close observation, radiographic imaging and laboratory tests can be helpful. The two most common imaging tests used are an ultrasound and computed tomography (CT scan). CT scan has been shown to be more accurate than ultrasound in detecting acute appendicitis. However, ultrasound may be preferred as the first imaging test in children and pregnant women because of the risks associated with radiation exposure from CT scans.

The standard treatment for acute appendicitis is surgical removal of the appendix. This may be done by an open incision in the abdomen (laparotomy) or through a few smaller incisions with the help of cameras (laparoscopy). Surgery decreases the risk of side effects or death associated with rupture of the appendix. Antibiotics may be equally effective in certain cases of non-ruptured appendicitis. It is one of the most common and significant causes of severe abdominal pain that comes on quickly. In 2015 about 11.6 million cases of appendicitis occurred which resulted in about 50,100 deaths. In the United States, appendicitis is the most common cause of acute abdominal pain requiring surgery. Each year in the United States, more than 300,000 people with appendicitis have their appendix surgically removed. Reginald Fitz is credited with being the first person to describe the condition in 1886.

Signs and Symptoms

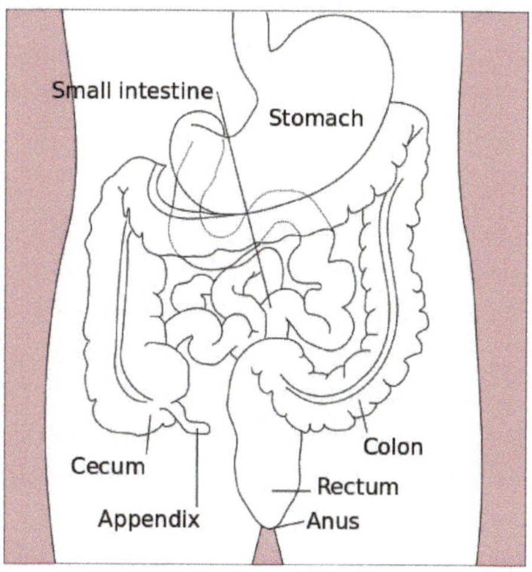

Location of the appendix in the digestive system

The presentation of acute appendicitis includes abdominal pain, nausea, vomiting, and fever. As the appendix becomes more swollen and inflamed, it begins to irritate the adjoining abdominal wall. This leads to the localization of the pain to the right lower quadrant. This classic migration of pain may not be seen in children under three years. This pain can be elicited through signs and can be severe. Signs include localized findings in the right iliac fossa. The abdominal wall becomes very sensitive to gentle pressure (palpation). There is severe pain on sudden release of deep pressure in the lower abdomen (rebound tenderness). If the appendix is retrocecal (localized behind the cecum), even deep pressure in the right lower quadrant may fail to elicit tenderness (silent appendix). This is because the cecum, distended with gas, protects the inflamed appendix from pressure. Similarly, if the appendix lies entirely within the pelvis, there is usually complete absence of abdominal rigidity. In such cases, a digital rectal examination elicits tenderness in the rectovesical pouch. Coughing causes point tenderness in this area (McBurney's point).

Causes

Acute appendicitis seems to be the end result of a primary obstruction of the appendix. Once this obstruction occurs, the appendix becomes filled with mucus and swells. This continued production of mucus leads to increased pressures within the lumen and the walls of the appendix. The increased pressure results in thrombosis and occlusion of the small vessels, and stasis of lymphatic flow. At this point spontaneous recovery rarely occurs. As the occlusion of blood vessels progresses, the appendix becomes ischemic and then necrotic. As bacteria begin to leak out through the dying walls, pus forms within and around the appendix (suppuration). The end result is appendiceal rupture (a 'burst appendix') causing peritonitis, which may lead to sepsis and eventually death. These events are responsible for the slowly evolving abdominal pain and other commonly associated symptoms.

The causative agents include bezoars, foreign bodies, trauma, intestinal worms, lymphadenitis and, most commonly, calcified fecal deposits that are known as appendicoliths or fecaliths. The occurrence of obstructing fecaliths has attracted attention since their presence in people with appendicitis is higher in developed than in developing countries. In addition an appendiceal fecalith is commonly associated with complicated appendicitis. Fecal stasis and arrest may play a role, as demonstrated by people with acute appendicitis having fewer bowel movements per week compared with healthy controls.

The occurrence of a fecalith in the appendix was thought to be attributed to a right-sided fecal retention reservoir in the colon and a prolonged transit time. However, a prolonged transit time was not observed in subsequent studies. From epidemiological data, it has been stated that diverticular disease and adenomatous polyps were unknown and colon cancer exceedingly rare in communities exempt from appendicitis. And acute appendicitis has been shown to occur antecedent to cancer in the colon and rectum. Several studies offer evidence that a low fiber intake is involved in the pathogenesis of appendicitis. This low intake of dietary fiber is in accordance with the occurrence of a right-sided fecal reservoir and the fact that dietary fiber reduces transit time.

Diagnosis

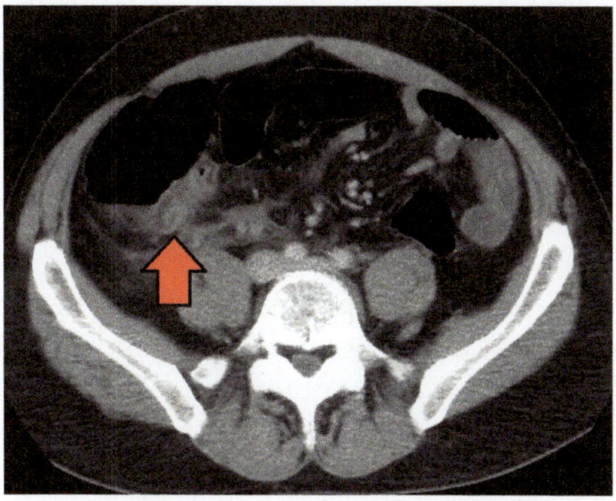

Appendicitis as seen on CT imaging

Diagnosis is based on a medical history (symptoms) and physical examination which can be supported by an elevation of neutrophilic white blood cells and imaging studies if needed. (Neutrophils are the primary white blood cells that respond to a bacterial infection.) Histories fall into two categories, typical and atypical.

Typical appendicitis includes several hours of generalized abdominal pain that begins in the region of the umbilicus with associated anorexia, nausea, or vomiting. The pain then "localizes" into the right lower quadrant where the tenderness increases in intensity. It is possible the pain could localize to the left lower quadrant in people with situs inversus totalis. The combination of pain, anorexia, leukocytosis, and fever is classic.

Atypical histories lack this typical progression and may include pain in the right lower quadrant as an initial symptom. Irritation of the peritoneum (inside lining of the abdominal wall) can lead to increased pain on movement, or jolting, for example going over speedbumps. Atypical histories often require imaging with ultrasound or CT scanning.

Clinical

- Aure-Rozanova's sign: Increased pain on palpation with finger in right Petit triangle (can be a positive Shchetkin-Bloomberg's).
- Bartomier-Michelson's sign: Increased pain on palpation at the right iliac region as the person being examined lies on his or her left side compared to when he/she lies on the back.
- Dunphy's sign: Increased pain in the right lower quadrant with coughing.
- Hamburger sign: The patient refuses to eat (anorexia is 80% specific for appendicitis)

- Kocher's (Kosher's) sign: From the person's medical history, the start of pain in the umbilical region with a subsequent shift to the right iliac region.
- Massouh sign: Developed in and popular in southwest England, the examiner performs a firm swish with his or her index and middle finger across the abdomen from the xiphoid process to the left and the right iliac fossa. A positive Massouh sign is a grimace of the person being examined upon a right sided (and not left) sweep.
- Obturator sign: The person being evaluated lies on her or his back with the hip and knee both flexed at ninety degrees. The examiner holds the person's ankle with one hand and knee with the other hand. The examiner rotates the hip by moving the person's ankle away from his or her body while allowing the knee to move only inward. A positive test is pain with internal rotation of the hip.
- Psoas sign, also known as "Obraztsova's sign", is right lower-quadrant pain that is produced with either the passive extension of the right hip or by the active flexion of the person's right hip while supine. The pain that is elicited is due to inflammation of the peritoneum overlying the iliopsoas muscles and inflammation of the psoas muscles themselves. Straightening out the leg causes pain because it stretches these muscles, while flexing the hip activates the iliopsoas and causes pain.
- Rovsing's sign: Pain in the lower right abdominal quadrant with continuous deep palpation starting from the left iliac fossa upwards (counterclockwise along the colon). The thought is there will be increased pressure around the appendix by pushing bowel contents and air toward the ileocaecal valve provoking right-sided abdominal pain.
- Sitkovskiy (Rosenstein)'s sign: Increased pain in the right iliac region as the person is being examined lies on his/her left side.

Blood and Urine Test

While there is no laboratory test specific for appendicitis, a complete blood count (CBC) is done to check for signs of infection. Although 70–90 percent of people with appendicitis may have an elevated white blood cell (WBC) count, there are many other abdominal and pelvic conditions that can cause the WBC count to be elevated. Due to its low sensitivity and specificity, on its own, WBC is not seen as a good indicator of appendicitis.

A urinalysis generally does not show infection, but it is important for determining pregnancy status, especially the possibility of an ectopic pregnancy in women of childbearing age. The urinalysis is also important for ruling out a urinary tract infection as the cause of abdominal pain. The presence of more than 20 WBC per high-power field in the urine is more suggestive of a urinary tract disorder.

Imaging

In children the clinical examination is important to determine which children with abdominal pain should receive immediate surgical consultation and which should receive diagnostic imaging. Because of the health risks of exposing children to radiation, ultrasound is the preferred first choice with CT scan being a legitimate follow-up if the ultrasound is inconclusive. CT scan is more accurate than ultrasound for the diagnosis of appendicitis in adults and adolescents. CT scan has a sensitivity of 94%, specificity of 95%. Ultrasonography had an overall sensitivity of 86%, a specificity of 81%.

Ultrasound

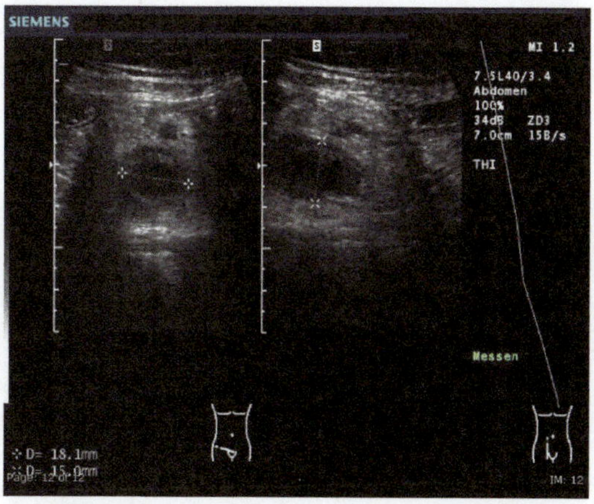

Ultrasound image of acute appendicitis

Ultrasonography and doppler sonography are useful to detect appendicitis, especially in children. Ultrasound can show free fluid collection in the right iliac fossa, along with a visible appendix with increased blood flow when using color Doppler, and noncompressibility of the appendix, as it is essentially a walled off abscess. Other secondary sonographic signs of acute appendicitis include the presence of echogenic mesenteric fat surrounding the appendix and the acoustic shadowing of an appendicolith. In some cases (approximately 5%), ultrasonography of the iliac fossa does not reveal any abnormalities despite the presence of appendicitis. This false negative finding is especially true of early appendicitis before the appendix has become significantly distended. In addition, false negative findings are more common in adults where larger amounts of fat and bowel gas make visualizing the appendix technically difficult. Despite these limitations, sonographic imaging in experienced hands can often distinguish between appendicitis and other diseases with similar symptoms. Some of these conditions include inflammation of lymph nodes near the appendix or pain originating from other pelvic organs such as the ovaries or Fallopian tubes.

Computed Tomography

Where it is readily available, computed tomography (CT) has become frequently used, especially in people whose diagnosis is not obvious on history and physical examination. Concerns about radiation tend to limit use of CT in pregnant women and children, especially with the increasingly widespread usage of MRI.

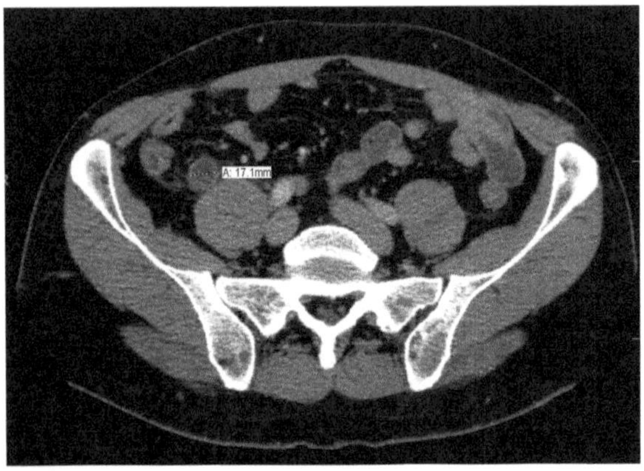

A CT scan demonstrating acute appendicitis (note the appendix has a diameter of 17.1 mm and there is surrounding fat stranding)

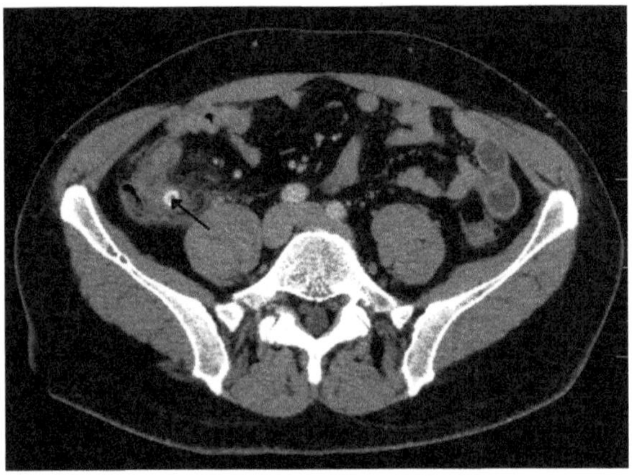

A fecalith marked by the arrow that has resulted in acute appendicitis.

The accurate diagnosis of appendicitis is multi-tiered, with the size of the appendix having the strongest positive predictive value, while indirect features can either increase or decrease sensitivity and specificity. A size of over 6 mm is both 95% sensitive and specific for appendicitis.

However, because the appendix can be filled with fecal material, causing intraluminal distention, this criterion has shown limited utility in more recent meta analyses. This is as opposed to ultrasound, in which the wall of the appendix can be more easily distinguished from intraluminal feces. In such scenarios, ancillary features such as increased wall enhancement as compared to adjacent bowel and inflammation of the surrounding fat, or fat stranding, can be supportive of the diagnosis, although their absence does not preclude it. In severe cases with perforation, an adjacent phlegmon or abscess can be seen. Dense fluid layering in the pelvis can also result, related to either pus or enteric spillage. When patients are thin or younger, the relative absence of fat can make the appendix and surrounding fat stranding difficult to see.

Magnetic Resonance Imaging

MRI use has become increasingly common for diagnosis of appendicitis in children and pregnant patients due to the radiation dosage that, while of nearly negligible risk in healthy adults, can be harmful to children or the developing fetus. In pregnancy, it has been found to be more useful during the second and third trimester, particularly as the enlargening uterus displaces the appendix, making it difficult to find by ultrasound. The periappendiceal stranding that is reflected on CT by fat stranding on MRI appears as increased fluid signal on T2 weighted sequences. First trimester pregnancies are usually not candidates for MRI, as the fetus is still undergoing organogenesis, and there are no long-term studies to date regarding its potential risks or side effects.

X-ray

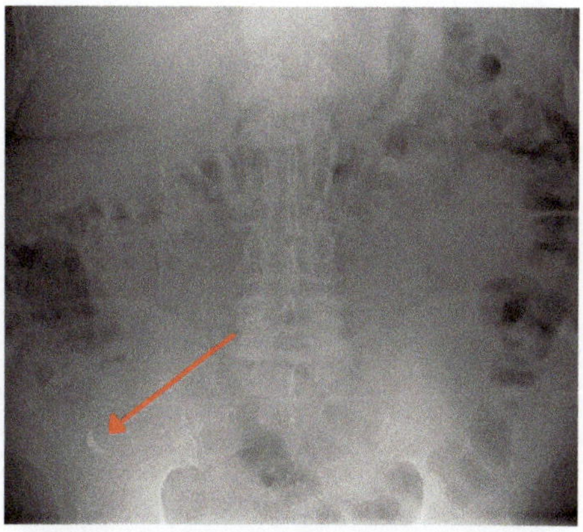

Appendicolith as seen on plain X-ray

In general, plain abdominal radiography (PAR) is not useful in making the diagnosis of appendicitis and should not be routinely obtained from a person being evaluated for appendicitis. Plain abdominal films may be useful for the detection of ureteral calculi, small bowel obstruction, or perforated ulcer, but these conditions are rarely confused with appendicitis. An opaque fecalith can be identified in the right lower quadrant in fewer than 5% of people being evaluated for appendicitis. A barium enema has proven to be a poor diagnostic tool for appendicitis. While failure of the appendix to fill during a barium enema has been associated with appendicitis, up to 20% of normal appendices do not fill.

Scoring Systems

Alvarado score	
Migratory right iliac fossa pain	1 point
Anorexia	1 point
Nausea and vomiting	1 point
Right iliac fossa tenderness	2 points

Rebound abdominal tenderness	1 point
Fever	1 point
High white blood cell count (leukocytosis)	2 points
Shift to left (segmented neutrophils)	1 point
Total score	**10 points**

No excellent scoring system exists to determine if a child has appendicitis. The Alvarado score and pediatric appendicitis score are useful but not definitive.

The Alvarado score is the most widely used scoring system. A score below 5 suggests against a diagnosis of appendicitis, whereas a score of 7 or more is predictive of acute appendicitis. In a person with an equivocal score of 5 or 6, a CT scan or ultrasound exam may be used to reduce the rate of negative appendectomy.

Pathology

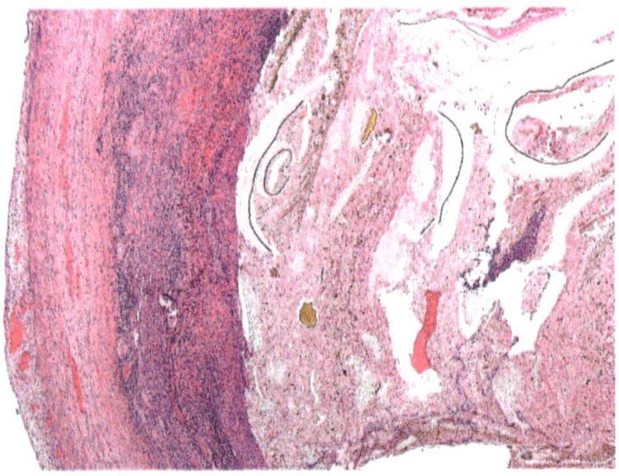

Micrograph of appendicitis and periappendicitis. H&E stain.

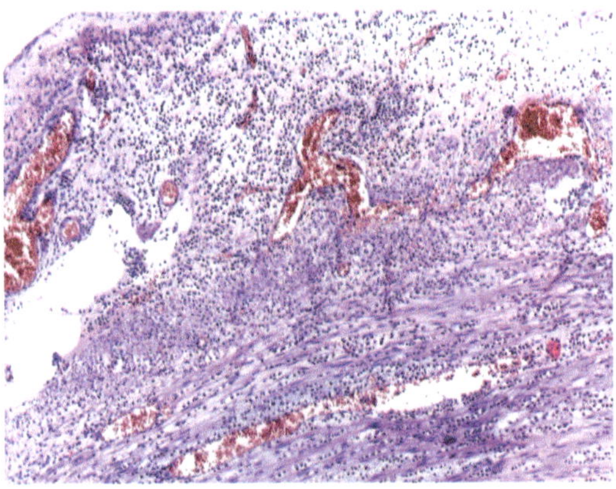

Micrograph of appendicitis showing neutrophils in the muscularis propria. H&E stain.

The definitive diagnosis is based on pathology. The histologic finding of appendicitis is neutrophilic infiltrate of the muscularis propria.

Periappendicitis, inflammation of tissues around the appendix, is often found in conjunction with other abdominal pathology.

Differential Diagnosis

Children: Gastroenteritis, mesenteric adenitis, Meckel's diverticulitis, intussusception, Henoch–Schönlein purpura, lobar pneumonia, urinary tract infection (abdominal pain in the absence of other symptoms can occur in children with UTI), new-onset Crohn's disease or ulcerative colitis, pancreatitis, and abdominal trauma from child abuse; distal intestinal obstruction syndrome in children with cystic fibrosis; typhlitis in children with leukemia.

Women: A pregnancy test is important for all women of childbearing age since an ectopic pregnancy can have signs and symptoms similar to those of appendicitis. Other obstetrical/gynecological causes of similar abdominal pain in women include pelvic inflammatory disease, ovarian torsion, menarche, dysmenorrhea, endometriosis, and Mittelschmerz (the passing of an egg in the ovaries approximately two weeks before menstruation).

Men: testicular torsion

Adults: new-onset Crohn's disease, ulcerative colitis, regional enteritis, renal colic, perforated peptic ulcer, pancreatitis, rectus sheath hematoma and epiploic appendagitis.

Elderly: diverticulitis, intestinal obstruction, colonic carcinoma, mesenteric ischemia, leaking aortic aneurysm.

The term "pseudoappendicitis" is used to describe a condition mimicking appendicitis. It can be associated with *Yersinia enterocolitica*.

Management

Acute appendicitis is typically managed by surgery. However, in uncomplicated cases, antibiotics are effective and safe. While antibiotics are effective for treating uncomplicated appendicitis, 26% of people had a recurrence within a year and required eventual appendectomy. They work less well if an appendicolith is present. Cost effectiveness of surgery versus antibiotics is unclear.

Pain

Pain medications (such as morphine) do not appear to affect the accuracy of the clinical diagnosis of appendicitis and therefore should be given early in the patient's care. Historically there were concerns among some general surgeons that analgesics would affect the clinical exam in children, and some recommended that they not be given until the surgeon was able to examine the person.

Surgery

The surgical procedure for the removal of the appendix is called an appendectomy. Appendectomy can be performed through open or laparoscopic surgery. Laparoscopic appendectomy has several advantages over open appendectomy as an intervention for acute appendicitis.

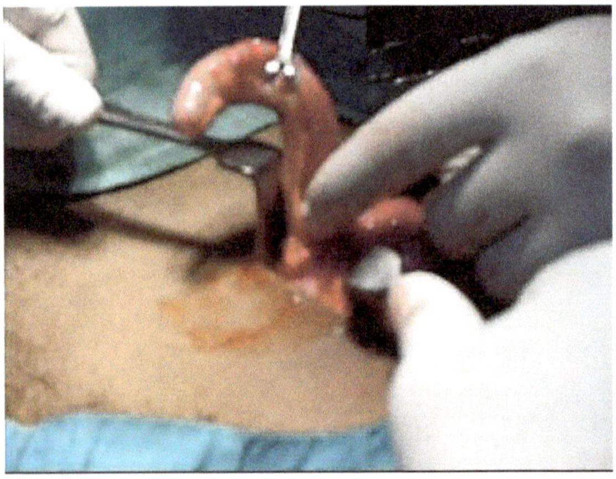

Inflamed appendix removal by open surgery

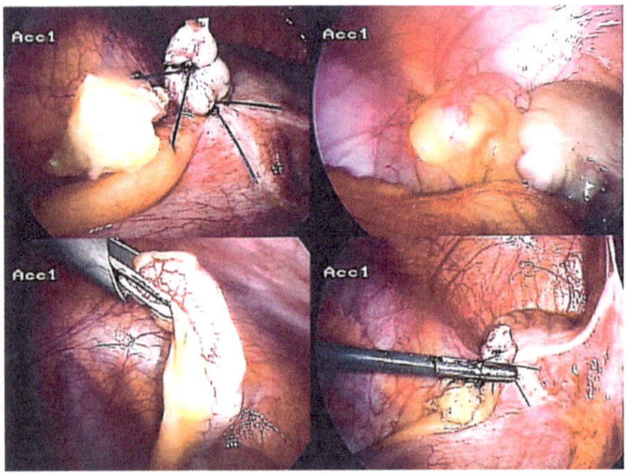

Laparoscopic appendectomy.

Open Appendectomy

For over a century, laparotomy (open appendectomy) was the standard treatment for acute appendicitis. This procedure consists of the removal of the infected appendix through a single large incision in the lower right area of the abdomen. The incision in a laparotomy is usually 2 to 3 inches (51 to 76 mm) long.

During an open appendectomy, the person with suspected appendicitis is placed under general anesthesia to keep the muscles completely relaxed and to keep the person unconscious. The incision is two to three inches (76 mm) long and it is made in the right lower abdomen, several inches above the hip bone. Once the incision opens the abdomen cavity and the appendix is identified, the surgeon removes the infected tissue and cuts the appendix from the surrounding tissue. After careful and close inspection of the infected area, and ensuring there are no signs that surrounding tissues are damaged or infected, the surgeon will start closing the incision. This means sewing the muscles and using surgical staples or stitches to close the skin up. To prevent infections, the incision is covered with a sterile bandage.

Laparoscopic Appendectomy

Laparoscopic appendectomy has become an increasingly prevalent intervention for acute appendicitis since its introduction in 1983. This surgical procedure consists of making three to four incisions in the abdomen, each 0.25 to 0.5 inches (6.4 to 12.7 mm) long. This type of appendectomy is made by inserting a special surgical tool called laparoscope into one of the incisions. The laparoscope is connected to a monitor outside the person's body and it is designed to help the surgeon to inspect the infected area in the abdomen. The other two incisions are made for the specific removal of the appendix by using surgical instruments. Laparoscopic surgery requires general anesthesia, and it can last up to two hours. Laparoscopic appendectomy has several advantages over open appendectomy, including a shorter post-operative recovery, less post-operative pain, and lower superficial surgical site infection rate. However, the occurrence of intra-abdominal abscess is almost three times more prevalent in laparoscopic appendectomy than open appendectomy.

Pre-surgery

The treatment begins by keeping the person who will be having surgery from eating or drinking for a given period, usually overnight. An intravenous drip is used to hydrate the person who will be having surgery. Antibiotics given intravenously such as cefuroxime and metronidazole may be administered early to help kill bacteria and thus reduce the spread of infection in the abdomen and postoperative complications in the abdomen or wound. Equivocal cases may become more difficult to assess with antibiotic treatment and benefit from serial examinations. If the stomach is empty (no food in the past six hours) general anaesthesia is usually used. Otherwise, spinal anaesthesia may be used.

Once the decision to perform an appendectomy has been made, the preparation procedure takes approximately one to two hours. Meanwhile, the surgeon will explain the surgery procedure and will present the risks that must be considered when performing an appendectomy. (With all surgeries there are risks that must be evaluated before performing the procedures.) The risks are different depending on the state of the appendix. If the appendix has not ruptured, the complication rate is only about 3% but if the appendix has ruptured, the complication rate rises to almost 59%. The most usual complications that can occur are pneumonia, hernia of the incision, thrombophlebitis, bleeding or adhesions. Recent evidence indicates that a delay in obtaining surgery after admission results in no measurable difference in outcomes to the person with appendicitis.

The surgeon will explain how long the recovery process should take. Abdomen hair is usually removed to avoid complications that may appear regarding the incision.

In most cases, patients going in for surgery experience nausea or vomiting that requires medication before surgery. Antibiotics along with pain medication may be administrated before appendectomies.

After Surgery

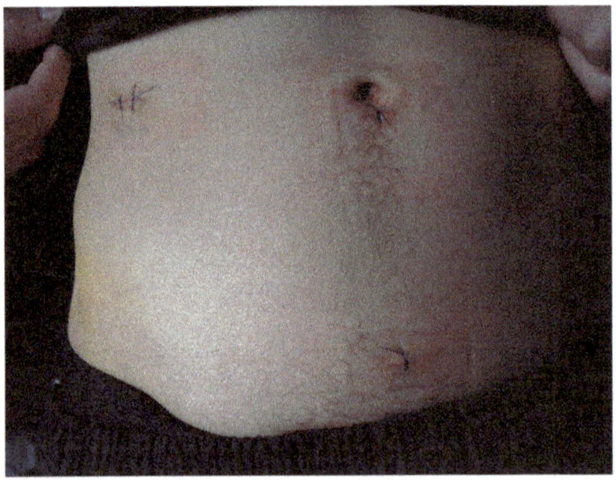

The stitches the day after having the appendix removed by laparoscopic surgery

Hospital lengths of stay typically range from a few hours to a few days but can be a few weeks if complications occur. The recovery process may vary depending on the severity of the condition: if the appendix had ruptured or not before surgery. Appendix surgery recovery is generally a lot faster if the appendix did not rupture. It is important that people undergoing surgery respect their doctor's advice and limit their physical activity so the tissues can heal faster. Recovery after an appendectomy may not require diet changes or a lifestyle change.

Length of hospital stays for appendicitis varies on the severity of the condition. A study from the United States found that in 2010, the average appendicitis hospital stay was 1.8 days. For stays where the person's appendix had ruptured, the average length of stay was 5.2 days.

After surgery, the patient will be transferred to a postanesthesia care unit so his or her vital signs can be closely monitored to detect anesthesia- or surgery-related complications. Pain medication may be administered if necessary. After patients are completely awake, they are moved to a hospital room to recover. Most individuals will be offered clear liquids the day after the surgery, then progress to a regular diet when the intestines start to function properly. Patients are recommended to sit up on the edge of the bed and walk short distances several times a day. Moving is mandatory and pain medication may be given if necessary. Full recovery from appendectomies takes about four to six weeks but can be prolonged to up to eight weeks if the appendix had ruptured.

Prognosis

Most people with appendicitis recover easily after surgical treatment, but complications can occur if treatment is delayed or if peritonitis occurs. Recovery time depends on age, condition, complications, and other circumstances, including the amount of alcohol consumption, but usually is between 10 and 28 days. For young children (around 10 years old), the recovery takes three weeks.

The possibility of peritonitis is the reason why acute appendicitis warrants speedy evaluation and treatment. People with suspected appendicitis may have to undergo a medical evacuation. Appendectomies have occasionally been performed in emergency conditions (i.e., not in a proper hospital), when a timely medical evacuation was impossible.

Typical acute appendicitis responds quickly to appendectomy and occasionally will resolve spontaneously. If appendicitis resolves spontaneously, it remains controversial whether an elective interval appendectomy should be performed to prevent a recurrent episode of appendicitis. Atypical appendicitis (associated with suppurative appendicitis) is more difficult to diagnose and is more apt to be complicated even when operated early. In either condition, prompt diagnosis and appendectomy yield the best results with full recovery in two to four weeks usually. Mortality and severe complications are unusual but do occur, especially if peritonitis persists and is untreated.

Another entity known as appendicular lump is talked about. It happens when the appendix is not removed early during infection and omentum and intestine adhere to it, forming a palpable lump. During this period, surgery is risky unless there is pus formation evident by fever and toxicity or by USG. Medical management treats the condition.

An unusual complication of an appendectomy is "stump appendicitis": inflammation occurs in the remnant appendiceal stump left after a prior incomplete appendectomy. Stump appendicitis can occur months to years after initial appendectomy and can be identified with imaging modalities like ultrasound.

Epidemiology

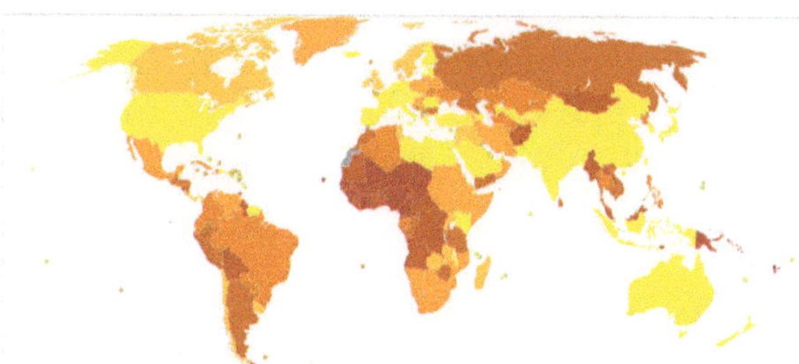

Appendicitis deaths per million persons in 2012

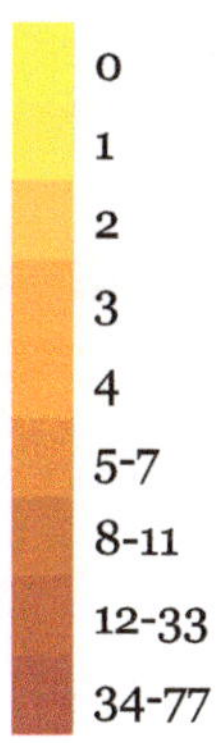

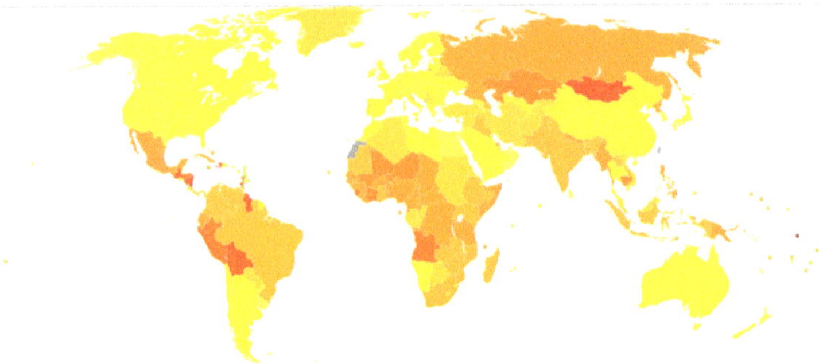

Disability-adjusted life year for appendicitis per 100,000 inhabitants in 2004.

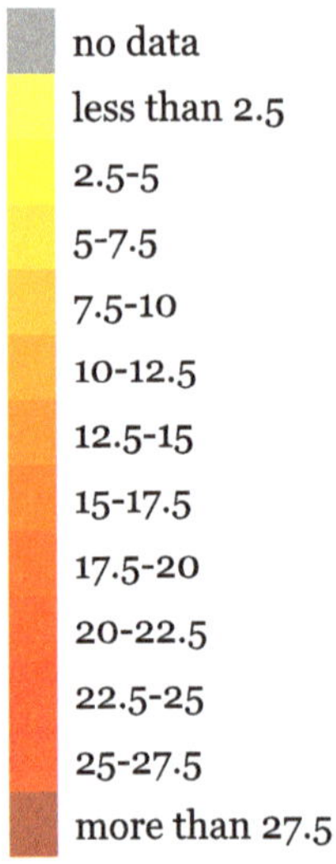

Appendicitis is most common between the ages of 5 and 40; the median age is 28. It tends to affect males, those in lower income groups and, for unknown reasons, people living in rural areas. In 2013 it resulted in 72,000 deaths globally down from 88,000 in 1990.

In the United States, there were nearly 293,000 hospitalizations involving appendicitis in 2010. Appendicitis is one of the most frequent diagnoses for emergency department visits resulting in hospitalization among children ages 5–17 years in the United States.

Acute Abdomen

An acute abdomen refers to a sudden, severe abdominal pain. It is in many cases a medical emergency, requiring urgent and specific diagnosis. Several causes need surgical treatment.

Causes

The differential diagnoses of acute abdomen include but are not limited to:

1. Acute appendicitis
2. Acute peptic ulcer and its complications
3. Acute cholecystitis
4. Acute pancreatitis
5. Acute intestinal ischemia
6. Acute diverticulitis
7. Ectopic pregnancy with tubal rupture
8. Ovarian torsion
9. Acute peritonitis (including hollow viscus perforation)
10. Acute ureteric colic
11. Bowel volvulus
12. Acute pyelonephritis
13. Adrenal crisis
14. Biliary colic
15. Abdominal aortic aneurysm
16. Familial Mediterranean fever
17. Hemoperitoneum
18. Ruptured spleen
19. Kidney stone
20. Sickle cell anaemia

Peritonitis

Acute abdomen is occasionally used synonymously with peritonitis. While this is not entirely incorrect, peritonitis is the more specific term, referring to inflammation of the peritoneum. It manifests on physical examination as rebound tenderness, or pain upon *removal* of pressure more than on *application* of pressure to the abdomen. Peritonitis may result from several of the above diseases, notably appendicitis and pancreatitis. While rebound tenderness is commonly associated with peritonitis, the most specific finding is rigidity.

Ischemic acute Abdomen

Vascular disorders are more likely to affect the small bowel than the large bowel. Arterial supply to the intestines is provided by the superior and inferior mesenteric arteries (SMA and IMA respectively), both of which are direct branches of the aorta.

The superior mesenteric artery supplies:

1. Small bowel
2. Ascending and proximal two-thirds of the transverse colon

The inferior mesenteric artery supplies:

1. Distal one-third of the transverse colon
2. Descending colon
3. Sigmoid colon

Of note, the splenic flexure, or the junction between the transverse and descending colon, is supplied by the most distal portions of both the inferior mesenteric artery and superior mesenteric artery, and is thus referred to medically as a watershed area, or an area especially vulnerable to ischemia during periods of systemic hypoperfusion, such as in shock.

Acute abdomen of the ischemic variety is usually due to:

1. A thromboembolism from the left side of the heart, such as may be generated during atrial fibrillation, occluding the SMA.
2. Nonocclusive ischemia, such as that seen in hypotension secondary to heart failure, may also contribute, but usually results in a mucosal or mural infarct, as contrasted with the typically transmural infarct seen in thromboembolus of the SMA.
3. Primary mesenteric vein thromboses may also cause ischemic acute abdomen, usually precipitated by hypercoagulable states such as polycythemia vera.

Clinically, patients present with diffuse abdominal pain, bowel distention, and bloody diarrhea. On physical exam, bowel sounds will be absent. Laboratory tests reveal a neutrophilic leukocytosis, sometimes with a left shift, and increased serum amylase. Abdominal radiography will show many air-fluid levels, as well as widespread edema.

Acute ischemic abdomen is a surgical emergency. Typically, treatment involves removal of the region of the bowel that has undergone infarction, and subsequent anastomosis of the remaining healthy tissue.

Workup

Stable patients presenting to A&E (accident and emergency department) or ER (emergency room) with severe abdominal pain will almost always have an abdominal x-ray and/or a CT scan. These tests can provide a differential diagnosis between simple and complex pathologies. However, in the unstable patient, fluid resuscitation and a FAST-ultrasound are done first, and if the latter is positive for free fluid, straight to surgery. They may also provide evidence to the doctor whether surgical intervention is necessary.

Patients will also most likely receive a complete blood count (or full blood count in the U.K.), looking for characteristic findings such as neutrophilia in appendicitis.

Traditionally, the use of opiates or other painkillers in patients with an acute abdomen has been discouraged before the clinical examination, because these would alter the examination. However, the scientific literature does not reveal any negative results from these alterations.

Neuropathic Pain

Neuropathic pain is pain caused by damage or disease affecting the somatosensory nervous system. Neuropathic pain may be associated with abnormal sensations called dysesthesia or pain from normally non-painful stimuli (allodynia). It may have continuous and/or episodic (paroxysmal) components. The latter resemble stabbings or electric shocks. Common qualities include burning or coldness, “pins and needles” sensations, numbness and itching.

Up to 7% to 8% of the European population is affected, and in 5% of persons it may be severe. Neuropathic pain may result from disorders of the peripheral nervous system or the central nervous system (brain and spinal cord). Thus, neuropathic pain may be divided into peripheral neuropathic pain, central neuropathic pain, or mixed (peripheral and central) neuropathic pain.

Cause

Central neuropathic pain is found in spinal cord injury, multiple sclerosis, and some strokes. Aside from diabetes and other metabolic conditions, the common causes of painful peripheral neuropathies are herpes zoster infection, HIV-related neuropathies, nutritional deficiencies, toxins, remote manifestations of malignancies, immune mediated disorders and physical trauma to a nerve trunk. Neuropathic pain is common in cancer as a direct result of cancer on peripheral nerves (e.g., compression by a tumor), or as a side effect of chemotherapy (chemotherapy-induced peripheral neuropathy), radiation injury or surgery.

Mechanisms

Peripheral

After a peripheral nerve lesion, aberrant regeneration may occur. Neurons become unusually sensitive and develop spontaneously pathological activity, abnormal excitability, and heightened sensitivity to chemical, thermal and mechanical stimuli. This phenomenon is called “peripheral sensitization”.

Central

The (spinal cord) dorsal horn neurons give rise to the spinothalamic tract (STT), which constitutes the major ascending nociceptive pathway. As a consequence of ongoing spontaneous activity arising in the periphery, STT neurons develop increased background activity, enlarged receptive fields and increased responses to afferent impulses, including normally innocuous tactile stimuli. This phenomenon is called central sensitization. Central sensitization is an important mechanism of persistent neuropathic pain.

Other mechanisms, however, may take place at the central level after peripheral nerve damage. The loss of afferent signals induces functional changes in dorsal horn neurons. A decrease in the large fiber input decreases the activity of interneurons inhibiting nociceptive neurons i.e. loss of afferent inhibition. Hypoactivity of the descending antinociceptive systems or loss of descending inhibition may be another factor. With the loss of neuronal input (deafferentation) the STT neurons begin to fire spontaneously, a phenomenon designated “deafferentation hypersensitivity.”

Neuroglia (“glial cells”) may play a role in central sensitization. Peripheral nerve injury induces glia to release proinflammatory cytokines and glutamate—which, in turn influence neurons.

Cellular

The phenomena described above are dependent on changes at the cellular and molecular levels. Altered expression of ion channels, changes in neurotransmitters and their receptors as well as altered gene expression in response to neural input are at play.

Treatments

Neuropathic pain can be very difficult to treat with only some 40-60% of people achieving partial relief.

Favored treatments are certain antidepressants (tricyclic antidepressant and serotonin–norepinephrine reuptake inhibitors), anticonvulsants (pregabalin and gabapentin), and topical lidocaine. Opioid analgesics are recognized as useful agents but are not recommended as first line treatments.

Anticonvulsants

Pregabalin and gabapentin may reduce pain associated with diabetic neuropathy. The anticonvulsants carbamazepine and oxcarbazepine are especially effective in trigeminal neuralgia. Gabapentin may reduce symptoms associated with neuropathic pain or fibromyalgia in some people. There is no predictor test to determine if it will be effective for a particular person. A short trial period of gabapentin therapy is recommended, to determine the effectiveness for that person. 62% of people taking gabapentin may have at least one adverse event, however the incidence of serious adverse events was found to be low.

Lamotrigine does not appear to be effective for neuropathic pain.

Antidepressants

Dual serotonin-norepinephrine reuptake inhibitors such as duloxetine, venlafaxine, and milnacipran, as well as tricyclic antidepressants such as amitriptyline, nortriptyline, and desipramine are considered first-line medications for this condition. While amitriptyline and desipramine have been used as first-line treatments, the quality of evidence to support their use is poor.

Bupropion has been found to have efficacy in the treatment of neuropathic pain.

Botulinum Toxin Type A

Botulinum toxin type A (BTX-A) is best known by its trade name, Botox. Local intradermal injection of BTX-A is helpful in chronic focal painful neuropathies. The analgesic effects are not dependent on changes in muscle tone. Benefits persist for at least 14 weeks from the time of administration.

The utility of BTX-A in other painful conditions remains unproven.

Cannabinoids

Cannabis and a number of cannabinoid receptor agonists appear to be effective for neuropathic pain.

The predominant adverse effects are CNS depression and cardiovascular effects—which are mild and well tolerated, but psychoactive side effects limit their use.

Long-term studies are needed to assess the probability of weight gain and possible harmful psychological effects.

Dietary Supplements

A 2007 review of studies found that injected (parenteral) administration of alpha lipoic acid (ALA) was found to reduce the various symptoms of peripheral diabetic neuropathy. While some studies on orally administered ALA had suggested a reduction in both the positive symptoms of diabetic neuropathy (dysesthesia including stabbing and burning pain) as well as neuropathic deficits (paresthesia), the meta-analysis showed "more conflicting data whether it improves sensory symptoms or just neuropathic deficits alone". There is some limited evidence that ALA is also helpful in some other non-diabetic neuropathies.

Benfotiamine is an oral prodrug of Vitamin B1 that has several placebo-controlled double-blind trials proving efficacy in treating neuropathy and various other diabetic comorbidities.

Neuromodulators

Neuromodulation is a field of science, medicine and bioengineering that encompasses both implantable and non-implantable technologies (electrical and chemical) for treatment purposes.

Implanted devices are expensive and carry the risk of complications. Available studies have focused on conditions having a different prevalence than neuropathic pain patients in general. More research is needed to define the range of conditions that they might benefit.

Deep Brain Stimulation

The best long-term results with deep brain stimulation have been reported with targets in the periventricular/periaqueductal grey matter (79%), or the periventricular/periaqueductal grey matter plus thalamus and/or internal capsule (87%). There is a significant complication rate, which increases over time.

Motor Cortex Stimulation

Stimulation of the primary motor cortex through electrodes placed within the skull but outside the thick meningeal membrane (dura) has been used to treat pain. The level of stimulation is below that for motor stimulation. As compared with spinal stimulation, which is associated with noticeable tingling (paresthesia) at treatment levels, the only palpable effect is pain relief.

Spinal Cord Stimulators and Implanted Spinal Pumps

Spinal cord stimulators use electrodes placed adjacent to but outside the spinal cord. The overall complication rate is one-third, most commonly due to lead migration or breakage but advancements in the past decade have driven complication rates much lower. Lack of pain relief occasionally prompts device removal.

Intrathecal pumps deliver medication directly to the fluid filled (subarachnoid) space surrounding the spinal cord. Opioids alone or opioids with adjunctive medication (either a local anesthetic or clonidine) or more recently ziconotide are infused. Complications such as serious infection (meningitis), urinary retention, hormonal disturbance and intrathecal granuloma formation have been noted with intrathecal infusion.

There are no randomized studies of infusion pumps. For selected patients 50% or greater pain relief is achieved in 38% to 56% at six months but declines with the passage of time. These results must be viewed skeptically since placebo effects cannot be evaluated.

NMDA Antagonism

The *N*-methyl-D-aspartate (NMDA) receptor seems to play a major role in neuropathic pain and in the development of opioid tolerance. Dextromethorphan is an NMDA antagonist at high doses. Experiments in both animals and humans have established that NMDA antagonists such as ketamine and dextromethorphan can alleviate neuropathic pain and reverse opioid tolerance. Unfortunately, only a few NMDA antagonists are clinically available and their use is limited by a very short half life (dextromethorphan), weak activity (memantine) or unacceptable side effects (ketamine).

Opioids

Opioids, also known as narcotics, are increasingly recognized as important treatment options for chronic pain. They are not considered first-line treatments for neuropathic pain but remain the most consistently effective class of drugs for this condition. Due to the risk of addiction or diversion, opioids must be used only in appropriate individuals and under close medical supervision.

Several opioids, particularly methadone and ketobemidone, possess NMDA antagonism in addition to their μ-opioid agonist properties. Methadone does so because it is a racemic mixture; only the l-isomer is a potent μ-opioid agonist. The d-isomer does not have opioid agonist action and acts as an NMDA antagonist; d-methadone is analgesic in experimental models of chronic pain. Clinical studies are in progress to test the efficacy of d-methadone in neuropathic pain syndromes.

There is little evidence to indicate that one strong opioid is more effective than another. Expert opinion leans toward the use of methadone for neuropathic pain, in part because of its NMDA antagonism. It is reasonable to base the choice of opioid on other factors. It is unclear if fentanyl gives pain relief to people with neuropathic pain.

Topical Agents

In some forms of neuropathy, especially post-herpetic neuralgia, the topical application of local anesthetics such as lidocaine is reported to provide relief. A transdermal patch containing lidocaine is available commercially in some countries.

Repeated topical applications of capsaicin, are followed by a prolonged period of reduced skin sensibility referred to as desensitization, or nociceptor inactivation. Capsaicin not only depletes substance P but also results in a reversible degeneration of epidermal nerve fibers. Nevertheless, benefits appear modest with standard (low) strength preparations, and topical capsaicin can itself induce pain.

Research Directions

- Gallium maltolate in a cream or ointment base has been studied in a case report as a treatment of refractory postherpetic trigeminal neuralgia.

Other topical agents such as amitriptyline, gabapentin, Citrullus colocynthis extract, nifedipine, and pentoxifylline are also under investigation.

History

The history of pain management can be traced back to ancient times. Galen also suggested nerve tissue as the transferring route of pain to the brain through the invisible psychic pneuma. The idea of origination of pain from the nerve itself, without any exciting pathology in other organs is presented by medieval medical scholars such as Rhazes, Haly Abbas and Avicenna. They named this type of pain specifically as "*vaja al asab*" [nerve originated pain], described its numbness, tingling and needling quality, discussed its etiology and the differentinting characteristics. The description of neuralgia was made by John Fothergill (1712-1780). In an medical article entitled "Clinical Lecture on Lead Neuropathy" published in 1924 the word "Neuropathy" was used for the first time by Gordon.

Phantom Pain

Phantom pain sensations are described as perceptions that an individual experiences relating to a limb or an organ that is not physically part of the body. Limb loss is a result of either removal by amputation or congenital limb deficiency. However, phantom limb sensations can also occur following nerve avulsion or spinal cord injury.

Sensations are recorded most frequently following the amputation of an arm or a leg, but may also occur following the removal of a breast or an internal organ. Phantom limb pain is the feeling of pain in an absent limb or a portion of a limb. The pain sensation varies from individual to individual.

Phantom limb sensation is the term given to any sensory phenomenon (except pain) which is felt at an absent limb or a portion of the limb. It has been known that at least 80% of amputees experience phantom sensations at some time of their lives. Some experience some level of this phantom pain and feeling in the missing limb for the rest of their lives.

The term "phantom limb" was first coined by American neurologist Silas Weir Mitchell in 1871. Mitchell described that "thousands of spirit limbs were haunting as many good soldiers, every now and then tormenting them". However, in 1551, French military surgeon Ambroise Paré recorded the first documentation of phantom limb pain when he reported that, "For the patients, long after the amputation is made, say that they still feel pain in the amputated part".

Types

There are various types of sensations that may be felt:

- Sensations related to the phantom limb's posture, length and volume e.g. feeling that the phantom limb is behaving just like a normal limb like sitting with the knee bent or feeling that the phantom limb is as heavy as the other limb. Sometimes, an amputee will experience a sensation called telescoping. This is the feeling that the phantom limb is gradually shortening over time.
- Sensations of movement (e.g. feeling that the phantom foot is moving).
- Sensations of touch, temperature, pressure and itchiness. Many amputees report of feeling heat, tingling, itchiness, and pain.

Signs and Symptoms

Phantom pain involves the sensation of pain in a part of the body that has been removed.

Epidemiology

Phantom limb pain and phantom limb sensations are linked, but must be differentiated from one another. While phantom limb sensations are experienced by those with congenital limb deficiency, spinal cord injury, and amputation, phantom limb pain occurs almost exclusively as a result of amputation. Almost immediately following the amputation of a limb, 90-98% of patients report experiencing a phantom sensation. Nearly 75% of individuals experience the phantom as soon as anesthesia wears off, and the remaining 25% of patients experience phantoms within a few days or weeks. Of those experiencing innocuous sensations, a majority of patients also report distinct painful sensations.

Age and gender have not been shown to affect the onset or duration of phantom limb pain. Although it has not been fully explored, one investigation of lower limb amputation observed that as stump length decreased, there was a greater incidence of moderate and severe phantom pain.

Pathophysiology

The neurological basis and mechanisms for phantom limb pain are all derived from experimental theories and observations. Little is known about the true mechanism causing phantom pains, and many theories highly overlap. Historically, phantom pains were thought to originate from neuromas located at the stump tip. Traumatic neuromas, or non-tumor nerve injuries, often arise from surgeries and result from the abnormal growth of injured nerve fibers. Although stump neuromas contribute to phantom pains, they are not the sole cause. This is because patients with congenital limb deficiency can sometimes, although rarely, experience phantom pains. This suggests that there is a central representation of the limb responsible for painful sensations. Currently, theories are based on altered neurological pathways and cortical reorganization.

Peripheral Mechanisms

Neuromas formed from injured nerve endings at the stump site are able to fire abnormal action potentials, and were historically thought to be the main cause of phantom limb pain. Although neuromas are able to contribute to phantom pain, pain is not completely eliminated when peripheral nerves are treated with conduction blocking agents. Physical stimulation of neuromas can increase C fiber activity, thus increasing phantom pain, but pain still persists once the neuromas have ceased firing action potentials. The peripheral nervous system is thought to have at most a modulation effect on phantom limb pain.

Spinal Mechanisms

In addition to peripheral mechanisms, spinal mechanisms are thought to have an influencing role in phantom pains. Peripheral nerve injury can lead to the degeneration of C fibers in the dorsal horn of the spinal cord, and terminating A fibers may subsequently branch into the same lamina. If this occurs, A fiber inputs could be reported as noxious stimuli. Substance P, involved in the transmission of pain signals, is usually expressed by Aδ and C fibers, but following peripheral nerve damage, substance P is expressed by Aβ fibers. This leads to hyperexcitability of the spinal cord, which usually occurs only in the presence of noxious stimuli. Because patients with complete spinal cord injury have experienced phantom pains, there must be an underlying central mechanism responsible for the generation of phantom pains.

Central Mechanisms and Cortical Remapping

Under ordinary circumstances, the genetically determined circuitry in the brain remains largely stable throughout life. It was thought, until about 30 years ago, that no new neural circuits could be formed in the adult mammalian brain. Recently, functional MRI studies in amputees have shown that almost all patients have experienced motor cortical remapping. The majority of motor reorganization has occurred as a downward shift of the hand area of the cortex onto the area of face representation, especially the lips. Sometimes there is a side shift of the hand motor cortex to the ipsilateral cortex. In patients with phantom limb pain, the reorganization was great enough to cause a change in cortical lip representation into the hand areas only during lip movements. It has also been found that there is a high correlation between the magnitude of phantom limb pain and the extent to which the shift of the cortical representation of the mouth into the hand area in motor and somatosensory cortical reorganization has occurred. Additionally, as phantom pains in upper extremity amputees increased, there was a higher degree of medial shift of the facial motor representation. There are multiple theories that try to explain how cortical remapping occurs in amputees, but none have been supported to a great extent.

The Neuromatrix

The neuromatrix theory proposes that there is an extensive network connecting the thalamus and the cortex, and the cortex and the limbic system. It is a theory that extends beyond body schema theory and incorporates the conscious awareness of oneself. This theory proposes that conscious awareness and the perception of self are generated in the brain via patterns of input that can be modified by different perceptual inputs. The network is genetically predetermined, and is modified throughout one's lifetime by various sensory inputs to create a neurosignature. It is the neurosignature of a specific body part that determines how it is consciously perceived. The input systems contributing to the neurosignature are primarily the somatosensory, limbic, and thalamocortical systems. The neuromatrix theory aims to explain how certain activities associated with pain lead to the conscious perception of phantom pain. The persistence of the neurosignature, even after limb amputation, may be the cause of phantom sensations and pain. Phantom pain may arise from abnormal reorganization in the neuromatrix to a pre-existing pain state.

Opposition to the neuromatrix theory exists largely because it fails to explain why relief from phantom sensations rarely eliminates phantom pains. It also does not address how sensations can spontaneously end and how some amputees do not experience phantom sensations at all. In addition, a major limitation of the neuromatrix theory is that it too broadly accounts for various aspects of phantom limb perception. It is also likely that it is too difficult to be tested empirically, especially when testing painless phantom sensations.

Management

Various methods have been used to treat phantom limb pain. Doctors may prescribe medications to reduce the pain. Some antidepressants or antiepileptics have been shown to have a beneficial effect on reducing phantom limb pain. Often physical methods such as light massage, electrical stimulation, and hot and cold therapy have been used with variable results.

There are many different treatment options for phantom limb pain that are actively being researched. Most treatments do not take into account the mechanisms underlying phantom pains, and are therefore ineffective. However, there are a few treatment options that have been shown to alleviate pain in some patients, but these treatment options usually have a success rate less than 30%. It is important to note that this rate of success does not exceed the placebo effect. It is also important to note that because the degree of cortical reorganization is proportional to phantom limb pains, any perturbations to the amputated regions may increase pain perception.

Nonsurgical Techniques

Mirror Box Therapy

Mirror box therapy allows for illusions of movement and touch in a phantom limb by inducing somatosensory and motor pathway coupling between the phantom and real limb. Many patients experience pain as a result of a clenched phantom limb, and because phantom limbs are not under voluntary control, unclenching becomes impossible. This theory proposes that the phantom limb feels paralyzed because there is no feedback from the phantom back to the brain to inform it otherwise. Vilayanur S. Ramachandran believes that if the brain received visual feedback that the limb had moved, then the phantom limb would become unparalyzed.

Although the use of mirror therapy has been shown to be effective in some cases there is still no widely accepted theory of how it works. In a 2010 study of phantom limb pain, Martin Diers and his colleagues found that "In a randomized controlled trial that used graded motor imagery...and mirror training, patients with complex regional pain syndrome or phantom limb pain showed a decrease in pain as well as an improvement in function post-treatment and at the 6-month follow-up. And it was shown that the order of treatment mattered." This study found that mirrored imagery produced no significant cortical activity in patients with phantom limb pain and concluded that "The optimal method to alter pain and brain representation, and the brain mechanisms underlying the effects [of] mirror training or motor imagery, are still unclear."

A number of small scale research studies have shown encouraging results, however there is no current consensus as to the effectiveness of mirror therapy. Recent reviews of the published research literature by Mosely and Ezendam concluded that much of the evidence supporting mirror therapy is anecdotal or comes from studies that had weak methodological quality. In 2011, a large scale review of the literature on mirror therapy by Rothgangel summarized the current research as follows:

> "For stroke there is a moderate quality of evidence that MT [Mirror Therapy] as an additional intervention improves recovery of arm function, and a low quality of evidence regarding lower limb function and pain after stroke. The quality of evidence in patients with complex regional pain syndrome and phantom limb pain is also low. Firm conclusions could not be drawn. Little is known about which patients are likely to benefit most from MT, and how MT should preferably be applied. Future studies with clear descriptions of intervention protocols should focus on standardized outcome measures and systematically register adverse effects."

Pharmacological Treatment

Pharmacological techniques are often continued in conjunction with other treatment options. Doses of pain medications needed often drop substantially when combined with other techniques, but rarely are discontinued completely. Tricyclic antidepressants, such as amitriptyline, and sodium channel blockers, mainly carbamazepine, are often used to relieve chronic pain, and recently have been used in an attempt to reduce phantom pains. Pain relief may also be achieved through use of opioids, ketamine, calcitonin, and lidocaine.

Surgical Techniques

Deep-brain Stimulation

Deep brain stimulation is a surgical technique used to alleviate patients from phantom limb pain. Prior to surgery, patients undergo functional brain imaging techniques such as PET scans and functional MRI to determine an appropriate trajectory of where pain is originating. Surgery is then carried out under local anesthetic, because patient feedback during the operation is needed. In the study conducted by Bittar et al., a radiofrequency electrode with four contact points was placed on the brain. Once the electrode was in place, the contact locations were altered slightly according to where the patient felt the greatest relief from pain. Once the location of maximal relief was determined, the electrode was implanted and secured to the skull. After the primary surgery, a secondary surgery under general anesthesia was conducted. A subcutaneous pulse generator was implanted into a pectoral pocket below the clavicle to stimulate the electrode. It was found that all three patients studied had gained satisfactory pain relief from the deep brain stimulation. Pain had not been completely eliminated, but the intensity had been reduced by over 50% and the burning component had completely vanished.

Psychogenic Pain

Psychogenic pain, also called psychalgia, is physical pain that is caused, increased, or prolonged by mental, emotional, or behavioral factors.

Headache, back pain, or stomach pain are some of the most common types of psychogenic pain. It may occur, rarely, in persons with a mental disorder, but more commonly it accompanies or is induced by social rejection, broken heart, grief, lovesickness, or other such emotional events.

Sufferers are often stigmatized, because both medical professionals and the general public tend to think that pain from psychological source is not “real”. However, specialists consider that it is no less actual or hurtful than pain from other sources.

The International Association for the Study of Pain defines pain as "an unpleasant sensory and emotional experience associated with actual or potential tissue damage, *or described in terms of such damage*" (emphasis added). In the note accompanying that definition, the following can be found about pain that happens for psychological reasons:

Many people report pain in the absence of tissue damage or any likely pathophysiological cause; usually this happens for psychological reasons. There is usually no way to distinguish their experience from that due to tissue damage if we take the subjective report. If they regard their experience as pain and if they report it in the same ways as pain caused by tissue damage, it should be accepted as pain.

Medicine refers also to psychogenic pain or psychalgia as a form of chronic pain under the name of *persistent somatoform pain disorder* or *functional pain syndrome*. Causes may be linked to stress, unexpressed emotional conflicts, psychosocial problems, or various mental disorders. Some specialists believe that psychogenic chronic pain exists as a protective distraction to keep dangerous repressed emotions such as anger or rage unconscious.

It remains controversial, however, that chronic pain might arise purely from emotional causes. Treatment may include psychotherapy, antidepressants, analgesics, and other remedies that are used for chronic pain in general.

Pain in Babies

Pain in babies, and whether babies feel pain, has been the subject of debate within the medical profession for centuries. Prior to the late nineteenth century it was generally considered that babies hurt more easily than adults. It was only in the last quarter of the 20th century that scientific techniques finally established babies definitely do experience pain – probably more than adults – and has developed reliable means of assessing and of treating it. As recently as 1999, it was commonly stated that babies could not feel pain until they were a year old, but today it is believed newborns and likely even fetuses beyond a certain age can experience pain.

Effects

There are a number of metabolic and homeostatic changes which result from untreated pain, including an increased requirement for oxygen, accompanied by a reduction in the efficiency of gas exchange in the lungs. This combination can lead to inadequate oxygen supply, resulting in potential hypoxemia. In addition, a rise in stomach acidity accompanies the stress reaction precipitated by pain, and there is a risk of aspirating this into the lungs, further endangering lung integrity and tissue oxygenation. In cases of acute, persistent pain, the metabolism becomes predominantly catabolic, causing reduced efficiency of the immune system and a breakdown of proteins caused by the action of the stress hormones. In combination, healing of damaged or infected tissue may be impaired, and morbidity and mortality increased.

The neuropsychological effect on the bonding between mother and child, on later contact with health professionals, and on personal and social psychological well-being is difficult to quantify. Research suggests that babies exposed to pain in the neonatal period have more difficulty in these areas. Professionals working in the field of neonatal pain have speculated that adolescent aggression and self-destructive behaviour, including suicide, may, in some cases, be attributed to the long-term effects of untreated neonatal pain.

Pathophysiology

The present understanding of pain in babies is largely due to the recognition that the fetal and newborn unmyelinated nerve fibres are capable of relaying information, albeit slower than would be the case with myelinated fibres. At birth a baby has developed the neural pathways for nociception and for experiencing pain, but the pain responses are an immature version of that of an adult. There are a number of differences in both nerve structure and in the quality and extent of nerve response which are considered to be pertinent to understanding neonatal pain.

The nerves of young babies respond more readily to noxious stimuli, with a lower threshold to stimulation, than those of adults. A baby's threshold for sensitization is also substantially decreased, whilst the process involves a much larger area of sensitization with each trauma. The neural pathways that descend from the brain to the spinal cord are not well developed in the newborn, resulting in the ability of the central nervous system to inhibit nociception being more limited than in the adult.

There are also indication that the neonate's nervous system may be much more active than that of an adult, in terms of transforming its connections and central nerve pathways in response to stimuli. The ongoing process of neural pathway development, involving both structural and chemical changes of the nervous system, have been shown to be affected by pain events, both in the short term and potentially into adult life.

Diagnosis

Some of the signs of pain in babies are obvious, requiring no special equipment or training. The baby is crying and irritable when awake, develops a disturbed sleep pattern, feeds poorly, and shows a fearful, distrustful reaction towards care-givers.

The classical International Association for the Study of Pain definition of pain as a subjective, emotional experience that is *described in terms of tissue damage*, depends on the sufferer being able to self-report pain, which is little use in diagnosing and treating pain in babies. More significant are non-verbal responses, of which there are two kinds:

gross physical movements and physiological response measurements. The former are simple direct observation, while the latter requires specific equipment to monitor blood pressure and stress hormone levels.

The cry response is increasingly important, as researchers are now able to differentiate between different kinds of cry: classed as "hungry", "angry", and "fearful or in pain". Interpretation is difficult, however, depending on the sensitivity of the listener, and varies significantly between observers.

Studies have sought additional, visible and easily definable indicators of pain and in particular the high level of pain detected in babies when hungry, compared to pain levels in further developed children. Combinations of crying with facial expressions, posture and movements, aided by physiological measurements, have been tested and found to be reliable indicators. A number of such observational scales have been published and verified Even with noticeable responses from an infant, the underlying problem may be hidden. Due to the inability to speak or the side effects of the illness, it may be difficult to receive a proper diagnosis, causing infant diagnosis to be one of the hardest to do in the medical field.

Children and Infants' Postoperative Pain Scale

The Children and Infants Postoperative Pain Scale (ChIPPS) is often used in the assessment of hospitalised babies. The scale requires no special measurements, and is therefore applicable across a wide range of circumstances.

Described in 2000, the scale uses a measurement of five items, each rated as 0, 1, or 2 based on the following parameters:

Item	Score 0	Score 1	Score 2
Crying	None	Moaning	Screaming
Facial expression	Relaxed smiling	Wry mouth	Grimacing
Posture of the trunk	Neutral	Variable	Rear up
Posture of the legs	Neutral	Kicking	Tightened
Motor restlessness	None	Moderate	Restless

Total score indicates how the baby should be managed according to the scale:

- 0 - 3 No requirement for treating pain,
- 4 - 10 Progressively greater need for analgesia.

All observations, both movement and physiological, tend to decrease when pain is persistent, thus rendering the scale unreliable in acute or prolonged cases. In addition, hyperalgesia and allodynia, occur more quickly and more extensively in babies than in adults. Day to day changes in the response to a specific injury may therefore become unpredictable and variable.

Treatment

Where the baby is to undergo some form of planned procedure, health professionals will take steps to reduce pain to a minimum, though in some circumstances it may be not be possible to remove all pain.

In case of illness, accident and post operative pain, a graded sequence of treatment is becoming established as standard practice. Research is making it easier and simpler to provide the necessary care, with a clearer understanding of the risks and possible side effects.

Measures not Involving Medication

Comforting

Touching, holding, stroking, keeping warm, talking and singing/music are ways in which adults have been comforting babies since the start of human history. This way of managing pain is shared with other primates, where the actions are performed both by female and male adults. Children who are able to verbalise pain report it to be an ineffective strategy and this is assumed to also be true of babies.

While the pain of a procedure may or may not be affected, the fear is visibly reduced. This works to ameliorate the negative effects of fear in health care situations. It is, therefore, considered good practice to involve parents or care-givers directly, having them present and in contact with the baby whenever possible before a minor painful procedure, such as the drawing of blood, or prior to giving a local anaesthetic injection.

Oral Stimulation

Breastfeeding, the use of a pacifier and the administration of sugar orally has been proven to reduce the signs of pain in babies. Electroencephalographic changes are reduced by sugar, but the mechanism for this remains unknown; it does not seem to be endorphin mediated. As in comforting, it is unknown whether the physical pain is reduced, or whether it is the level of anxiety which is affected. However, the reduction in pain behaviour is assumed to be accompanied by a reduction in pain-related disorders, both immediate and longer term.

Oral Sugar

Sugar taken orally reduces the total crying time but not the duration of the first cry in newborns undergoing a painful procedure (a single lancing of the heel). It does not moderate the effect of pain on heart rate and a recent single study found that sugar did not significantly affect pain-related electrical activity in the brains of newborns one second after the heel lance procedure. Sweet oral liquid moderately reduces the incidence and duration of crying caused by immunization injection in children between one and twelve months of age.

Sensorial Saturation

It is based on the competition of various gentle stimuli with pain transmission to the central nervous system: the so-called gate control theory of pain (proposed by Patrick David Wall and Ronald Melzack in 1965). Sensorial saturation follows a "3Ts" rule: using touch, taste and talk to distract the baby and antagonize pain. In babies treated with Sensorial Saturation, a reduction in crying time and pain score were noted, with respect to a control group and with respect to groups in which only oral sugar, only sucking, or a combination of the two was used. The "3Ts" stimuli (touch, talk, and taste)given throughout the painful procedure increase the well-known analgesic effect of oral sugar. Sensorial Saturation has been included in several international guidelines for analgesia

Other Techniques

Other "old fashioned" techniques are being tested with some success. "Facilitated tucking", swaddling and "kangaroo care" have been shown to reduce the response of babies to painful or distressful circumstances, while a comprehensive technique of nursing, called "developmental care", has been developed for managing pre-term infants.

Measures Involving Medication

Local Anaesthetics

A variety of *topical anaesthetic* creams have been developed, ranging from single agents with good skin penetration, to eutectic mixtures of agents and technologically modern formulations of lignocaine in microspheres. They are effective in suitable procedures, if correctly and timeously applied. Disadvantages are the slow onset of adequate anaesthesia, inadequate analgesia for larger procedures, and toxicity of absorbed medication.

Local infiltration anaesthesia, the infiltration of anaesthetic agent directly into the skin and subcutaneous tissue where the painful procedure is to be undertaken, may be effectively used to reduce pain after a procedure under general anaesthesia. To reduce the pain of the initial injection, a topical anaesthetic ointment may be applied.

Regional anaesthesia requires the injection of local anaesthetic around the nerve trunks that supply a limb, or into the epidural space surrounding the spinal cord. It is used for pain relief after surgery, but requires special facilities for observation of the baby until the effect has worn out.

Analgesics

As the site of pain in babies is difficult to confirm, analgesics are often advised against until a proper diagnosis has been performed. For all analgesic drugs, the immaturity of the baby's nervous system and metabolic pathways, the different way in which the drugs are distributed, and the reduced ability of the baby to excrete the drugs though the kidneys make the prescription of dosage important. The potentially harmful side effects of analgesic drugs are the same for babies as they are for adults and are both well known and manageable.

There are three forms of analgesia suitable for the treatment of pain in babies: paracetamol (acetaminophen), the non-steroidal anti-inflammatory drugs, and the opioids. Paracetamol is safe and effective if given in the correct dosage. The same is true of the non-steroidal anti-inflammatory drugs, such as ibuprofen (aspirin is seldom used). Of the opioids, morphine and fentanyl are most often used in a hospital setting, while codeine is effective for use at home.

History

Pre Late 19th Century

Before the late nineteenth century, babies were considered to be more sensitive to pain than adults. Doris Cope quotes paediatric surgeon Felix Würtz of Basel, writing in 1656:

> *If a new skin in old people be tender, what is it you think in a newborn Babe? Doth a small thing pain you so much on a finger, how painful is it then to a Child, which is tormented all the body over, which hath but a tender new grown flesh?*

Late 19th Century

In the late nineteenth, and first half of the twentieth century, doctors were taught that babies did not experience pain, and were treating their young patients accordingly. From needle sticks to tonsillectomies to heart operations were done with no anaesthesia or analgesia, other than muscle relaxation for the surgery. The belief was that in babies the expression of pain was reflexive and, owing to the immaturity of the infant brain, the pain could not really matter.

Cope considers it probable that the belief arose from misinterpretation of discoveries made in the new science of embryology. Dr Paul Flechsig equated the non-myelinisation of much of a baby's nervous system with an inability to function.

It was generally believed that babies would not remember any pain that they happened to feel, and that lack of conscious memory meant lack of long-term harm. Scientific studies on animals with various brain lesions were interpreted as supporting the idea that the responses seen in babies were merely spinal reflexes. Furthermore, the whole effort of relieving pain was considered futile since it was thought to be impossible to measure the child's pain.

This, coupled with a concern that use of opiates would lead to addiction, and the time and effort needed to provide adequate analgesia to the newborn, contributed to the medical profession's continued practice of not providing pain relief for babies.

Mid 1980s

In the United States, a major change in practice was brought about by events surrounding one operation. Infant Jeffrey Lawson underwent open heart surgery in 1985. His mother, Jill R. Lawson, subsequently discovered that he had been operated on without any anaesthesia, other than a muscle relaxant. She started a vigorous awareness campaign which created such a public, and medical, reaction that by 1987 medical opinion had come full circle.

A number of studies on the measurement of pain in young children, and on ways of reducing the injury response began, and publications on the hormonal and metabolic responses of babies to pain stimuli began to appear, confirming that the provision of adequate anaesthesia and analgesia was better medicine on both humanitarian and physiological grounds.

It is now accepted that *the neonate responds more extensively to pain* than the adult does, and that exposure to severe pain, without adequate treatment, can have long-term consequences. Despite the difficulty of assessing how much pain a baby is experiencing, and the practical problem of prescribing the correct dosage or technique for treatment, modern medicine is firmly committed to improving the quality of pain relief for the very young.

The effective treatment of pain benefits the baby immediately, reduces some medium-term negative consequences, and likely prevents a number of adult psycho-physiological problems.

References

- Debono, DJ; Hoeksema, LJ; Hobbs, RD (August 2013). "Caring for Patients with Chronic Pain: Pearls and Pitfalls". Journal of the American Osteopathic Association. 113 (8): 620–627. doi:10.7556/jaoa.2013.023. PMID 23918913
- The neurobiology of pain: Symposium of the Northern Neurobiology Group, held at Leeds on 18 April 1983. Manchester: Manchester University Press; 1984. ISBN 0-7190-0996-0. Cutaneous nociceptors. p. 106
- Leiter, Brian (1 January 2015). "Nietzsche's Moral and Political Philosophy". The Stanford Encyclopedia of Philosophy. Metaphysics Research Lab, Stanford University. Retrieved 26 November 2016
- Why patients use alternative medicine: Results of a national study. Journal of the American Medical Association. 1998;279(19):1548–1553. doi:10.1001/jama.279.19.1548. PMID 9605899
- Pathophysiology of somatic, visceral, and neuropathic cancer pain. In: Sykes N, Bennett MI & Yuan C-S. Clinical pain management: Cancer pain. 2 ed. London: Hodder Arnold; ISBN 978-0-340-94007-5. p. 3–12
- Chiu, HY; Hsieh, YJ; Tsai, PS (Feb 7, 2016). "Systematic review and meta-analysis of acupuncture to reduce cancer-related pain". Eur J Cancer Care. doi:10.1111/ecc.12457. PMID 26853524. Retrieved 9 March 2016

- The high prevalence of pain in emergency medical care. American Journal of Emergency Medicine. 2002;20(3):165–9. doi:10.1053/ajem.2002.32643. PMID 11992334
- Beecher, HK (1959). Measurement of subjective responses. New York: Oxford University Press. cited in Melzack, R; Wall, PD (1996). The challenge of pain (2 ed.). London: Penguin. p. 7. ISBN 978-0-14-025670-3
- "Do Invertebrates Feel Pain?" Archived 6 January 2010 at the Wayback Machine., The Senate Standing Committee on Legal and Constitutional Affairs, The Parliament of Canada Web Site. Retrieved 11 June 2008
- Katz, Joel; Rosenbloom, Brittany N; Fashler, Samantha (2 February 2017). "Chronic Pain, Psychopathology, and DSM-5 Somatic Symptom Disorder". Canadian Journal of Psychiatry. Revue
- Taylor, Carol (2015). Fundamentals of nursing : the art and science of person-centered nursing care. Philadelphia: Wolters Kluwer Health. p. 241. ISBN 9781451185614
- Kreitler S; Niv D (2007). "Cognitive impairment in chronic pain" (pdf). Pain: Clinical Updates. International Association for the Study of Pain. XV (4): 1–4. Retrieved 2008-04-15
- Paice, JA (Jul–Aug 2003). "Mechanisms and management of neuropathic pain in cancer" (PDF). Journal of supportive oncology. 1 (2): 107–20. PMID 15352654
- Cousins and Bridenbaugh's Neural Blockade in Clinical Anesthesia and Pain Medicine. Hagerstwon, MD: Lippincott Williams & Wilkins; 2008. ISBN 0-7817-7388-1
- "Academic continuity through online collaboration: Mathematics teachers support the learning of pupils with chronic illness during school absence". ResearchGate. Retrieved 2017-03-28
- Manners, Prudence Joan; Bower, Carol (2002-07-01). "Worldwide prevalence of juvenile arthritis why does it vary so much?". The Journal of Rheumatology. 29 (7): 1520–1530. ISSN 0315-162X. PMID 12136914
- Coda, BA; Bonica, JJ (2001). "General considerations of acute pain". In Loeser, D; Bonica, JJ. Bonica's management of pain (3 ed.). Philadelphia: Lippincott Williams & Wilkins. ISBN 0-443-05683-8
- "Back Pain Information Page: National Institute of Neurological Disorders and Stroke (NINDS)". Ninds.nih.gov. 2010-05-19. Archived from the original on 6 June 2010. Retrieved 2010-06-02

3

Pain Scale and Assessment

Pain scale is the measurement of pain that a patient is suffering. The measurement can be done by observing the patient, self-report or physiological data. Schmidt sting pain index, pain tolerance, pain assessment, pain ladder, etc. are some of the other indicators of pain and its management. The aspects elucidated in this chapter are of vital importance, and provide a better understanding of pain scale and assessment.

Pain Scale

A pain scale measures a patient's pain intensity or other features. Pain scales are based on self-report, observational (behavioral), or physiological data. Self-report is considered primary and should be obtained if possible. Pain measurements help determine the severity, type, and duration of the pain, and are used to make an accurate diagnosis, determine a treatment plan, and evaluate the effectiveness of treatment. Pain scales are available for neonates, infants, children, adolescents, adults, seniors, and persons whose communication is impaired. Pain assessments are often regarded as "the 5th Vital Sign".

Partial List of Pain Measurement Scales

- Alder Hey Triage Pain Score
- Behavioral Pain Scale (BPS)
- Brief Pain Inventory (BPI)
- Checklist of Nonverbal Pain Indicators (CNPI)
- Clinical Global Impression (CGI)
- Critical-Care Pain Observation Tool (CPOT)
- COMFORT scale
- Dallas Pain Questionnaire
- Descriptor differential scale (DDS)
- Dolorimeter Pain Index (DPI)

- Edmonton Symptom Assessment System
- Faces Pain Scale – Revised (FPS-R)
- Face Legs Activity Cry Consolability scale
- Lequesne algofunctional index: a composite measure of pain and disability, with separate self-report questionnaires for hip and knee OA (osteoarthritis):
    - Original index (1987)
    - 1991 revision
    - 1997 revision
- McGill Pain Questionnaire (MPQ)
- Neck Pain and Disability Scale –NPAD
- Numerical 11 point box (BS-11)
- Numeric Rating Scale (NRS-11)
- OSWESTRY Index
- Palliative Care Outcome Scale (PCOS)
- Roland-Morris Back Pain Questionnaire
- Support Team Assessment Schedule (STAS)
- Wong-Baker FACES Pain Rating Scale
- Visual analog scale (VAS)

Specialized Tests

- Disease-Specific Pain Scale: $DSPI = (\Sigma X \cdot Y) \cdot 100$ where X is the highest pain level on a 0–10 scale and Y is the percentage of this pain level in the group. The DSPI is different from the simple numeric 0–10 scale in that it is measured for a group of patients with a specific diagnosis whereas the numeric 0–10 pain scale is administered individually.
- Pediatric Pain Questionnaire (PPQ) for measuring pain in children
- Premature Infant Pain Profile (PIPP) for measuring pain in premature infants
- Schmidt Sting Pain Index and Starr sting pain scale both for insect stings
- Colorado Behavioral Numerical Pain Scale (for sedated patients)

- AUSCAN: Disease-Specific, to assess hand osteoarthritis outcomes.
- WOMAC : Disease-Specific, to assess knee osteoarthritis outcomes.
- Osteoarthritis Research Society International-Outcome Measures in Rheumatoid Arthritis Clinical Trials (OARSI-OMERACT) Initiative, New OA Pain Measure: Disease-Specific, Osteoarthritis Pain.

Numeric Rating Scale

The Numeric Rating Scale (NRS-11) is an 11-point scale for patient self-reporting of pain. It is for adults and children 10 years old or older.

Rating	Pain Level
0	No Pain
1–3	Mild Pain (nagging, annoying, interfering little with ADLs)
4–6	Moderate Pain (interferes significantly with ADLs)
7–10	Severe Pain (disabling; unable to perform ADLs)

In Endometriosis

The most common pain scale for quantification of endometriosis-related pain is the visual analogue scale (VAS). A review came to the conclusion that VAS and numerical rating scale (NRS) were the best adapted pain scales for pain measurement in endometriosis. For research purposes, and for more detailed pain measurement in clinical practice, the review suggested use of VAS or NRS for each type of typical pain related to endometriosis (dysmenorrhea, deep dyspareunia and non-menstrual chronic pelvic pain), combined with the clinical global impression (CGI) and a quality of life scale.

Cold Pressor Test

The cold pressor test is a cardiovascular test performed by immersing the hand into an ice water container, usually for one minute, and measuring changes in blood pressure and heart rate. These changes relate to vascular response and pulse excitability.

Other measures can also be obtained from the cold pressor such as pain threshold and pain tolerance. This is done by requiring a participant to place their hand in the cold pressor for as long as they can. Once pain is present, they let the researcher know. Once the pain is unbearable, the participant removes his/her hand. This provides a measure of threshold (first feeling pain) and tolerance (total time minus threshold). This method is the most frequently used application of the cold pressor task. Comparable in terms of pain elicitation is the hot water immersion test, the equivalent to the cold pressor using hot water. The hot water immersion test (HIT) is equally capable of triggering a pain response without the confounding of baroreflex activation.

Physiology

Sensory afferent nerves trigger a systemic sympathetic activation leading to marked vasoconstriction. The result is an elevated pulse pressure (normal is 40mm Hg), due to catecholamine release. This increased pressure fills the ventricle to a greater extent, but stroke volume decreases due to an increase in afterload.

Dolorimeter

A dolorimeter is an instrument used to measure pain threshold and pain tolerance. Dolorimetry has been defined as "the measurement of pain sensitivity or pain intensity". Several types of dolorimeter have been developed. Dolorimeters apply steady pressure, heat, or electrical stimulation to some area, or move a joint or other body part and determine what level of heat or pressure or electric current or amount of movement produces a sensation of pain. Sometimes the pressure is applied using a blunt object, or by locally increasing the air pressure on some area of the body, and sometimes by pressing a sharp instrument against the body.

History

In 1940, James D. Hardy, Harold G. Wolff and Helen Goodell of Cornell University introduced the first dolorimeter as a method for evaluating the effectiveness of analgesic medications. They did their work at New York Hospital. They focused the light of a 100 watt projection lamp with a lens on an area of skin that had been blackened. They found that most people expressed a pain sensation when the skin temperature reached 113 °F (45 °C). They also found that after the skin temperature reached 152 °F (67 °C), the pain sensations did not intensify even if the heat was increased. They developed a pain scale, called the "Hardy-Wolff-Goodell" scale, with 10 gradations, or 10 levels. They assigned the name of "dols" to these levels. Unfortunately, other researchers were not able to reproduce the results of Hardy, Wolff and Goodell and the device and the approach was abandoned. Harvard Medical School Professor and Massachusetts General Hospital Anaesthetist Henry K. Beecher (1957) expressed skepticism about this method of measuring pain.

In 1945, *Time* magazine reported that Cleveland's Dr. Lorand Julius Bela Gluzek had developed a dolorimeter that measured pain in grams. Dr. Gluzek claimed that his dolorimeter was 97% accurate.

Palpometer

A dolorimeter known as the *Sonic Palpometer* was developed at the University of Victoria in British Columbia, Canada. Patents have been applied for worldwide. The Sonic Palpometer uses ultrasound and computer technology to automate the physician's technique of palpation to determine sensitivity of some part of the patient's body.

The related pressure controlled palpometer (PCP) uses a pressure-sensitive piece of plastic film to determine how much pressure is being applied in palpation. This technique appears to be more reliable than unaided palpation.

Algorimeter and Other Methods

Techniques Using Lasers

Svensson et al. (1997) describe the use of a CO_2 laser or a contact thermode to heat the skin and elicit a pain response.

A laser-based dolorimeter called a *Dolorimeter Analgesia meter* is marketed by IITC Life Sciences.

Techniques Using Heat Lamps

Another pain measurement device uses heat from a 500 watt lamp which is delivered to a small area of skin.

Other Dolorimeters

- Björnström's algesimeter measures sensitivity of the skin to pain.
- Boas' algesimeter measures sensitivity over the epigastrium
- The AlgiScan, used for measuring the analgesia level in patients during anesthesia, quantifies within seconds the reflex papillary dilatation through an integrated nociceptive stimulator.

Other terms for similar instruments include *algesiometer*, *algesichronometer* (which also takes time into consideration), *analgesia meter*, *algometer*, *algonometer*, *prick-algesimeter*, *pressure-algometer*.

Dolorimetry for Animals

Dolorimetry in animals involves application of pain to various body parts. It is occasionally used as a diagnostic tool, and routinely used in basic pain research and in the testing of analgetics.

Tail

- Tail-withdrawal tests
- Tail-pinch tests
- Tail flick test

Paw

- Randall-Selitto test (paw pressure test)
- Hot plate test

Schmidt Sting Pain Index

The Schmidt sting pain index is a pain scale rating the relative pain caused by different hymenopteran stings. It is mainly the work of Justin O. Schmidt (born 1947), an entomologist at the Carl Hayden Bee Research Center in Arizona. Schmidt has published a number of papers on the subject, and claims to have been stung by the majority of stinging Hymenoptera.

His original paper in 1983 was an attempt to systematize and compare the hemolytic properties of insect venoms. The index contained in the paper started from 0 for stings that are completely ineffective against humans, progressed through 2, a familiar pain such as a common bee or wasp sting and finished at 4 for the most painful stings. *Synoeca septentrionalis*, along with other wasps in the *Synoeca* genus, bullet ants and tarantula hawks were the only species to attain this ranking. In the conclusion, some descriptions of the most painful examples were given, e.g.: "*Paraponera clavata* stings induced immediate, excruciating pain and numbness to pencil-point pressure, as well as trembling in the form of a totally uncontrollable urge to shake the affected part."

Subsequently, Schmidt has refined his scale, culminating in a paper published in 1990, which classifies the stings of 78 species and 41 genera of Hymenoptera. Schmidt described some of the experiences in vivid detail.

An entry in *The Straight Dope* reported that "implausibly exact numbers" which do not appear in any of Schmidt's published scientific papers were "wheedled out of him" by *Outside* magazine for an article it published in 1996.

In September 2015 Schmidt was co-awarded the Ig Nobel Physiology and Entomology prize with Michael Smith, for their Hymenoptera research.

Schmidt's pain scale of Hymenopteran stings is organized into levels, ranging between below 1 to 4, with 4 being the most painful. However, insect stings that feel very differently can be put into the same level. Thus, Schmidt always includes a brief description of his experience being stung by each type of insect. On that note, these stings are based on Schmidt's subjective perspective, and insect stings can vary person to person, so the scale is not universal.

Pain Level 1

Some of the insect stings Schmidt considers to be at a pain level of 1 include the Southern fire ant, the Elongate twig ant, the Western paper wasp, the white-faced bee, and most small bees. The duration of the pain of insect stings categorized into Pain Level 1 generally is five minutes or less.

Since many small bees are categorized into a pain level of 1, it should be noted that the most toxic polypeptides in bee venom are melittin, apamin, and MCD peptide. Melittin is the main toxin of bee venom, and it damages red blood cells and white blood cells. Apamin is a neurotoxin that augments polysynaptic reflexes. MCD peptide destroys mast cells.

Feeling only slight pain, Schmidt has described the sting of the Anthophorid bee, categorized into Pain Level 1, as "almost pleasant, a lover just bit your earlobe a little too hard." Also rated into Pain Level 1, Schmidt has described the sting of the sweat bee as "light, ephemeral, almost fruity. A tiny spark has singed a single hair on your arm."

Pain Level 2

Schmidt sets the sting of the Western honey bee at a pain level of 2 to be the anchoring value, basing his categorization of all other stings off of it. He has categorized a variety of wasps, bees, and ants into Pain Level 2, including the yellowjacket, the Asiatic honey bee, and the trap-jaw ant. The duration of the stings in this level is generally between five to ten minutes long. Schmidt categorized the majority of Hymenopteran stings as having a pain level of 2.

The sting of a termite-raiding ant, categorized as a pain level of 2, has a similar feeling as "the debilitating pain of a migraine contained in the tip of your finger," according to Schmidt. On the contrary, the yellowjacket's sting was described as being "hot and smoky, almost irreverent. Imagine W. C. Fields extinguishing a cigar on your tongue." Though the sting was a different feeling, the yellowjacket was also rated at a pain level of 2.

Pain Level 3

Most insects that are characterized as having a pain level of 3 are wasps, including the red paper wasp, the metricus paper wasp, and the velvet ant (which is actually a wasp, not an ant). The duration of the sting pain can range anywhere from one minute (such as the sting of the red paper wasp) to half an hour (such as the sting of the velvet ant). Wasp venom uniquely contains wasp kinin that exhibit kininlike activity. One of the kinins found in wasp kinin, polistes kinin 3, is found to lead to similar effects on smooth musculature and circulation as bradykinin.

Some ants are also rated at a Pain Level 3, including the giant bull ant and the Maricopa harvester ant. Schmidt considered the sting of the Maricopa harvester ant as having a pain level of 3, describing it as such: "After eight unrelenting hours of drilling into that ingrown toenail, you find the drill wedged into the toe."

Pain Level 4

Pain Level 4 is the highest level in the Schmidt sting pain index. Schmidt gave the sting of the tarantula hawk a rating of a 4, which he described as "blinding, fierce [and] shockingly electric." The composition of the tarantula hawk sting is unknown, though the duration of the sting is short-lived, lasting only approximately 5 minutes.

Schmidt rated the sting of the bullet ant as a 4-plus. This sting can last between 5 to 24 hours. Schmidt has described the sting as "pure, intense, brilliant pain...like walking over flaming charcoal with a three-inch nail embedded in your heel." The bullet ant's venom primarily contains poneratoxin, a paralyzing neurotoxic peptide.

Schmidt has considered the stings of the tarantula hawk and the bullet ant to be the most painful stings.

Evolution from Painful to Toxic Stings

The Schmidt Sting Pain Index arose from the pursuit of a larger hypothesis: that the evolution of sociality in *Hymenoptera* was dependent on the evolution of venom that was both painful and toxic. Pain is an advertisement of damage in the body, but molecules that produce pain and those that are toxic, and actively cause damage, are not the same. Although the painful signal acts as a deterrent, intelligent predators will learn the dishonesty of this signal with repeated exposure – that there is no real damage being done. For the early *Hymenoptera* that were primarily solitary, the pain alone would allow them the chance to escape. Furthermore, solitary insects do not provide a high energy reward for predators, and therefore predators do not expend significant effort to hunt them. However, with the evolution of sociality where many *Hymenoptera* cluster together in colonies, nests become a nutritionally rich and therefore worthwhile target. If there were no defenses, predators would devour the defenseless society, leaving few surviving individuals and eliminating social reproduction. Sociality would therefore not be beneficial. In order for sociality to evolve, *Hymenoptera* needed a defense beyond a painful sting to protect their whole colony. Their sting was an advertisement of damage, and toxicity evolved as its truth. With a toxic sting, and thus the ability to protect against predators, *Hymenoptera* were able to progress towards sociality and its associated evolutionary benefits of the shared raising of youth, individual task specialization, inter-colony communication, and food storage.

To approach studying this evolutionary connection between toxicity and sociality, Schmidt recognized there needed to be a quantitative measure with which to score the painfulness of stings. Assays for toxicity are already well characterized and can be quantified, but without the Schmidt Sting Pain Index, there would be no way to relate the amount of sociality to the level of pain, and therefore this hypothesis could not have been studied.

Threshold of Pain

The threshold of pain or pain threshold is the point along a curve of increasing perception of a stimulus at which pain begins to be felt. It is an entirely subjective phenomenon. A distinction must be maintained between the stimulus (an external thing that can be directly measured, such as with a thermometer) and the person or animal's resulting pain perception (an internal, subjective thing that can sometimes be measured indirectly, such as with a visual analog scale). Although an IASP document defines "pain threshold" as "the minimum intensity of a stimulus that is perceived as painful", it then goes on to say (contradictorily in letter although not in spirit) that:

> Traditionally the threshold has often been defined, as we defined it formerly, as the least stimulus intensity at which a subject perceives pain. Properly defined, the threshold is really the experience of the patient, whereas the intensity measured is an external event. It has been common usage for most pain research workers to define the threshold in terms of the stimulus, and that should be avoided... The stimulus is not pain (q.v.) and cannot be a measure of pain.

Although the phrasing may not convey it perfectly, the distinction clearly meant is the aforementioned one between the stimulus and the perception of it. The intensity at which a stimulus (e.g., heat, pressure) begins to evoke pain is thus called by a separate term, *threshold intensity*. So, if a hotplate on a person's skin begins to hurt at 42°C (107°F), that is the *pain threshold temperature* for that bit of skin at that time. It is not the pain threshold (which is internal/subjective) but the temperature at which the pain threshold was crossed (which is external/objective).

The intensity at which a stimulus begins to evoke pain varies from individual to individual and for a given individual over time.

Heat

The temperature at which heat becomes painful for a recipient is called the *heat pain threshold* for that person at that time. One study showed that morning oriented people have higher pain threshold for heat as compared to evening oriented individuals.

Hearing

The pressure at which sound becomes painful for a listener is the *pain threshold pressure* for that person at that time. The threshold pressure for sound varies with frequency and can be age-dependent. Additionally, people who have been exposed to more noise/music usually have a higher threshold pressure. *Threshold shift* can also cause threshold pressure to vary. Prolonged exposure to sound at levels evoking pain can cause physical damage, potentially leading to hearing impairment.

The volume in acoustics refers to loudness. It is a common term for the amplitude of sound, the sound pressure level or the sound pressure. Different values for pain threshold pressure level and pain threshold pressure are found in the literature:

Pain Tolerance

Pain tolerance is the maximum level of pain that a person is able to tolerate. Pain tolerance is distinct from pain threshold (the point at which pain begins to be felt).

Factors

Clinical studies by the journal of *Psychosomatic Medicine* found that "men had higher pain thresholds and tolerances and lower pain ratings than women" when they are exposed to cold pressor pain. The study asked participants to submerge their hands in ice water (the cold pressor pain procedure) and told members of the experimental group (as opposed to the control group) that they would be compensated financially for keeping their hand submerged. Suggested explanations for this difference include, "men are more motivated to tolerate and suppress expressions of pain because of the masculine sex role, whereas the feminine sex role encourages pain expression and produces lower motivation to tolerate pain among women."

A similar study published in the same books focused on the effects of having individuals perform the ice water procedure if they are accompanied by another participant. Their results revealed, "Participants in the active support and passive support conditions reported less pain than participants in the alone and interaction conditions, regardless of whether they were paired with a friend or stranger. These data suggest that the presence of an individual who provides passive or active support reduces experimental pain."

Other factors that affect pain tolerance are association and disassociation. These two cognitive strategies have been found to increase pain tolerance.

Exposure as Tolerance Booster

It is widely believed that regular exposure to painful stimuli will increase pain tolerance: increases the ability of the individual to handle pain by becoming more conditioned to it. However, in some cases, there is evidence to support the theory that greater exposure to pain will result in more painful future exposures. Repeated exposure bombards pain synapses with repetitive input, increasing their responsiveness to later stimuli, through a process similar to learning. Therefore, although the individual may learn cognitive methods of coping with pain, such methods may not be sufficient to cope with the boosted response to future painful stimuli. "An intense barrage of painful stimuli potentiates the cells responsive to pain so that they respond more vigorously to minor stimulation in the future."

Thus, trauma victims (or patients in pain) are given painkillers (such as morphine) as soon as possible to prevent pain sensitization.

Kalat suggests that morphine should be taken before surgery; "People who begin taking morphine before surgery need less of it afterward."

Grimace Scale (Animals)

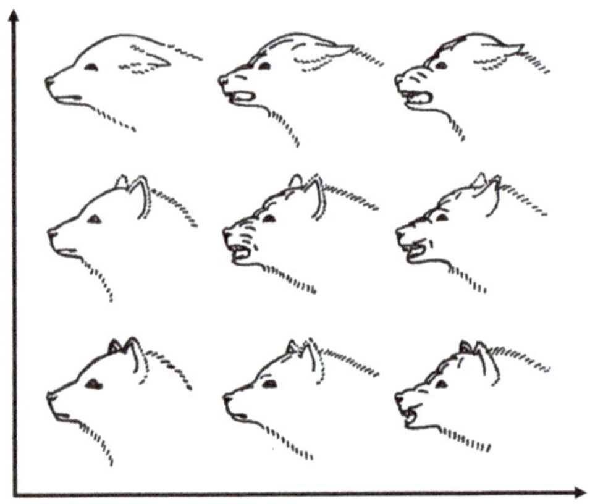

A drawing by Konrad Lorenz showing facial expressions of a dog

The grimace scale (GS), sometimes called the grimace score, is a method of assessing the occurrence or severity of pain experienced by non-human animals according to objective and blinded scoring of facial expressions, as is done routinely for the measurement of pain in non-verbal humans. Observers score the presence or prominence of "facial action units" (FAU), e.g. Orbital Tightening, Nose Bulge, Ear Position and Whisker Change. These are scored by observing the animal directly in real-time, or post hoc from photographs or screen-grabs from videos. The facial expression of the animals is sometimes referred to as the pain face.

The GS method of pain assessment is highly applicable to laboratory rodents as these are usually prey species which tend to inhibit the expression of pain to prevent appearing vulnerable to predators. For this reason, behavioural changes in these species are mainly observed with acute pain (hours) but are less pronounced in longer-lasting pain (days).

For mice at least, the GS has been shown to be a highly accurate, repeatable and reliable means of assessing pain requiring only a short period of training for the observer. Across species, GS are proven to have high accuracy and reliability, and are considered useful for indicating both procedural and postoperative pain, and for assessing the efficacy of analgesics.

The overall accuracy of GS is reported as 97% for mice, 84% for rabbits, 82% for rats and 73.3% for horses.

History

Facial expressions have long been considered as indicators of emotion in both human and non-human animals. The biologist, Charles Darwin, considered that non-human animals exhibit similar facial expressions to emotional states as do humans. The assessment of changes in human anatomy during facial expressions were successfully translated from humans to non-human primates, such as the chimpanzee (ChimpFACS) and rhesus macaque (MaqFACS), but were not originally applied to assess pain in these species. In 2010, a team of researchers successfully developed the first method to assess pain using changes in facial expression in any non-human animal species. Broadly speaking, GS quantify spontaneous pain according to objective and blinded scoring of facial expressions, as is done routinely for the measurement of pain in non-verbal humans. Observers score the presence and extent of "facial action units" (FAU), e.g. Orbital Tightening, Nose Bulge, Ear Position and Whisker Change. These are scored in real-time by observing the animal directly, or, post hoc from photographs or screen-grabs from videos.

This method of pain assessment highly applicable to prey animals which tend to inhibit the overt expression of pain to prevent appearing vulnerable to predators. For this reason, behavioural changes in these species are mainly observed with acute pain (hours) but are less pronounced in longer-lasting pain (days).

GS offer advantages over other methods of pain assessment. For example, the analgesic morphine reduces pain but can affect other aspects of behaviour in pain-free animals, for example, excitement, increased activity or sedation, which can hamper traditional behavioural assessment of its action on pain. Morphine not only reduces the frequency of "pain faces" but has no effect on GS in baseline, pain-free mice.

In Mice

The GS for mice usually consists of five FAU, i.e. Orbital Tightening, Nose Bulge, Cheek Bulge, Ear position and Whisker Change. These are scored on a 0-2 scale where 0=the criterion is absent, 1=moderately present and 2=obviously present. In mice, the GS offers a means of assessing post-operative pain that is as effective as manual behavioural-based scoring, without the limitations of such approaches.

Facial grimacing by mice after undergoing laparotomy surgery indicates postoperative pain lasts for 36 to 48 h (and at relatively high levels for 8 to 12 h) with relative exacerbation during the early dark (active) photo-phase. Furthermore, the grimacing indicates that buprenorphine is fully efficacious at recommended doses against early postoperative pain, but carprofen and ketoprofen are efficacious only at doses much higher than currently recommended: acetaminophen is not efficacious.

A study in 2014 examined postoperative pain in mice following surgical induction of myocardial infarction. The effectiveness of the GS at identifying pain was compared with a traditional welfare scoring system based on behavioural, clinical and procedure-specific criteria. It was reported that post hoc GS (but not real-time GS) indicated a significant proportion of the mice were in low-level pain at 24 h which were not identified as such by traditional assessment methods. Importantly, those mice identified as experiencing low-level pain responded to analgesic treatment, indicating the traditional methods of welfare assessment were insensitive in this aspect of pain recognition.

Mice with induced sickle cell disease and their controls exhibited a "pain face" when tested on a cold plate, but sickle mice showed increased intensity compared to controls; this was confirmed using Von Frey filaments a traditional method of pain assessment. GS have also been used to assess pain and methods of its alleviation in pancreatitis. GS have also been used to test the degree of pain caused as a side-effect of therapeutic drugs and methods of mitigating the pain.

The mouse GS has been shown to be a highly accurate, repeatable and reliable means of assessing pain, requiring only a short period of training for the observer.

Sex and Strain Effects

It has been noted that DBA/2 strain mice, but not CBA strain mice, show an increase in GS score following only isoflurane anaesthesia, which should be taken into account when using the GS to assess pain. Administration of a common analgesic, buprenorphine, had no effect on the GS of either strain.

There are interactions between the sex and strain of mice in their GS and also the method that is used to collect the data (i.e. real-time or post hoc), which indicates scorers need to consider these factors.

Effects of Non-painful Procedures

It is important to establish whether methods of pain assessment in laboratory animals are influenced by other factors, especially those which are a normal part of routine procedures or husbandry. There is no difference in GS scores between mice handled using a tube compared with mice picked up by the tail, indicating these handling techniques are not confounding factors in GS assessment. A similar study reported there was no difference between GS scores at baseline and immediately post ear notching (a method frequently used to identify laboratory mice), potentially indicating that the pain associated with ear notching is either too acute to assess using the GS tool or the practice is not painful.

In Rats

There are differences between the "pain face" of mice and rats. In mice, the nose and cheek at baseline have a smooth appearance, but in the presence of pain, change to distinct bulges in both the nose and cheek regions. By contrast, in rats at baseline, the nose and cheek regions show distinct bulging, and with pain, the bridge of the nose flattens and elongates causing the whisker pads to flatten. As a consequence of these differences, the GS for rats sometimes use four FAU, i.e. Orbital Tightening, Nose/Cheek Flattening, Ear Changes and Whisker Changes. Nose/Cheek Flattening, appears to show the highest correlation with the presence of pain in the rat.

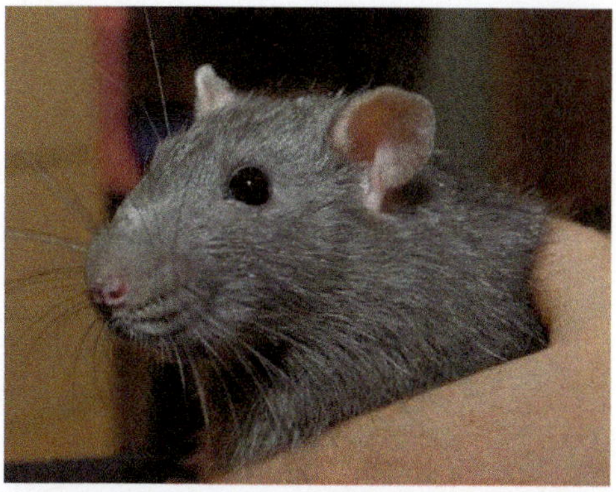

Closeup of the face of an agouti Russian blue rat

GS for rats has been used to assess pain due to surgery, orthodontic tooth movement, and the efficacy of analgesics for these procedures and other painful conditions. Furthermore, GS have been used to examine the effects of postoperative analgesia on the reduction of post-operative cognitive dysfunction in aged rats.

As with mice, studies have examined the extent of agreement in assessing pain between rat GS and the use of von Frey filaments. Good agreement has been found between these in relation to three models of pain (intraplantar carrageenan, intraplantar complete Freund's adjuvant and plantar incision). The GS score significantly increased in all pain models and the peak GS score also coincided with the development of paw hypersensitivity, although hypersensitivity persisted after GS scores returned to baseline.

For rats, software (Rodent Face Finder®) has been developed which successfully automates the most labour-intensive step in the process of quantifying the GS, i.e. frame-grabbing individual face-containing frames from digital video, which is hindered by animals not looking directly at the camera or poor images due to motion blurring.

In Rabbits

A GS for rabbits using four FAU, i.e. Orbital Tightening, Cheek Flattening, Nose Shape, Whisker Position (Ear Position is excluded from the analysis) has been developed and used to assess the effectiveness of an analgesic cream for rabbits having undergone ear-tattooing. Similarly, a GS has been used to evaluate wellness in the post-procedural monitoring of rabbits.

In Horses

A GS for horses has been developed from post-operative (castration) individuals. This is based on six FAU, i.e. Stiffly Backwards Ears, Orbital Tightening, Tension Above the Eye Area, Prominent Strained Chewing Muscles, Mouth Strained and Pronounced Chin, Strained Nostrils and Flattening of the Profile.

A related study stated that the equine "pain face" involves low and/or asymmetrical ears, an angled appearance of the eyes, a withdrawn and/or tense stare, medio-laterally dilated nostrils and tension of the lips, chin and certain mimetic muscles and can potentially be incorporated to improve existing pain evaluation tools.

In Cats

Observers shown facial images from painful and pain-free cats had difficulty in identifying pain-free from painful cats, with only 13% of observers being able to discriminate more than 80% of painful cats.

In Sheep

A GS for sheep has been developed to detect pain caused by naturally occurring diseases such as footrot and mastitis. A GS has been used to assess pain due to the routine husbandry procedure of tail-docking in lambs. There was high reliability between and within the observers, and high accuracy. Restraint of the lambs during the tail-docking caused changes in facial expression, which needs to be taken into account in use of the GS.

Nociception Assay

A nociception assay (nocioception or nocioperception assay) evaluates the ability of an animal, usually a rodent, to detect a noxious stimulus such as the feeling of pain, caused by stimulation of nociceptors. These assays measure the existence of pain through behaviors such as withdrawal, licking, immobility, and vocalization. The sensation of pain is not a unitary concept; therefore, a researcher must be conscious as to which nociception assay to use.

Formalin

The formalin assay is the most popular chemical assay of nociception. It entails the injection of a dilute solution of formalin into the surface of the rodent's hindpaw, followed by the scoring of stereotypical behaviors such as flinching, licking, and biting of the affected hindpaw. The behaviors last for approximately 1 hour, with the early or acute stage (directly after injection) reflecting direct activation of nociceptors and the late or tonic phase (15 to 20 minutes after the injection) reflecting inflammation.

Typically, the formalin assay is used on rats; however, formalin concentrations and scoring methods can be modified as to suit mice. One major advantage of the formalin assay over other models of inflammatory pain is the limited duration (approximately 1 hour) of the response. Additionally, as described before, this assay produces a response in two discrete stages, allowing researchers to model both acute and tonic pain using a single noxious chemical.

Von Frey

The Von Frey assay, introduced by Maximilian von Frey and modified by Weinstein, uses Von Frey hair or fibers, which are small pieces of nylon rod, approximately 50 mm in length, and of varying diameters, to test a rodent's sensitivity to a mechanical stimulus. It is unclear whether the process is really considered noxious versus simply annoying, so this assay is a test of mechanical nociception or simply mechanical sensibility. In this test, the animal stands on an elevated mesh platform, and the Von Frey hairs are inserted through the mesh to poke the animal's hindpaw. Normal reactions for the animal include withdrawing or licking or shaking the paw, and possible vocalization, but these can depend on variability within the experiment. For example, the ventral surface of the hind paw is typically associated with lower withdrawal thresholds compared to the dorsal surface, and the exact force of the fiber is determined by its thickness. It is also important to note that thresholds usually are initially decreasing during successive tests, but do become stable after about 3 sessions. Algorithms such as up-down or Bruceton analysis are available to concentrate testing into the most dynamic part of the range, and subsequent curve fitting and parameter estimation can be similarly standardised. Alternatively, automated von Frey systems have recently been discovered that gradually increase the force of a single probe so that a researcher can observe when withdrawal responses occur.

Thermal Assays

Sensitivity to acute thermal stimulation is the most common test used in live species pain research. The behavioral reflex evoked by noxious heat stimuli is a relatively good predictor of pain sensitivity and its reduction through various analgesics. One significant limitation of thermal assays lies in the specificity and validity of results in animals as models of human pain. Very little is known about the functional mechanics of nociceptive afferents in murine subjects, thus the translation of any pain response observed from these animals to humans is questionable.

Tail Withdrawal

Two versions of the tail withdrawal assay are commonly employed in pain sensitivity testing. In the classic radiant heat test, a heat source is targeted onto a small area of the tail, and the latency to withdraw the tail away from the heat source is measured. In the tail-immersion test, a container of liquid is heated or cooled to a nociceptive temperature – normally 50–55 °C or below 0 °C. The animal subject is then placed with its tail immersed in the liquid, and the latency to withdraw the tail from the liquid is measured.

Animal subjects used must be restrained to a fairly high degree when performing the tail withdrawal test due to the exact positioning necessary to direct the noxious stimuli. Restraint is usually accomplished by placing the subjects in small Plexiglas tubes or cloth/cardboard pockets that the subjects can either be habituated to or voluntarily enter.

The primary advantage of tail withdrawal assays to other forms of thermal nociception testing, such as the hot-plate test or Hargreaves test, is the relative stability of results with repeated observations. Pain-reflex latency observations from other tests are usually much more variable both across and within subjects than those obtained from the tail withdrawal assay.

Hot Plate

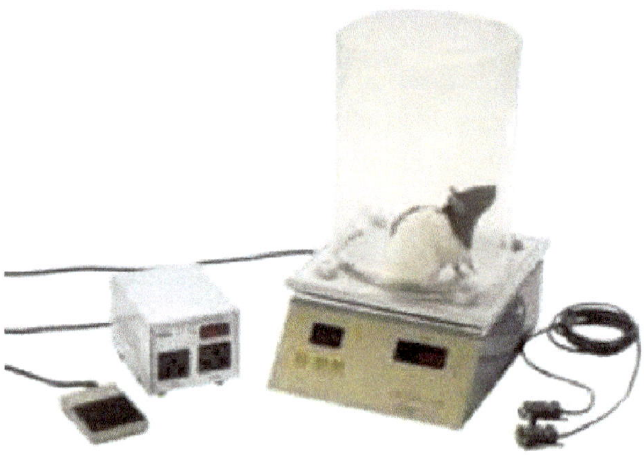

Example of a hot plate assay performed on a rat

A heat-conductive surface, such as porcelain or metal, is heated to a temperature that will induce a nociceptive response in an animal subject – normally 50–56 °C. The subject is then placed onto the surface and prevented from leaving the platform by blockades. The latency to pain-reflex behavior is measured. One complication of this assay is its unsuitability for repeated testing. Animals that have been subjected to the hot-plate test in the past display a behavioral tolerance phenomenon, which is characterized by decreased latencies and reduced sensitivities to antinociceptive agents. Another complication of the hot-plate test is determining what constitutes a behavioral pain response; is it the lifting/licking of paws, vocalization, attempting to climb out of the cylinder, etc. Also, delivering the heat stimulus in a controlled fashion presents difficulties due to each section having varying temperatures based upon surface area exposure and whether the animal is moving or not.

Tail Flick

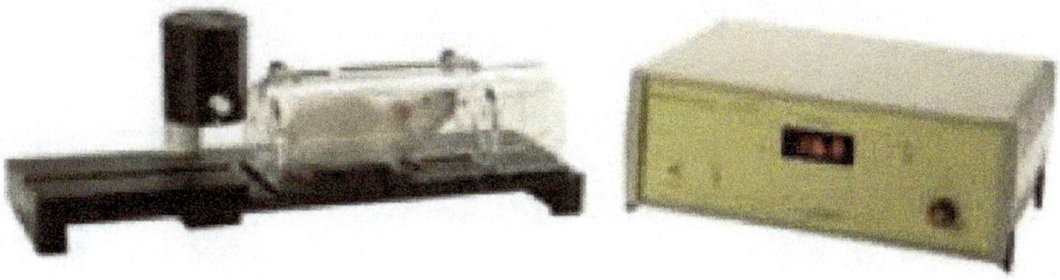

Example of a traditional set-up for the tail flick assay

The tail flick assay or tail flick test uses a high-intensity beam of light aimed at a rodent's tail to detect nociception. In normal rodents, the noxious heat sensation induced by the beam of light causes a prototypical movement of the tail via the flexor withdrawal reflex. An investigator normally measures the time it takes for the reflex to be induced, a factor influenced by a rodent's sex, age and body weight. The most critical parameter for the tail flick assay is the beam intensity; stimuli producing latencies of larger than 3–4 seconds generally create more variable results. Another important factor to consider is the level of restraint used; rodents held too tightly may exhibit greater tail flick latencies due to heightened stress levels.

Hargreaves

The Hargreaves assay uses a high-intensity beam of light directed at the hindpaw rather than the tail to induce pain; an investigator then measures the time it takes for the animal to withdraw its hindpaw. In contrast to the tail flick assay, rodents are often unrestrained while the radiant heat source is focused on the hindpaw. Cut-off latency for the Hargreaves assay is commonly set at 10 seconds. The main advantage of this test over the tail flick assay is that it allows independent assessment of treatment effects on both sides of the body.

Applications

One of the most common applications of nociception assays is to test the effectiveness of new pain medications and drugs of the like. One can then perform comparative tests to measure the differences in the effects of the drug on varying populations, such as men versus women, or young versus old. These tests can also identify certain harmful diseases or abnormalities in subjects if they display atypical nociception test responses. Additionally, nociception tests can be used to test the heritability of nociception itself. One can also use nociception assays to assess the physiology of the "pain" pathways. The role capsaicin receptors play in the pain pathways has been measured by comparing results from nociception assays in mice with and without the receptor. In addition, they are useful in other tests to make sure control subjects have normal nociception responses.

Hot Plate Test

The hot plate test is a test of the pain response in animals, similar to the tail flick test. It is used in basic pain research and in testing the effectiveness of analgesics by observing the reaction to pain caused by heat.

It was proposed by Eddy and Leimbach in 1953. They used a behavioral model of nociception where behaviors such as jumping and hind paw-licking are elicited following a noxious thermal stimulus. Licking is a rapid response to painful thermal stimuli that is a direct indicator of nociceptive threshold. Jumping represents a more elaborated response, with a latency, and encompasses an emotional component of escaping.

Procedure

- A transparent glass cylinder is used to keep the animal on the heated surface of the plate.
- The temperature of the hot plate is set using a thermoregulated water-circulated pump.
- The time of latency is defined as the time period between the zero point, when the animal is placed on the hot plate surface, and the time when the animal licks its paw or jumps off to avoid thermal pain.

Research Findings

Sex Studies Using Antidepressants

Significant differences in pain sensitivity in male and female mice have been observed in laboratory studies. The SSRI antidepressant paroxetine did not display a gender difference in antinociceptive effects in mice.

Ion Channels

Voltage-gated ion channels are implicated in pain sensation and transmission signaling mechanisms within both peripheral nociceptors and the spinal cord. Specific ion channel isoforms such as Nav1.7 and Nav1.8 sodium channels and Cav3.2 T-type calcium channels have distinct pro-nociceptive roles.

Opioid Receptors

Activation of the μ-opioid receptor (MOR) and norepinephrine reuptake inhibition (NRI) are mechanisms of acute and chronic pain. OPRM1 knockout mice were used to determine the relative contribution of MOR activation to tapentadol and morphine induced analgesia. Wild-type mice exhibited an antinociceptive effect ten times that of OPM1 knockouts. However, the OPRM1 knockouts still exhibited a slight analgesic effect to tapentadol but not to morphine. This indicated that the antinociceptive effect of tapentadol is based on a combined mechanism of action involving both MOR and NRI.

Benzodiazepines and GABA Receptors

Diazepam is a GABAA receptor benzodiazepine ligand that is an anxiety modulator. Studies using diazepam with the hot plate test showed that diazepam modified the behavioral structure of the pain response not from pain modulation but rather by reducing anxiety levels.

Ethics

The Ethical Committee of the International Association for the Study of Pain has developed guidelines for the ethical use of this procedure. In the United States, such experiments must be approved by an Institutional Animal Care and Use Committee.

Nociceptor

A nociceptor is a type of sensory receptor at the end of a sensory neuron's axon that responds to damaging or potentially damaging stimuli by sending signals of pain to the spinal cord and brain. This process is called nociception.

History

Nociceptors were discovered by Charles Scott Sherrington in 1906. In earlier centuries, scientists believed that animals were like mechanical devices that transformed the energy of sensory stimuli into motor responses. Sherrington used many different styles of experiments to demonstrate that different types of stimulation to an afferent nerve fiber's receptive field led to different responses. Some intense stimuli trigger reflex withdrawal, autonomic responses and pain. The specific receptors for these intense stimuli were called nociceptors.

Location

In mammals, nociceptors are sensory neurons that are found in any area of the body that can sense noxious stimuli either externally or internally. External examples are in tissues such as skin (cutaneous nociceptors), cornea and mucosa. Internal nociceptors are in a variety of organs, such as the muscle, joint, bladder, gut and continuing along the digestive tract. The cell bodies of these neurons are located in either the dorsal root ganglia or the trigeminal ganglia. The trigeminal ganglia are specialized nerves for the face, whereas the dorsal root ganglia associate with the rest of the body. The axons extend into the peripheral nervous system and terminate in branches to form receptive fields.

Development

Nociceptors develop from neural crest stem cells. The neural crest is responsible for a large part of early development in vertebrates. More specifically it is responsible for development of the peripheral nervous system. The neural crest stem cells split off from the neural tube as it closes, and nociceptors grow from the dorsal part of this neural crest tissue. They form late during neurogenesis. Earlier forming cells from this region can become non-pain sensing receptors; either proprioceptors or low-threshold mechanoreceptors. All neurons derived from neural crest, including embryonic nociceptors, express the TrkA which is a receptor to nerve growth factor (NGF). However, transcription factors that determine the type of nociceptor remain unclear.

Following sensory neurogenesis, differentiation occurs and two different types of nociceptors are formed. They are classified as either peptidergic or nonpeptidergic nociceptors. The sets of receptors express distinct repertoires of ion channels and receptors. With their specialization, it allows the receptors to innervate different peripheral and central targets. This differentiation occurs in both perinatal and postnatal periods. The nonpeptidergic nociceptors switch off the TrkA and begin expressing Ret. Ret is a transmembrane signaling component which allows for the expression of another growth factor—glial cell-derived growth factor (GDNF). This transition is assisted by Runx1 which has proven to be vital in the development of nonpeptidergic nociceptors. On the contrary, the peptidergic nociceptors continue to use TrkA and they express a completely different type of growth factor. Currently there is a lot of research being done to determine more specifically what creates the differences between nociceptors.

Types and Functions

The peripheral terminal of the mature nociceptor is where the noxious stimuli are detected and transduced into electrical energy. When the electrical energy reaches a threshold value, an action potential is induced and driven towards the central nervous system (CNS). This leads to the train of events that allows for the conscious awareness of pain. The sensory specificity of nociceptors is established by the high threshold only to particular features of stimuli. Only when the high threshold has been reached by either chemical, thermal, or mechanical environments are the nociceptors triggered. The majority of nociceptors are classified by which of the environmental modalities they respond to. Some nociceptors respond to more than one of these modalities and are consequently designated polymodal. Other nociceptors respond to none of these modalities (although they may respond to stimulation under conditions of inflammation) and are referred to as sleeping or silent.

Nociceptors have two different types of axons. The first are the Aδ fiber axons. They are myelinated and can allow an action potential to travel at a rate of about 20 meters/second towards the CNS. The other type is the more slowly conducting C fiber axons. These only conduct at speeds of around 2 meters/second. This is due to the light or non-myelination of the axon. As a result, pain comes in two phases. The first phase is mediated by the fast-conducting Aδ fibers and the second part due to (Polymodal) C fibers. The pain associated with the Aδ fibers can be associated to an initial extremely sharp pain. The second phase is a more prolonged and slightly less intense feeling of pain as a result of the acute damage. If there is massive or prolonged input to a C fiber, there is a progressive build up in the spinal cord dorsal horn; this phenomenon is similar to tetanus in muscles but is called wind-up. If wind-up occurs there is a probability of increased sensitivity to pain.

Thermal

Thermal nociceptors are activated by noxious heat or cold at various temperatures. There are specific nociceptor transducers that are responsible for how and if the specific nerve ending responds to the thermal stimulus. The first to be discovered was TRPV1, and it has a threshold that coincides with the heat pain temperature of 42 °C. Other temperature in the warm–hot range is mediated by more than one TRP channel. Each of these channels express a particular C-terminal domain that corresponds to the warm–hot sensitivity. The interactions between all these channels and how the temperature level is determined to be above the pain threshold are unknown at this time. The cool stimuli are sensed by TRPM8 channels. Its C-terminal domain differs from the heat sensitive TRPs. Although this channel corresponds to cool stimuli, it is still unknown whether it also contributes in the detection of intense cold. An interesting finding related to cold stimuli is that tactile sensibility and motor function deteriorate while pain perception persists.

Mechanical

Mechanical nociceptors respond to excess pressure or mechanical deformation. They also respond to incisions that break the skin surface. The reaction to the stimulus is processed as pain by the cortex, just like chemical and thermal responses. These mechanical nociceptors frequently have polymodal characteristics. So it is possible that some of the transducers for thermal stimuli are the same for mechanical stimuli. The same is true for chemical stimuli, since TRPA1 appears to detect both mechanical and chemical changes.

Chemical

Chemical nociceptors have TRP channels that respond to a wide variety of spices. The one that sees the most response and is very widely tested is capsaicin. Other chemical stimulants are environmental irritants like acrolein, a World War I chemical weapon and a component of cigarette smoke. Apart from these external stimulants, chemical nociceptors have the capacity to detect endogenous ligands, and certain fatty acid amines that arise from changes in internal tissues. Like in thermal nociceptors, TRPV1 can detect chemicals like capsaicin and spider toxins.

Sleeping/silent

Although each nociceptor can have a variety of possible threshold levels, some do not respond at all to chemical, thermal or mechanical stimuli unless injury actually has occurred. These are typically referred to as silent or sleeping nociceptors since their response comes only on the onset of inflammation to the surrounding tissue.

Polymodal

Many neurons perform only a single function, therefore neurons that perform these functions in combination are given the classification "polymodal."

Pathway

Afferent nociceptive fibers (those that send information *to*, rather than *from* the brain) travel back to the spinal cord where they form synapses in its dorsal horn. This nociceptive fiber (located in the periphery) is a first order neuron. The cells in the dorsal horn are divided into physiologically distinct layers called laminae. Different fiber types form synapses in different layers, and use either glutamate or substance P as the neurotransmitter. Aδ fibers form synapses in laminae I and V, C fibers connect with neurons in lamina II, Aβ fibers connect with lamina I, III, & V. After reaching the specific lamina within the spinal cord, the first order nociceptive project to second order neurons that cross the midline at the anterior white commissure. The second order neurons then send their information via two pathways to the thalamus: the dorsal column medial-lemniscal system and the anterolateral system. The first is reserved more for regular non-painful sensation, while the lateral is reserved for pain sensation. Upon reaching the thalamus, the information is processed in the ventral posterior nucleus and sent to the cerebral cortex in the brain via fibers in the posterior limb of the internal capsule. As there is an ascending pathway to the brain that initiates the conscious realization of pain, there also is a descending pathway which modulates pain sensation. The brain can request the release of specific hormones or chemicals that can have analgesic effects which can reduce or inhibit pain sensation. The area of the brain that stimulates the release of these hormones is the hypothalamus.

This effect of descending inhibition can be shown by electrically stimulating the periaqueductal grey area of the midbrain. The periaqueductal grey in turn projects to other areas involved in pain regulation, such as the nucleus raphes magnus which also receives similar afferents from the nucleus reticularis paragigantocellularis (NPG). In turn the nucleus raphe magnus projects to the substantia gelatinosa region of the dorsal horn and mediates the sensation of spinothalamic inputs. The periaqueductal grey also contains opioid receptors which explains one of the mechanisms by which opioids such as morphine and diacetylmorphine exhibit an analgesic effect.

Sensitivity

Nociceptor neuron sensitivity is modulated by a large variety of mediators in the extracellular space. Peripheral sensitization represents a form of functional plasticity of the nociceptor. The nociceptor can change from being simply a noxious stimulus detector to a detector of non-noxious stimuli. The result is that low intensity stimuli from regular activity, initiates a painful sensation. This is commonly known as hyperalgesia. Inflammation is one common cause that results in the sensitization of nociceptors. Normally hyperalgesia ceases when inflammation goes down, however, sometimes genetic defects and/or repeated injury can result in allodynia: a completely non-noxious stimulus like light touch causes extreme pain. Allodynia can also be caused when a nociceptor is damaged in the peripheral nerves. This can result in deafferentation, which means the development of different central processes from the surviving afferent nerve. With this situation, surviving dorsal root axons of the nociceptors can make contact with the spinal cord, thus changing the normal input.

Other Animals

Nociception has been documented in non-mammalian animals, including fish and a wide range of invertebrates, including leeches, nematode worms, sea slugs, and fruit flies. Although these neurons may have different pathways and relationships to the central nervous system than mammalian nociceptors, nociceptive neurons in non-mammals often fire in response to similar stimuli as mammals, such as high temperature (40 degrees C or more), low pH, capsaicin, and tissue damage.

Terminology

Due to historical understandings of pain, nociceptors are also called *pain receptors*. This usage is not consistent with the modern definition of pain as a subjective experience.

Pain Catastrophizing

Pain catastrophizing is the tendency to describe a pain experience in more exaggerated terms than the average person, to ruminate on it more (e.g., "I kept thinking 'this is terrible'"), and/or to feel more helpless about the experience ("I thought it was never going to get better"). People who report a large number of such thoughts during a pain experience are more likely to rate the pain as more intense than those who report fewer such thoughts.

It is generally assumed that the tendency to catastrophize plays a causal role in the pain experience – that is, it *causes* the person to experience the pain as more intense. One suggestion is that catastrophizing influences pain perception through altering attention and anticipation, and heightening emotional responses to pain. However, we cannot yet rule out the possibility that at least some aspects of catastrophization may actually be the *product* of an intense pain experience, rather than its cause. That is, the more intense the pain feels to the person, the more likely they are to have thoughts about it that fit the definition of catastrophization.

Measurement

The components of catastrophizing that are considered primary were long under debate until the development of the pain catastrophizing scale (PCS). The pain catastrophizing scale is a 13-item self-report scale to measure pain catastrophizing created by Michael J. L. Sullivan, Scott R. Bishop and Jayne Pivik. In the PCS, each item is rated on a 5-point scale: 0 (Not at all) to 4 (all the time). It is broken into three subscales being magnification, rumination, and helplessness. The scale was developed as a self-report measurement tool that provided a valid index of catastrophizing in clinical and non-clinical populations. It is hypothesized that pain catastrophizing is related to various levels of pain, physical disability and psychological disability in clinical and non-clinical populations.

1. I worry all the time about whether the pain will end. (H)
2. I feel I can't go on. (H)
3. It's terrible and I think it's never going to get any better. (H)
4. It's awful and I feel that it overwhelms me. (H)
5. I feel I can't stand it anymore. (H)
6. I become afraid that the pain may get worse. (M)
7. I think of other painful experiences. (M)
8. I anxiously want the pain to go away. (R)
9. I can't seem to keep it out of my mind. (R)
10. I keep thinking about how much it hurts. (R)
11. I keep thinking about how badly I want the pain to stop. (R)
12. There is nothing I can do to reduce the intensity of the pain. (H)
13. I wonder whether something serious may happen. (M)

(Note: For the listed items above, (R) Rumination, (M) Magnification, and (H) Helplessness.)

Before the development of the PCS there had been no other self-report measurement tool that focused primarily on catastrophizing. Other self-report measurement tools such as: the Coping Strategies Questionnaire (CSQ), the Pain-Related Self-Statements Scale (PRSS) and the Cognitive Coping Strategy Inventory (CCS) had subscales for assessing catastrophizing but failed to explore specific dimensions of catastrophizing.

Studies of the PCS have generally used a self-report design. Participants are asked about pain experiences in their past; they then rate how well various statements fit their thoughts and feelings at the time. Several such studies have shown the PCS to be invariant, with most accuracy in the three oblique factor structure, across genders and both clinical and non-clinical groups. The gender focused study expressed that female subjects report more frequent experiences of pain, varied intensity with increased persistence, and lower pain tolerances and thresholds. However, it is important to remember that these studies ask participants to report on pain experiences from their past; the overall level of pain experienced is not controlled across genders. If female participants have, on average, experienced more intense and/or persistent pain in their past than male participants, this could also explain their higher endorsement of items relating to pain catastrophizing. Further, more controlled studies are urgently needed to tease apart these issues of cause and effect.

With minimal modification, to address the subject of the catastrophizing, the PCS can also be applied to pain catastrophizing in a social context. The social aspects studied were parents of disabled children and spouses of individuals with chronic pain. Specifically it has been shown to determine illness related stress and depression issues that arise from parent's catastrophizing about their child's pain in regards to a disability or illness. Similarly with respect to pain catastrophizing between romantic partners, spouse catastrophizing about a partner's chronic pain was related to depressive and pain severity levels in both spouses.

Applications

Research on pain catastrophizing has found that catastrophic thinking is associated with a more intense experience of pain. It is generally believed that the catastrophic thoughts cause the person to experience pain more intensely. This may in turn lead to increased use of health care and longer hospital stays. Following this logic, if the catastrophic thinking can be addressed, then the person's pain experience might also be reduced, which in turn might reduce health care utilization. The use of scales such as the PCS may be useful for measuring pain catastrophizing in these contexts.

Treatment

The primary treatment for pain catastrophizing is cognitive behavior therapy for chronic pain. This is typically delivered in individual psychotherapy sessions, or in group pain coping skills classes. These sessions and classes typically span 6 to 12 weeks, and cover a variety of psychobehavioral topics in addition to pain catastrophizing. In 2014, researchers at Stanford University found that a single-session class that they developed specifically to treat pain catastrophizing was effective. However, to date, there have been no studies that meet the usual standards required for medical treatment intervention studies (for example, where patients are randomly allocated to a treatment or an appropriate control condition, and patients are unaware of which condition is expected to be associated with the better outcome).

Pain Catastrophizing Scale

Catastrophic thinking has widely been recognized in the development and maintenance of hypochondriasis and anxiety disorders. This broadly accepted understanding has classified catastrophizing as a tendency to misinterpret and exaggerate situations that may be threatening. Pain is an undesirable sensory and emotional experience in response to potential or actual tissue damage. A general consensus of pain catastrophizing involves an exaggerated negative perception to painful stimuli. The components of catastrophizing that are considered primary were long under debate until the development of the Pain Catastrophizing Scale (PCS) by Michael J. L. Sullivan and Scott R. Bishop of Dalhousie University in 1995. The PCS is a 13 item scale, with each item rated on a 5-point scale: 0 (Not at all) to 4 (all the time). The PCS is broken into three subscales being magnification, rumination, and helplessness. The scale was developed as a self-report measurement tool that provided a valid index of catastrophizing in clinical and non-clinical populations. The results of the initial development and validation studies indicated that the PCS is a reliable and valid measurement tool for catastrophizing. The high test-retest relationships concluded that individuals may possess enduring beliefs with regards to the threat value of painful stimuli. It was also found that from a clinical perspective, the PCS may be useful in identifying individuals that may be more susceptible to high distress responses from aversive medical procedures such as chemotherapy or surgery.

Items

1. I worry all the time about whether the pain will end. (H)
2. I feel I can't go on. (H)
3. It's terrible and I think it's never going to get any better. (H)
4. It's awful and I feel that it overwhelms me. (H)
5. I feel I can't stand it anymore. (H)
6. I become afraid that the pain may get worse. (M)
7. I think of other painful experiences. (M)
8. I anxiously want the pain to go away. (R)

9. I can't seem to keep it out of my mind. (R)
10. I keep thinking about how much it hurts. (R)
11. I keep thinking about how badly I want the pain to stop. (R)
12. There is nothing I can do to reduce the intensity of the pain. (H)
13. I wonder whether something serious may happen. (M)

(Note: For the listed items above, (R) Rumination, (M) Magnification, and (H) Helplessness.)

Further Psychometric Evaluation

A secondary study was conducted by Augustine Osman of the University of Northern Iowa to replicate the findings found in the development and validation studies of Sullivan and Bishop. At the time of the study there was a great deal of interest in understanding the cognitive factors involving pain and an individual's response to persistent pain experiences. Before the development of the Pain Catastrophizing Scale (PCS) there had been no other self-report measurement tool that focused primarily on catastrophizing. Other self-report measurement tools such as: the Coping Strategies Questionnaire (CSQ), the Pain-Related Self-Statements Scale (PRSS) and the Cognitive Coping Strategy Inventory (CCS) had subscales for assessing catastrophizing but failed to explore specific dimensions of catastrophizing. Osman conducted a series of experiments to replicate the findings of Sullivan and Bishop, as well as evaluated the validity of the PCS's ability to effectively differentiate between adult outpatient and nonclinical community samples using adult subjects. The study that Osman conducted effectively replicated the findings of Sullivan and Bishop. The Study confirmed the ability of the PCS to isolate general catastrophizing characterized by the three primary related factors (rumination, magnification, and helplessness). The PCS was found to effectively differentiate between clinical and nonclinical samples, through verifying a clear distinction between overall and subscale scores of the PCS of the tested subjects. The findings of the study provided empirical support for the PCS in future studies.

As the Pain Catastrophizing Scale has been developed, the goal of studies has shifted to its usability as a universal scale. Through various studies the PCS was shown to be invariant (with most accuracy in the three oblique factor structure) across genders and both clinical and non-clinical groups. The gender focused study expressed that female subjects report more frequent experiences of pain, varied intensity with increased persistence, and lower pain tolerances and thresholds. With minimal modification (to address the subject of the catastrophizing) the PCS can also be applied to pain catastrophizing in a social context. The social aspects studied were parents of disabled children and spouses of individuals with chronic pain. Specifically it has been shown to determine illness related stress and depression issues that arise from parent's catastrophizing about their child's pain in regards to a disability or illness. Similarly with respect to pain catastrophizing between romantic partners, spouse catastrophizing about a partner's chronic pain was related to depressive and pain severity levels in both spouses.

Applications

Research of pain catastrophizing has found that catastrophic thinking can result in a more intense experience of Pain. By this association, catastrophizing has led to over predictions of pain, increased use of health care and longer hospital stays. The use of the PCS in clinical and nonclinical settings can provide a more specific tool for healthcare professionals to better care for their patients. A greater understanding of a person's experience of pain can allow for a better care regiment to beimplemented helping reduce problems that have previously come from catastrophizing.

Pain Assessment

Pain is often regarded as the fifth vital sign in regard to healthcare because it is accepted now in healthcare that pain, like other vital signs, is an objective sensation rather than subjective. As a result nurses are trained and expected to assess pain.

Regulation

Pain assessment and re-assessment after administration of analgesics or pain management is regulated in healthcare facilities by accreditation bodies, like the Joint Commission. The Joint Commission began setting standards for pain assessment in 2001 stating that the route of analgesic administration dictates the times for pain reassessment, as different routes require different amounts of time for the medication to have a therapeutic effect. Oral: 45–69 minutes. Intramuscular: 30 minutes. Intravascular: 15 minutes.

Types of Assessment

Most pain assessments are done in the form of a scale. The scale is explained to the patient, who then chooses a score. A rating is taken before administering any medication and after the specified time frame to rate the efficacy of treatment.

Number Scale

Patients rate pain on a scale from 0-10, 0 being no pain and 10 being the worst pain imaginable.

Faces Scale

A scale with corresponding faces depicting various levels of pain is shown to the patient and they select one.

Special Considerations

Patients who cannot verbalize/comprehend pain scales are assessed with different types of scales.

FLACC

Used for neonates/infants:

Assessment	0	1	2
Face	Smiling/expression-less	Frowning	Clenched jaw/Anguish
Legs	Normal movement/ Relaxed	Restless/Tense	Legs drawn up/Kicking
Activity	None/Lying quietly	Squirming/Tense movements	Arched back/Rigid/Jerk-ing
Cry	None	Occasional whim-per	Crying constantly/ Screaming
Consolability	Relaxed	Easily distracted or reassured	Difficult to distract/reas-sure

The scores are added together to achieve a 0-10 pain score.

Physiological Measurement of Pain

fMRI brain scanning has been used to measure pain, giving good correlations with self-reported pain.

Long-term Pain

Hedonic adaptation means that actual long-term suffering due to physical illness is often much lower than expected.

Legal Awards for Pain and Suffering

One area where assessments of pain and suffering are required to be made effectively is in legal awards. In the Western world these are typically discretionary awards made by juries and are regarded as difficult to predict, variable and subjective, for instance in the US, UK, Australia and New Zealand.

Addiction

Many patients who use drugs and are on opioids, analgesics, benzodiazepines, stimulants, barbiturates, and sedative-hypnotics have the potential to become addicted. Many people with chronic illnesses, injury, and history of mental illness are prescribed these drugs. As a nurse it is difficult to assess whether the pain is real or whether the patient is seeking the narcotic. Adult patients display pain and emotions differently. Many patients become dependent physically and mentally on these drugs.

1. name 2. age 3. sex 4. occupation 5. address 6. chief complaint of patient 7. history of patient:- present illness history past illness history medical history family history personal history 8. pain site of pain nature of pain quantity of pain on v.a.s scale type of pain 9. examination active movement passive movement 10. observation gait posture r.o.m palpation aggravating factor relieving factor tenderness 11. treatment

Nurse Pain Assessment

- Does the patient show nonverbal signs of pain such as crying or grimacing?
- Does the patient watch the clock and ask for the pain medication or sedative at the exact time it's due?
- Does the patient continually ask for the medication?
- Does the patient continually ask the physician to increase pain medication?
- What is the dose of the medication and how often does the patient ask for it?
- How long has the patient been taking the drug?
- Does the patient have a change in mood and behavior if they don't receive the medication at the exact time?
- Have a conversation with the patient. Do they want the medication because they are in pain or because they can't sleep?
- Do they want the medication because they are anxious?
- What is going on in the patient's life?
- What are their social circumstances?
- Is the nursing staff performing three non-drug interventions before administering a sedative, hypnotic, or anti anxiety medication?
- How many different medications is the patient on?
- Is the patient gradually asking for less medication as time goes on or are they asking for more?

Assessment Findings

If the patient is continually asking for the physician to increase their pain medication or increase the frequency, they need further evaluation by both a nurse and a physician. There is a good possibility the patient is in pain. There is also a possibility that they are becoming addicted to prescribed medication. The patient's history must be taken into account as well. Medical conditions such as cancer and rheumatoid arthritis are chronic conditions and can be very painful.

In long-term care facilities, three non-drug interventions need to be attempted before administering anti-anxiety or anti-psychotic medications. These interventions can consist of giving the patient food, drinks, one on one care, back rub, changing the patient's position in bed, adjusting the temperature, and redirecting the patient's mental focus. Many times these interventions work, but many times the medication may still need to be administered.

The patient's history and diagnosis are helpful in deciding whether or not the patient is developing a substance abuse problem. A patient having social or relationship problems may need to meet with a crisis counselor.

During every shift that a nurse is on duty, they must do an assessment of the patient. If they suspect the patient is becoming addicted, they must notify the physician.

Pain Ladder

"Pain ladder", or analgesic ladder, was created by the World Health Organization (WHO) as a guideline for the use of drugs in the management of pain. Originally published in 1986 for the management of cancer pain, it is now widely used by medical professionals for the management of all types of pain.

The general principle is to start with first step drugs, and then to climb the ladder if pain is still present. The medications range from common, over-the-counter drugs at the lowest rung, to strong opioids.

The Ladder

The WHO guidelines recommend prompt oral administration of drugs ("by the mouth") when pain occurs, starting, if the patient is not in severe pain, with non-opioid drugs such as paracetamol (acetaminophen) or aspirin, with or without "adjuvants" such as non-steroidal anti-inflammatory drugs (NSAIDs) including COX-2 inhibitors. Then, if complete pain relief is not achieved or disease progression necessitates more aggressive treatment, a weak opioid such as codeine, dihydrocodeine or tramadol is added to the existing non-opioid regime. If this is or becomes insufficient, a weak opioid is replaced by a strong opioid, such as morphine, diamorphine, fentanyl, buprenorphine, oxymorphone, oxycodone, or hydromorphone, while continuing the non-opioid therapy, escalating opioid dose until the patient is pain free or at the maximum possible relief without intolerable side effects. If the initial presentation is severe pain, this stepping process should be skipped and a strong opioid should be started immediately in combination with a non-opioid analgesic.

The guideline directs that medications should be given at regular intervals ("by the clock") so that continuous pain relief occurs, and ("by the individual") dosing by actual relief of pain rather than fixed dosing guidelines. It recognizes that breakthrough pain may occur and directs immediate rescue doses be provided.

The usefulness of the second step (weak opioid) is being debated in the clinical and research communities. Some authors challenge the pharmacological validity of the step and, pointing to their higher toxicity and low efficacy, argue that a weak opioid, with the possible exception of tramadol due to its unique action, could be replaced by smaller doses of a strong opioid.

Not all pain yields completely to classic analgesics, and drugs that are not traditionally considered analgesics, but which reduce pain in some cases, such as steroids or bisphosphonates, may be employed concurrently with analgesics at any stage. Tricyclic antidepressants, class I antiarrhythmics, or anticonvulsants are the drugs of choice for neuropathic pain. Up to 90 percent of cancer patients, immediately preceding death, use such adjuvants. Many adjuvants carry a significant risk of serious complications.

References

- Schmidt, Justin (22 March 2014). "Evolutionary responses of solitary and social Hymenoptera to predation by primates and overwhelmingly powerful vertebrate predators". Journal of Human Evolution. 71: 12-19
- Schmidt, Justin (2016). The Sting of the Wild. Baltimore, Maryland: Johns Hopkins University Press. ISBN 978-1-4214-1929-9
- Guesgen, M.; Leach, M. (2014). "Assessing pain using the lamb grimace scale (LGS)" (PDF). RSPCA. Retrieved January 11, 2015
- Jankowski, K.S. (2014). Morning types are less sensitive to pain than evening types all day long. European Journal of Pain, 17, 1068–1073
- Carter, Matt; Shieh, Jennifer C. (2010). "Nociception". Guide to Research Techniques in Neuroscience. Burlington, MA: Academic Press. pp. 51–2. ISBN 978-0-12-374849-2
- Miller, A.L.; Leach, M.C. (2015). "The mouse grimace scale: a clinically useful tool?". PLOS ONE. 10 (9): e0136000. doi:10.1371/journal.pone.0136000. PMC 4583436. PMID 26406227
- Mogil, Jeffrey; Wilson, Sonya; Wan, You (2001). "Methods in Pain Research". Frontiers in Neuroscience. 20012652. doi:10.1201/9781420042566-c2. ISBN 978-0-8493-0035-6

- Franks, John R.; Stephenson, Mark R.; Merry, Carol J., eds. (June 1996). Preventing Occupational Hearing Loss - A Practical Guide (PDF). National Institute for Occupational Safety and Health. p. 88. Retrieved 2009-07-15
- Bannon, Anthony W.; Malmberg, Annika B. (2007). "Current Protocols in Neuroscience". doi:10.1002/0471142301.ns0809s41. ISBN 978-0-471-14230-0
- Holden, E., Calvo, G., Collins, M., Bell, A., Reid, J., Scott, E.M. and Nolan, A.M. (2014). "Evaluation of facial expression in acute pain in cats". Journal of Small Animal Practice. 55 (12): 615–621. doi:10.1111/jsap.12283
- Jessell, Thomas M.; Kandel, Eric R.; Schwartz, James H. (1991). Principles of neural science. Norwalk, CT: Appleton & Lange. pp. 472–79. ISBN 0-8385-8034-3
- Pastor J.; Soria B.; Belmonte C. (1996). "Properties of the nociceptive neurons of the leech segmental ganglion". Journal of Neurophysiology. 75: 2268–2279
- D'Eon J. L.; Harris C. A.; Ellis J. A. (2004). "Testing Factorial Validity And Gender Invariance Of The Pain Catastrophizing Scale". Journal of Behavioral Medicine. 27 (4): 361–372. doi:10.1023/b:jobm.0000042410.34535.64

4

Analgesic: An Integrated Study

Analgesics or painkillers, are drugs given to patients to reduce their pain. These medicines are prescribed to the patient on the bases of the type of pain. Analgesics mainly include morphine, opioid drugs and nonsteroidal anti-inflammatory drugs. This chapter will provide an integrated understanding of analgesic.

Analgesic

An analgesic or painkiller is any member of the group of drugs used to achieve analgesia, relief from pain.

Analgesic drugs act in various ways on the peripheral and central nervous systems. They are distinct from anesthetics, which temporarily affect, and in some instances completely eliminate, sensation. Analgesics include paracetamol (known in North America as acetaminophen or simply APAP), the nonsteroidal anti-inflammatory drugs (NSAIDs) such as the salicylates, and opioid drugs such as morphine and oxycodone.

When choosing analgesics, the severity and response to other medication determines the choice of agent; the World Health Organization (WHO) pain ladder specifies mild analgesics as its first step.

Analgesic choice is also determined by the type of pain: For neuropathic pain, traditional analgesics are less effective, and there is often benefit from classes of drugs that are not normally considered analgesics, such as tricyclic antidepressants and anticonvulsants.

Uses

Topical nonsteroidal anti-inflammatory drugs provided pain relief in common conditions such as muscle sprains and overuse injuries. Since the side effects are also lesser, topical preparations could be preferred over oral medications in these conditions.

Contradictions

Each different type of analgesic has its own associated side effects.

Classification

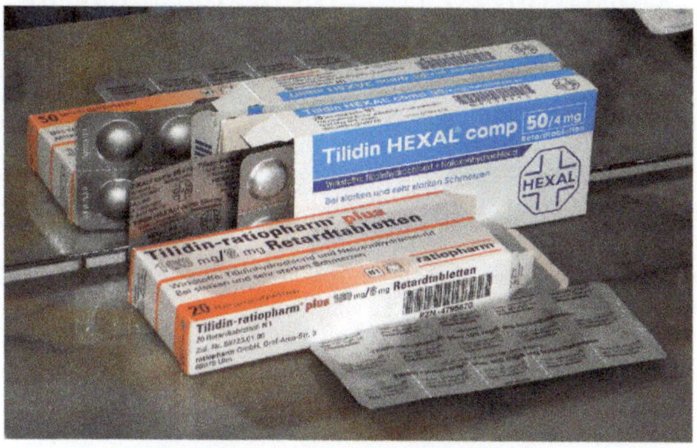

Tilidine, a type of painkiller

Drugs for pain are typically classified by chemical structure.

They may also be classified in other ways. Sometimes they are classified by use for various classes of medical condition. Other times they are sorted by the needs of special populations who would use them. They might be listed by availability in a geographical area, perhaps to prevent recommending a drug which is illegal in one place even if it is easily available elsewhere.

Paracetamol/acetaminophen

Paracetamol, also known as acetaminophen or APAP, is a medication used to treat pain and fever. It is typically used for mild to moderate pain. In combination with opioid pain medication, paracetamol is used for more severe pain such as cancer pain and after surgery. It is typically used either by mouth or rectally but is also available intravenously. Effects last between two and four hours. Paracetamol is classified as a mild analgesic. Paracetamol is generally safe at recommended doses.

NSAIDs

Nonsteroidal anti-inflammatory drugs (usually abbreviated to NSAIDs), are a drug class that groups together drugs that provide analgesic (pain-killing) and antipyretic (fever-reducing) effects, and, in higher efficacies, anti-inflammatory effects. The most prominent members of this group of drugs, aspirin, ibuprofen and naproxen, are all available over the counter in most countries.

COX-2 Inhibitors

These drugs have been derived from NSAIDs. The cyclooxygenase enzyme inhibited by NSAIDs was discovered to have at least 2 different versions: COX1 and COX2. Research suggested most of the adverse effects of NSAIDs to be mediated by blocking the COX1 (constitutive) enzyme, with the analgesic effects being mediated by the COX2 (inducible) enzyme. Thus, the COX2 inhibitors were developed to inhibit only the COX2 enzyme (traditional NSAIDs block both versions in general). These drugs (such as rofecoxib, celecoxib, and etoricoxib) are equally effective analgesics when compared with NSAIDs, but cause less gastrointestinal hemorrhage in particular.

After widespread adoption of the COX-2 inhibitors, it was discovered that most of the drugs in this class increase the risk of cardiovascular events by 40% on average. This led to the withdrawal of rofecoxib and valdecoxib, and warnings on others. Etoricoxib seems relatively safe, with the risk of thrombotic events similar to that of non-coxib NSAID diclofenac.

Opioids

Morphine, the archetypal opioid, and other opioids (e.g., codeine, oxycodone, hydrocodone, dihydromorphine, pethidine) all exert a similar influence on the cerebral opioid receptor system. Buprenorphine is a partial agonist of the μ-opioid receptor, and tramadol is a serotonin norepinephrine reuptake inhibitor (SNRI) with weak μ-opioid receptor agonist properties. Tramadol is structurally closer to venlafaxine than to codeine and delivers analgesia by not only delivering "opioid-like" effects (through mild agonism of the mu receptor) but also by acting as a weak but fast-acting serotonin releasing agent and norepinephrine reuptake inhibitor. Tapentadol, with some structural similarities to tramadol, presents what is believed to be a novel drug working through two (and possibly three) different modes of action in the fashion of both a traditional opioid and as a SNRI. The effects of serotonin and norepinephrine on pain, while not completely understood, have had causal links established and drugs in the SNRI class are commonly used in conjunction with opioids (especially tapentadol and tramadol) with greater success in pain relief. Dosing of all opioids may be limited by opioid toxicity (confusion, respiratory depression, myoclonic jerks and pinpoint pupils), seizures (tramadol), but opioid-tolerant individuals usually have higher dose ceilings than patients without tolerance.

Opioids, while very effective analgesics, may have some unpleasant side-effects. Patients starting morphine may experience nausea and vomiting (generally relieved by a short course of antiemetics such as phenergan). Pruritus (itching) may require switching to a different opioid. Constipation occurs in almost all patients on opioids, and laxatives (lactulose, macrogol-containing or co-danthramer) are typically co-prescribed.

When used appropriately, opioids and other central analgesics are otherwise safe and effective, however risks such as addiction and the body's becoming used to the drug (tolerance) can occur. The effect of tolerance means that frequent use of the drug may result in its diminished effect so, when safe to do so, the dosage may need to be increased to maintain effectiveness. This may be of particular concern regarding patients suffering with chronic pain. Opioid tolerance is often addressed with "opioid rotation therapy" in which a patient is routinely switched between two or more non-cross-tolerant opioid medications in order to prevent exceeding safe dosages in the attempt to achieve an adequate analgesic effect.

Alcohol

Describing the effects of using alcohol to treat pain is difficult. Alcohol has biological, mental, and social effects which influence the consequences of using alcohol for pain. Moderate use of alcohol can lessen certain types of pain in certain circumstances. Attempting to use alcohol to treat pain has also been observed to lead to negative outcomes including excessive drinking and alcohol use disorder.

Medical Cannabis

Medical cannabis or medical marijuana, can refer to the use of cannabis and its cannabinoids to treat disease or improve symptoms. There is evidence suggesting that cannabis can be used to treat chronic pain and muscle spasms; with some trials indicating improved relief of neuropathic pain over opioids.

Combinations

Analgesics are frequently used in combination, such as the paracetamol and codeine preparations found in many non-prescription pain relievers. They can also be found in combination with vasoconstrictor drugs such as pseudoephedrine for sinus-related preparations, or with antihistamine drugs for allergy sufferers.

While the use of paracetamol, aspirin, ibuprofen, naproxen, and other NSAIDS concurrently with weak to mid-range opiates (up to about the hydrocodone level) has been said to show beneficial synergistic effects by combatting pain at multiple sites of action, several combination analgesic products have been shown to have few efficacy benefits when compared to similar doses of their individual components. Moreover, these combination analgesics can often result in significant adverse events, including accidental overdoses, most often due to confusion that arises from the multiple (and often non-acting) components of these combinations.

Alternative Medicine

Many people use alternative medicine treatments including drugs for pain relief. There is some evidence that some treatments using alternative medicine can relieve some types of pain more effectively than placebo. The available research concludes that more research would be necessary to better understand the use of alternative medicine.

Psychotropic Agents

Other psychotropic analgesic agents include ketamine (an NMDA receptor antagonist), clonidine and other α_2-adrenoreceptor agonists, and mexiletine and other local anaesthetic analogues.

Other Drugs

Drugs that have been introduced for uses other than analgesics are also used in pain management. Both first-generation (such as amitriptyline) and newer anti-depressants (such as duloxetine) are used alongside NSAIDs and opioids for pain involving nerve damage and similar problems. Other agents directly potentiate the effects of analgesics, such as using hydroxyzine, promethazine, carisoprodol, or tripelennamine to increase the pain-killing ability of a given dose of opioid analgesic.

Adjuvant analgesics, also called atypical analgesics, include nefopam, orphenadrine, pregabalin, gabapentin, cyclobenzaprine, scopolamine, and other drugs possessing anticonvulsant, anticholinergic, and/or antispasmodic properties, as well as many other drugs with CNS actions. These drugs are used along with analgesics to modulate and/or modify the action of opioids when used against pain, especially of neuropathic origin.

Dextromethorphan has been noted to slow the development of tolerance to opioids and exert additional analgesia by acting upon the NMDA receptors; some analgesics such as methadone and ketobemidone and perhaps piritramide have intrinsic NMDA action.

High-alcohol liquor, two forms of which were found in the US Pharmacopoeia up until 1916 and in common use by physicians well into the 1930s, has been used in the past as an agent for dulling pain, due to the CNS depressant effects of ethyl alcohol, a notable example being the American Civil War. However, the ability of alcohol to relieve severe pain is likely inferior to many analgesics used today (e.g., morphine, codeine). As such, in general, the idea of alcohol for analgesia is considered a primitive practice in virtually all industrialized countries today.

The use of adjuvant analgesics is an important and growing part of the pain-control field and new discoveries are made practically every year. Many of these drugs combat the side-effects of opioid analgesics, an added bonus. For example, antihistamines including orphenadrine combat the release of histamine caused by many opioids. Stimulants such as methylphenidate, caffeine, ephedrine, dextroamphetamine, methamphetamine, and cocaine work against heavy sedation and may elevate mood in distressed patients as do the antidepressants. The use of medicinal cannabis remains a debated issue.

In patients with chronic or neuropathic pain, various other substances may have analgesic properties. Tricyclic antidepressants, especially clomipramine and amitriptyline, have been shown to improve pain in what appears to be a central manner. Nefopam is used in Europe for pain relief with concurrent opioids. The exact mechanism of carbamazepine, gabapentin, and pregabalin is similarly unclear, but these anticonvulsants are used to treat neuropathic pain with differing degrees of success. Anticonvulsants are most commonly used for neuropathic pain as their mechanism of action tends to inhibit pain sensation.

Flupirtine is a centrally acting K+ channel opener with weak NMDA antagonist properties. It is used in Europe for moderate to strong pain and migraine and its muscle-relaxant properties. It has no anticholinergic properties and is believed to be devoid of any activity on dopamine, serotonin, or histamine receptors. It is not addictive, and tolerance usually does not develop. However, tolerance may develop in single cases.

Other Classification Systems

Topical analgesia is generally recommended to avoid systemic side-effects. Painful joints, for example, may be treated with an ibuprofen- or diclofenac-containing gel (The labeling for topical diclofenac has been updated to warn about drug-induced hepatotoxicity.); capsaicin also is used topically. Lidocaine, an anesthetic, and steroids may be injected into painful joints for longer-term pain relief. Lidocaine is also used for painful mouth sores and to numb areas for dental work and minor medical procedures. In February 2007 the FDA notified consumers and healthcare professionals of the potential hazards of topical anesthetics entering the blood stream when applied in large doses to the skin without medical supervision. These topical anesthetics contain anesthetic drugs such as lidocaine, tetracaine, benzocaine, and prilocaine in a cream, ointment, or gel.

Etymology

The word *analgesic* derives from Greek *an-* (without), *álgos* (pain), and *-ikos*. Such drugs were usually known as anodynes before the 20th century.

Research

Some novel and investigational analgesics include subtype-selective voltage-gated sodium channel blockers such as funapide and raxatrigine, as well as multimodal agents such as ralfinamide.

Nonsteroidal Anti-inflammatory Drug

Nonsteroidal anti-inflammatory drugs (NSAIDs) are a drug class that groups together drugs that provide analgesic (pain-killing) and antipyretic (fever-reducing) effects, and, in higher doses, anti-inflammatory effects.

The term *nonsteroidal* distinguishes these drugs from steroids, which, among a broad range of other effects, have a similar eicosanoid-depressing, anti-inflammatory action. First used in 1960, the term served to distance new drugs from steroid-related iatrogenic tragedies.

The most prominent members of this group of drugs are aspirin, ibuprofen and naproxen, all available over the counter in most countries. Paracetamol (acetaminophen) is generally not considered an NSAID because it has only little anti-inflammatory activity. It treats pain mainly by blocking COX-2 mostly in the central nervous system, but not much in the rest of the body.

Most NSAIDs inhibit the activity of cyclooxygenase-1 (COX-1) and cyclooxygenase-2 (COX-2), and thereby the synthesis of prostaglandins and thromboxanes. It is thought that inhibiting COX-2 leads to the anti-inflammatory, analgesic and antipyretic effects and that those NSAIDs also inhibiting COX-1, particularly aspirin, may cause gastrointestinal bleeding and ulcers.

Medical Uses

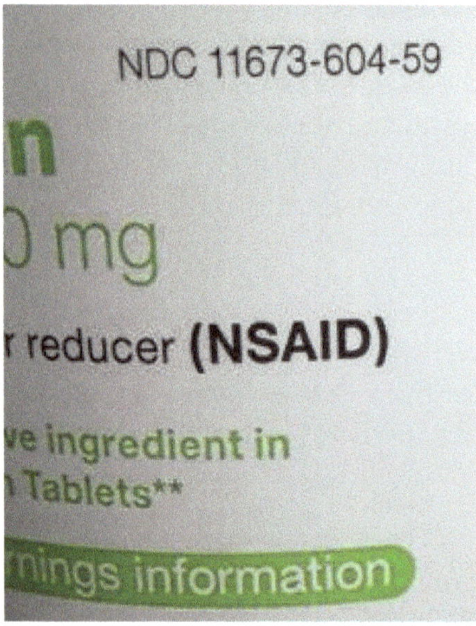

NSAID identification on label of generic ibuprofen, an OTC NSAID

NSAIDs are usually used for the treatment of acute or chronic conditions where pain and inflammation are present.

NSAIDs are generally used for the symptomatic relief of the following conditions:

- Osteoarthritis
- Rheumatoid arthritis
- Mild-to-moderate pain due to inflammation and tissue injury
- Low back pain
- Inflammatory arthropathies (e.g., ankylosing spondylitis, psoriatic arthritis, reactive arthritis)

- Tennis elbow
- Headache
- Migraine
- Acute gout
- Dysmenorrhoea (menstrual pain)
- Metastatic bone pain
- Postoperative pain
- Muscle stiffness and pain due to Parkinson's disease
- Pyrexia (fever)
- Ileus
- Renal colic
- They are also given to neonate infants whose ductus arteriosus is not closed within 24 hours of birth
- Macular edema

Aspirin, the only NSAID able to irreversibly inhibit COX-1, is also indicated for inhibition of platelet aggregation. This is useful for the management of arterial thrombosis and prevention of adverse cardiovascular events. Aspirin inhibits platelet aggregation by inhibiting the action of thromboxane A_2.

NSAIDs are useful in the management of post-operative dental pain following invasive dental procedures such as dental extraction. When not contra-indicated they are favoured over the use of paracetamol alone due to the anti-inflammatory effect they provide. When used in combination with paracetamol the analgesic effect has been proven to be improved. A 2012 Cochrane review found that there is some weak evidence suggesting that taking pre-operative analgesia can reduce the length of post operative pain associated with placing orthodontic spacers under local anaesthetic.

Contraindications

NSAIDs may be used with caution by people with the following conditions:

- Irritable bowel syndrome
- Persons who are over age 50, and who have a family history of GI (gastrointestinal) problems

- Persons who have had past GI problems from NSAID use

NSAIDs should usually be avoided by people with the following conditions:

- Peptic ulcer or stomach bleeding
- Uncontrolled hypertension
- Kidney disease
- People that suffer with inflammatory bowel disease (Crohn's disease or ulcerative colitis)
- Past transient ischemic attack (excluding ibuprofen)
- Past stroke (excluding ibuprofen)
- Past myocardial infarction (excluding ibuprofen)
- Coronary artery disease (excluding ibuprofen)
- Undergoing coronary artery bypass surgery
- Taking ibuprofen for heart
- Congestive heart failure (excluding low-dose ibuprofen)
- In third trimester of pregnancy
- Persons who have undergone gastric bypass surgery
- Persons who have a history of allergic or allergic-type NSAID hypersensitivity reactions, e.g. aspirin-induced asthma

Adverse Effects

The widespread use of NSAIDs has meant that the adverse effects of these drugs have become increasingly common. Use of NSAIDs increases risk of having a range of gastrointestinal (GI) problems. When NSAIDs are used for pain management after surgery they cause increased risk of kidney problems.

An estimated 10–20% of NSAID patients experience dyspepsia. In the 1990s high doses of prescription NSAIDs were associated with serious upper gastrointestinal adverse events, including bleeding. Over the past decade, deaths associated with gastric bleeding have declined.

NSAIDs, like all drugs, may interact with other medications. For example, concurrent use of NSAIDs and quinolones may increase the risk of quinolones' adverse central nervous system effects, including seizure.

There is an argument over the benefits and risks of NSAIDs for treating chronic musculoskeletal pain. Each drug has a benefit-risk profile and balancing the risk of no treatment with the competing potential risks of various therapies is the clinician's responsibility.

Combinational Risk

If a COX-2 inhibitor is taken, a traditional NSAID (prescription or over-the-counter) should not be taken at the same time. In addition, people on daily aspirin therapy (e.g., for reducing cardiovascular risk) must be careful if they also use other NSAIDs, as these may inhibit the cardioprotective effects of aspirin.

Rofecoxib (Vioxx) was shown to produce significantly fewer gastrointestinal adverse drug reactions (ADRs) compared with naproxen. This study, the VIGOR trial, raised the issue of the cardiovascular safety of the coxibs. A statistically significant increase in the incidence of myocardial infarctions was observed in patients on rofecoxib. Further data, from the APPROVe trial, showed a statistically significant relative risk of cardiovascular events of 1.97 versus placebo—which caused a worldwide withdrawal of rofecoxib in October 2004.

Use of methotrexate together with NSAIDS in rheumatoid arthritis is safe, if adequate monitoring is done.

Cardiovascular

NSAIDs aside from aspirin, both selective COX-2 inhibitors and traditional anti-inflammatories, increase the risk of myocardial infarction and stroke. This occurs at least within a week of use. They are not recommended in those who have had a previous heart attack as they increase the risk of death or recurrent MI. Evidence indicates that naproxen may be the least harmful out of these.

NSAIDs aside from (low-dose) aspirin are associated with a doubled risk of heart failure in people without a history of cardiac disease. In people with such a history, use of NSAIDs (aside from low-dose aspirin) was associated with a more than 10-fold increase in heart failure. If this link is proven causal, researchers estimate that NSAIDs would be responsible for up to 20 percent of hospital admissions for congestive heart failure. In people with heart failure, NSAIDs increase mortality risk (hazard ratio) by approximately 1.2–1.3 for naproxen and ibuprofen, 1.7 for rofecoxib and celecoxib, and 2.1 for diclofenac.

On 9 July 2015, the FDA toughened warnings of increased heart attack and stroke risk associated with nonsteroidal anti-inflammatory drugs (NSAID). Aspirin is an NSAID but is not affected by the new warnings.

Possible Erectile Dysfunction Risk

A 2005 Finnish study linked long term (over 3 months) use of NSAIDs with an increased risk of erectile dysfunction. This study was correlational only, and depended solely on self-reports (questionnaires).

A 2011 publication in *The Journal of Urology* received widespread publicity. According to this study, men who used NSAIDs regularly were at significantly increased risk of erectile dysfunction. A link between NSAID use and erectile dysfunction still existed after controlling for several conditions. However, the study was observational and not controlled, with low original participation rate, potential participation bias, and other uncontrolled factors. The authors warned against drawing any conclusion regarding cause.

Gastrointestinal

The main adverse drug reactions (ADRs) associated with NSAID use relate to direct and indirect irritation of the gastrointestinal (GI) tract. NSAIDs cause a dual assault on the GI tract: the acidic molecules directly irritate the gastric mucosa, and inhibition of COX-1 and COX-2 reduces the levels of protective prostaglandins. Inhibition of prostaglandin synthesis in the GI tract causes increased gastric acid secretion, diminished bicarbonate secretion, diminished mucus secretion and diminished trophic effects on the epithelial mucosa.

Common gastrointestinal ADRs include:

- Nausea/vomiting
- Dyspepsia
- Gastric ulceration/bleeding
- Diarrhea

Clinical NSAID ulcers are related to the systemic effects of NSAID administration. Such damage occurs irrespective of the route of administration of the NSAID (e.g., oral, rectal, or parenteral) and can occur even in patients with achlorhydria.

Ulceration risk increases with therapy duration, and with higher doses. To minimize GI ADRs, it is prudent to use the lowest effective dose for the shortest period of time—a practice that studies show is often not followed. Recent studies show that over 50% of patients who take NSAIDs have sustained some mucosal damage to their small intestine.

There are also some differences in the propensity of individual agents to cause gastrointestinal ADRs. Indomethacin, ketoprofen and piroxicam appear to have the highest prevalence of gastric ADRs, while ibuprofen (lower doses) and diclofenac appear to have lower rates.

Certain NSAIDs, such as aspirin, have been marketed in enteric-coated formulations that manufacturers claim reduce the incidence of gastrointestinal ADRs. Similarly, some believe that rectal formulations may reduce gastrointestinal ADRs. However, consistent with the systemic mechanism of such ADRs, and in clinical practice, these formulations have not demonstrated a reduced risk of GI ulceration.

Commonly, gastric (but not necessarily intestinal) adverse effects can be reduced through suppressing acid production, by concomitant use of a proton pump inhibitor, e.g., omeprazole, esomeprazole, or the prostaglandin analog misoprostol. Misoprostol is itself associated with a high incidence of gastrointestinal ADRs (diarrhea). While these techniques may be effective, they are expensive for maintenance therapy.

Inflammatory Bowel Disease

NSAIDs should be used with caution in individuals with inflammatory bowel disease (e.g., Crohn's disease or ulcerative colitis) due to their tendency to cause gastric bleeding and form ulceration in the gastric lining. Pain relievers such as paracetamol (also known as acetaminophen) or drugs containing codeine (which slows down bowel activity) are safer medications for pain relief in IBD.

Renal

NSAIDs are also associated with a fairly high incidence of renal adverse drug reactions (ADRs). The mechanism of these renal ADRs is due to changes in renal hemodynamics (kidney blood flow), ordinarily mediated by prostaglandins, which are affected by NSAIDs. Prostaglandins normally cause vasodilation of the afferent arterioles of the glomeruli. This helps maintain normal glomerular perfusion and glomerular filtration rate (GFR), an indicator of renal function. This is particularly important in renal failure where the kidney is trying to maintain renal perfusion pressure by elevated angiotensin II levels. At these elevated levels, angiotensin II also constricts the afferent arteriole into the glomerulus in addition to the efferent arteriole it normally constricts. Prostaglandins serve to dilate the afferent arteriole; by blocking this prostaglandin-mediated effect, particularly in renal failure, NSAIDs cause unopposed constriction of the afferent arteriole and decreased RPF (renal perfusion flow).

Common ADRs associated with altered renal function include:

- Salt (Sodium) and fluid retention
- Hypertension (high blood pressure)

These agents may also cause kidney impairment, especially in combination with other nephrotoxic agents. Kidney failure is especially a risk if the patient is also concomitantly taking an ACE inhibitor (which removes angiotensin II's vasoconstriction of the efferent arteriole) and a diuretic (which drops plasma volume, and thereby RPF)—the so-called "triple whammy" effect.

In rarer instances NSAIDs may also cause more severe kidney conditions:

- Interstitial nephritis
- Nephrotic syndrome
- Acute kidney failure
- Acute tubular necrosis
- Renal papillary necrosis

NSAIDs in combination with excessive use of phenacetin or paracetamol (acetaminophen) may lead to analgesic nephropathy.

Photosensitivity

Photosensitivity is a commonly overlooked adverse effect of many of the NSAIDs. The 2-arylpropionic acids are the most likely to produce photosensitivity reactions, but other NSAIDs have also been implicated including piroxicam, diclofenac and benzydamine.

Benoxaprofen, since withdrawn due to its hepatotoxicity, was the most photoactive NSAID observed. The mechanism of photosensitivity, responsible for the high photoactivity of the 2-arylpropionic acids, is the ready decarboxylation of the carboxylic acid moiety. The specific absorbance characteristics of the different chromophoric 2-aryl substituents, affects the decarboxylation mechanism. While ibuprofen has weak absorption, it has been reported as a weak photosensitising agent.

During Pregnancy

NSAIDs are not recommended during pregnancy, particularly during the third trimester. While NSAIDs as a class are not direct teratogens, they may cause premature closure of the fetal ductus arteriosus and renal ADRs in the fetus. Additionally, they are linked with premature birth and miscarriage. Aspirin, however, is used together with heparin in pregnant women with antiphospholipid antibodies. Additionally, Indomethacin is used in pregnancy to treat polyhydramnios by reducing fetal urine production via inhibiting fetal renal blood flow.

In contrast, paracetamol (acetaminophen) is regarded as being safe and well-tolerated during pregnancy, but Leffers et al. released a study in 2010 indicating that there may be associated male infertility in the unborn. Doses should be taken as prescribed, due to risk of hepatotoxicity with overdoses.

In France, the country's health agency contraindicates the use of NSAIDs, including aspirin, after the sixth month of pregnancy.

Allergy/allergy-like Hypersensitivity Reactions

A variety of allergic or allergic-like NSAID hypersensitivity reactions follow the ingestion of NSAIDs. These hypersensitivity reactions differ from the other adverse reactions listed here which are toxicity reactions, i.e. unwanted reactions that result from the pharmacological action of a drug, are dose-related, and can occur in any treated individual; hypersensitivity reactions are idiosyncratic reactions to a drug. Some NSAID hypersensitivity reactions are truly allergic in origin: 1) repetitive IgE-mediated urticarial skin eruptions, angioedema, and anaphylaxis following immediately to hours after ingesting one structural type of NSAID but not after ingesting structurally unrelated NSAIDs; and 2) Comparatively mild to moderately severe T cell-mediated delayed onset (usually more than 24 hour), skin reactions such as maculopapular rash, fixed drug eruptions, photosensitivity reactions, delayed urticaria, and contact dermatitis; or 3) far more severe and potentially life-threatening t-cell-mediated delayed systemic reactions such as the DRESS syndrome, acute generalized exanthematous pustulosis, the Stevens–Johnson syndrome, and toxic epidermal necrolysis. Other NSAID hypersensitivity reactions are allergy-like symptoms but do not involve true allergic mechanisms; rather, they appear due to the ability of NSAIDs to alter the metabolism of arachidonic acid in favor of forming metabolites that promote allergic symptoms. Afflicted individuals may be abnormally sensitive to these provocative metabolites or overproduce them and typically are susceptible to a wide range of structurally dissimilar NSAIDs, particularly those that inhibit COX1. Symptoms, which develop immediately to hours after ingesting any of various NSAIDs that inhibit COX-1, are: 1) exacerbations of asthmatic and rhinitis symptoms in individuals with a history of asthma or rhinitis and 2) exacerbation or first-time development of wheals or angioedema in individuals with or without a history of chronic urticarial lesions or angioedema.

Common adverse drug reactions (ADR), other than listed above, include: raised liver enzymes, headache, dizziness. Uncommon ADRs include: hyperkalaemia, confusion, bronchospasm, rash. Rapid and severe swelling of the face or body. Ibuprofen may also rarely cause irritable bowel syndrome symptoms. NSAIDs are also implicated in some cases of Stevens–Johnson syndrome.

Most NSAIDs penetrate poorly into the central nervous system (CNS). However, the COX enzymes are expressed constitutively in some areas of the CNS, meaning that even limited penetration may cause adverse effects such as somnolence and dizziness.

In very rare cases, ibuprofen can cause aseptic meningitis.

As with other drugs, allergies to NSAIDs might exist. While many allergies are specific to one NSAID, up to 1 in 5 people may have unpredictable cross-reactive allergic responses to other NSAIDs as well.

Drug Interactions

NSAIDs reduce renal blood flow and thereby decrease the efficacy of diuretics, and inhibit the elimination of lithium and methotrexate.

NSAIDs cause hypocoagulability, which may be serious when combined with other drugs that also decrease blood clotting, such as warfarin.

NSAIDs may aggravate hypertension (high blood pressure) and thereby antagonize the effect of antihypertensives, such as ACE Inhibitors.

NSAIDs may interfere and reduce efficiency of SSRI antidepressants.

Various widely used nonsteroidal anti-inflammatory drugs (NSAIDs) enhance endocannabinoid signaling by blocking the anandamide-degrading membrane enzyme fatty acid amide hydrolase (FAAH).

Mechanism of Action

Most NSAIDs act as nonselective inhibitors of the enzyme cyclooxygenase (COX), inhibiting both the cyclooxygenase-1 (COX-1) and cyclooxygenase-2 (COX-2) isoenzymes. This inhibition is competitively reversible (albeit at varying degrees of reversibility), as opposed to the mechanism of aspirin, which is irreversible inhibition. COX catalyzes the formation of prostaglandins and thromboxane from arachidonic acid (itself derived from the cellular phospholipid bilayer by phospholipase A_2). Prostaglandins act (among other things) as messenger molecules in the process of inflammation. This mechanism of action was elucidated by John Vane (1927–2004), who received a Nobel Prize for his work.

COX-1 is a constitutively expressed enzyme with a "house-keeping" role in regulating many normal physiological processes. One of these is in the stomach lining, where prostaglandins serve a protective role, preventing the stomach mucosa from being eroded by its own acid. COX-2 is an enzyme facultatively expressed in inflammation, and it is inhibition of COX-2 that produces the desirable effects of NSAIDs.

When nonselective COX-1/COX-2 inhibitors (such as aspirin, ibuprofen, and naproxen) lower stomach prostaglandin levels, ulcers of the stomach or duodenum internal bleeding can result.

NSAIDs have been studied in various assays to understand how they affect each of these enzymes. While the assays reveal differences, unfortunately, different assays provide differing ratios.

The discovery of COX-2 led to research to the development of selective COX-2 inhibiting drugs that do not cause gastric problems characteristic of older NSAIDs.

Paracetamol (acetaminophen) is not considered an NSAID because it has little anti-inflammatory activity. It treats pain mainly by blocking COX-2 mostly in the central nervous system, but not much in the rest of the body.

However, many aspects of the mechanism of action of NSAIDs remain unexplained, and for this reason, further COX pathways are hypothesized. The COX-3 pathway was believed to fill some of this gap but recent findings make it appear unlikely that it plays any significant role in humans and alternative explanation models are proposed.

NSAIDs interact with the endocannabinoid system and its endocannabinoids, as COX2 have been shown to utilize endocannabinoids as substrates, and may have a key role in both the therapeutic and adverse effects of NSAIDs, as well as in NSAIDs-induced placebo responses.

NSAIDs are also used in the acute pain caused by gout because they inhibit urate crystal phagocytosis besides inhibition of prostaglandin synthase.

Antipyretic Activity

NSAIDS have antipyretic activity and can be used to treat fever. Fever is caused by elevated levels of prostaglandin E2, which alters the firing rate of neurons within the hypothalamus that control thermoregulation. Antipyretics work by inhibiting the enzyme COX, which causes the general inhibition of prostanoid biosynthesis (PGE2) within the hypothalamus. PGE2 signals to the hypothalamus to increase the body's thermal set point. Ibuprofen has been shown more effective as an antipyretic than paracetamol (acetaminophen). Arachidonic acid is the precursor substrate for cyclooxygenase leading to the production of prostaglandins F, D & E.

Classification

NSAIDs can be classified based on their chemical structure or mechanism of action. Older NSAIDs were known long before their mechanism of action was elucidated and were for this reason classified by chemical structure or origin. Newer substances are more often classified by mechanism of action.

Salicylates

- Aspirin (acetylsalicylic acid)
- Diflunisal (Dolobid)
- Salicylic acid and other salicylates
- Salsalate (Disalcid)

Propionic Acid Derivatives

- Ibuprofen
- Dexibuprofen
- Naproxen
- Fenoprofen
- Ketoprofen
- Dexketoprofen
- Flurbiprofen
- Oxaprozin
- Loxoprofen

Acetic Acid Derivatives

- Indomethacin
- Tolmetin
- Sulindac
- Etodolac
- Ketorolac
- Diclofenac
- Aceclofenac
- Nabumetone (drug itself is non-acidic but the active, principal metabolite has a carboxylic acid group)

Enolic Acid (Oxicam) Derivatives

- Piroxicam
- Meloxicam
- Tenoxicam
- Droxicam
- Lornoxicam
- Isoxicam (withdrawn from market 1985)
- Phenylbutazone (Bute)

Anthranilic Acid Derivatives (Fenamates)

The following NSAIDs are derived from fenamic acid. which is a derivative of anthranilic acid, which in turn is a nitrogen isostere of salicylic acid, which is the active metabolite of aspirin.

- Mefenamic acid
- Meclofenamic acid
- Flufenamic acid
- Tolfenamic acid

Selective COX-2 Inhibitors (Coxibs)

- Celecoxib (FDA alert)
- Rofecoxib (withdrawn from market)
- Valdecoxib (withdrawn from market)
- Parecoxib FDA withdrawn, licensed in the EU
- Lumiracoxib TGA cancelled registration
- Etoricoxib not FDA approved, licensed in the EU
- Firocoxib used in dogs and horses

Sulfonanilides

- Nimesulide (systemic preparations are banned by several countries for the potential risk of hepatotoxicity)

Others

- Clonixin
- Licofelone acts by inhibiting LOX (lipooxygenase) & COX and hence known as 5-LOX/COX inhibitor
- H-harpagide in Figwort or Devil's Claw

Chirality

Most NSAIDs are chiral molecules (diclofenac is a notable exception). However, the majority are prepared in a racemic mixture. Typically, only a single enantiomer is pharmacologically active. For some drugs (typically profens), an isomerase enzyme *in vivo* converts the inactive enantiomer into the active form, although its activity varies widely in individuals. This phenomenon is likely responsible for the poor correlation between NSAID efficacy and plasma concentration observed in older studies, when specific analysis of the active enantiomer was not performed.

Ibuprofen and ketoprofen are now available in single, active enantiomer preparations (dexibuprofen and dexketoprofen), which purport to offer quicker onset and an improved side-effect profile. Naproxen has always been marketed as the single active enantiomer.

Main Practical Differences

NSAIDs within a group tend to have similar characteristics and tolerability. There is little difference in clinical efficacy among the NSAIDs when used at equivalent doses. Rather, differences among compounds usually relate to dosing regimens (related to the compound's elimination half-life), route of administration, and tolerability profile.

Regarding adverse effects, selective COX-2 inhibitors have lower risk of gastrointestinal bleeding, and there is no significant increase in risk of myocardial infarction. With the exception of naproxen, nonselective NSAIDs increase the risk of having a heart attack. Some data also supports that the partially selective nabumetone is less likely to cause gastrointestinal events.

A consumer report noted that ibuprofen, naproxen, and salsalate are less expensive than other NSAIDs, and essentially as effective and safe when used appropriately to treat osteoarthritis and pain.

Pharmacokinetics

Most nonsteroidal anti-inflammatory drugs are weak acids, with a pKa of 3–5. They are absorbed well from the stomach and intestinal mucosa. They are highly protein-bound in plasma (typically >95%), usually to albumin, so that their volume of distribution typically approximates to plasma volume. Most NSAIDs are metabolized in the liver by oxidation and conjugation to inactive metabolites that typically are excreted in the urine, though some drugs are partially excreted in bile. Metabolism may be abnormal in certain disease states, and accumulation may occur even with normal dosage.

Ibuprofen and diclofenac have short half-lives (2–3 hours). Some NSAIDs (typically oxicams) have very long half-lives (e.g. 20–60 hours).

History

From the era of Greek medicine to the mid-19th century, the discovery of medicinal agents was classed as an empirical art; folklore and mythological guidance were combined in deploying the vegetable and mineral products that made up the expansive pharmacopeia of the time. Myrtle leaves were in use by 1500 BCE. Hippocrates (460–377 BCE) first reported using willow bark and in 30 BCE Celsus described the signs of inflammation and also used willow bark to mitigate them. On 25 April 1763, Edward Stone wrote to the Royal Society describing his observations on the use of willow bark-based medicines in febrile patients. The active ingredient of willow bark, a glycoside called salicin, was first isolated by Johann Andreas Buchner in 1827. By 1829, French chemist Henri Leroux had improved the extraction process to obtain about 30g of purified salicin from 1.5 kg of bark.

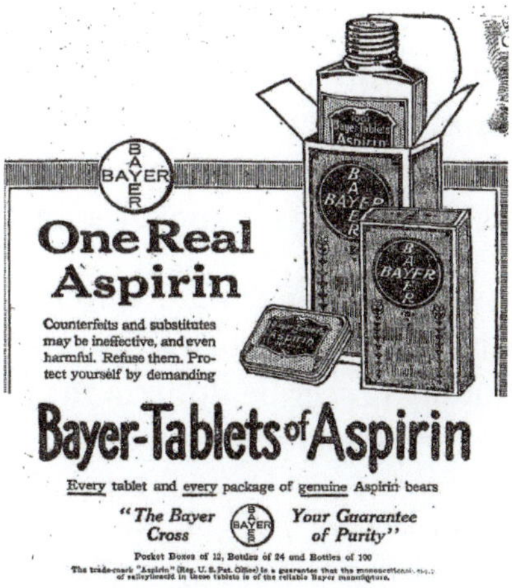

One of the first advertisements for Bayer Aspirin, published in *The New York Times* in 1917

By hydrolysis, salicin releases glucose and salicylic alcohol which can be converted into salicylic acid, both in vivo and through chemical methods. The acid is more effective than salicin and, in addition to its fever-reducing properties, is anti-inflammatory and analgesic. In 1869, Hermann Kolbe synthesised salicylate, although it was too acidic for the gastric mucosa. The reaction used to synthesise aromatic acid from a phenol in the presence of CO2 is known as the Kolbe-Schmitt reaction.

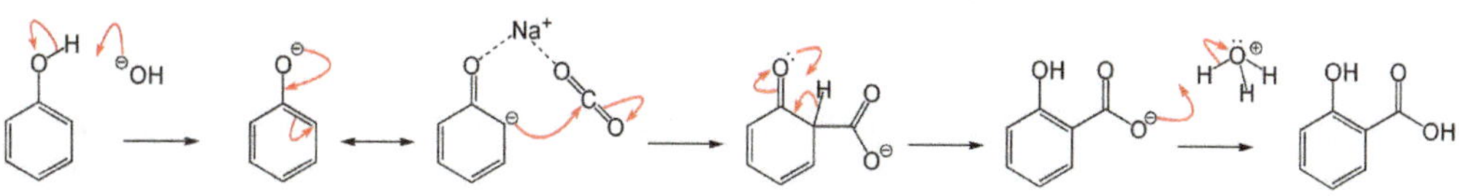

By 1897 the German chemist Felix Hoffmann and the Bayer company prompted a new age of pharmacology by converting salicylic acid into acetylsalicylic acid—named aspirin by Heinrich Dreser. Other NSAIDs were developed from the 1950s forward. In 2001, NSAIDs accounted for 70,000,000 prescriptions and 30 billion over-the-counter doses sold annually in the United States.

Research

While studies have been conducted to see if various NSAIDs can improve behavior in transgenic mouse models of Alzheimer's disease and observational studies in humans have shown promise, there is no good evidence from randomized clinical trials that NSAIDs can treat or prevent Alzheimer's in humans; clinical trials of NSAIDs for treatment of Alzheimer's have found more harm than benefit. Non-Steroidal Anti-Inflammatory Drugs (NSAIDs) coordinate with Metal ions affecting the cellular function .

Veterinary Use

Research supports the use of NSAIDs for the control of pain associated with veterinary procedures such as dehorning and castration of calves. The best effect is obtained by combining a short-term local anesthetic such as lidocaine with an NSAID acting as a longer term analgesic. However, as different species have varying reactions to different medications in the NSAID family, little of the existing research data can be extrapolated to animal species other than those specifically studied, and the relevant government agency in one area sometimes prohibits uses approved in other jurisdictions.

For example, ketoprofen's effects have been studied in horses more than in ruminants but, due to controversy over its use in racehorses, veterinarians who treat livestock in the United States more commonly prescribe flunixin meglumine, which, while labeled for use in such animals, is not indicated for post-operative pain.

In the United States, meloxicam is approved for use only in canines, whereas (due to concerns about liver damage) it carries warnings against its use in cats except for one-time use during surgery. In spite of these warnings, meloxicam is frequently prescribed "off-label" for non-canine animals including cats and livestock species. In other countries, for example The European Union (EU), there is a label claim for use in cats.

COX-2 Inhibitor

Selective COX-2 inhibitors are a type of non-steroidal anti-inflammatory drug (NSAID) that directly targets cyclooxygenase-2, COX-2, an enzyme responsible for inflammation and pain. Targeting selectivity for COX-2 reduces the risk of peptic ulceration, and is the main feature of celecoxib, rofecoxib and other members of this drug class. After several COX-2 inhibiting drugs were approved for marketing, data from clinical trials revealed that COX-2 inhibitors caused a significant increase in heart attacks and strokes, with some drugs in the class having worse risks than others. Rofecoxib (commonly known as Vioxx) was taken off the market in 2004 because of these concerns and celecoxib and traditional NSAIDs received boxed warnings on their labels.

Medical Uses

Some COX-2 inhibitors are used in a single dose to treat pain after surgery.

Etoricoxib appears as good as if not better than other pain medications. Celecoxib appears to be about as useful as ibuprofen.

NSAIDs are often used in treatment of acute gout attacks. COX-2 inhibitors appear to work as well as nonselective NSAIDS. They have not been compared to other treatment options such as colchicine or glucocorticoids.

Cancer

COX-2 appears to be related to cancers and abnormal growths in the intestinal tract. COX inhibitors have been shown to reduce the occurrence of cancers and pre-cancerous growths. The National Cancer Institute has done some studies on COX-2 and cancer. The FDA has approved Celebrex for treatment of familial adenomatous polyposis (FAP). COX-2 inhibitors are currently being studied in breast cancer and appear to be beneficial.

Neuropsychiatric Disorders

COX-2 inhibitors have been found to be effective in suppressing inflammatory neurodegenerative pathways in mental illness, with beneficial results in trials for major depressive disorder as well as schizophrenia.

Other Targets

The inhibition of COX-2 is paramount for the anti-inflammatory and analgesic function of the selective COX-2 inhibitor celecoxib. However, with regard to this drug's promise for the therapy of advanced cancers, it is unclear whether the inhibition of COX-2 plays a dominant role, and this has become a controversial and intensely researched issue. In recent years, several additional intracellular components (besides COX-2) were discovered that appear to be important for mediating the anticancer effects of celecoxib in the absence of COX-2. Moreover, a recent study with various malignant tumor cells showed that celecoxib could inhibit the growth of these cells, even though some of these cancer cells didn't even contain COX-2.

Additional support for the idea that other targets besides COX-2 are important for celecoxib's anticancer effects has come from studies with chemically modified versions of celecoxib. Several dozen analogs of celecoxib were generated with small alterations in their chemical structures. Some of these analogs retained COX-2 inhibitory activity, whereas many others didn't. However, when the ability of all these compounds to kill tumor cells in cell culture was investigated, it turned out that the antitumor potency did not at all depend on whether or not the respective compound could inhibit COX-2, showing that inhibition of COX-2 was not required for the anticancer effects. One of these compounds, 2,5-dimethyl-celecoxib, which entirely lacks the ability to inhibit COX-2, actually turned out to display stronger anticancer activity than celecoxib itself and this anticancer effect could also be verified in highly drug-resistant tumor cells and in various animal tumor models.

Adverse Effects

Analysis of clinical trial data revealed that there was a significant increase in the rate of vascular events with COX-2 inhibitors compared with placebo; "vascular events" are non-fatal myocardial infarction (MI) or heart attack, non-fatal stroke, and death from a vascular event such as MI or stroke. These results led Merck to voluntarily withdraw (Rofecoxib) from the market in September 2004 and to regulatory authorities imposing a boxed warning on the label of celecoxib. Traditional NSAIDs were also found to have cardiovascular risks, leading to similar boxed warnings.

The cause of the cardiovascular problems became, and remains, a subject of intensive research. As of 2012 results have been converging on the hypothesis that the adverse cardiovascular effects are most likely due to inhibition of COX-2 in blood vessels, which leads to a decrease in the production of prostacyclin in them. Prostacyclin usually prevents platelet aggregation and vasoconstriction, so its inhibition can lead to excess clot formation and higher blood pressure.

Research

Research History

The COX-2 enzyme was discovered in 1988 by Daniel Simmons, a Brigham Young University researcher. The mouse COX-2 gene was cloned by UCLA scientist Dr. Harvey Herschman, a finding published in 1991.

The basic research leading to the discovery of COX-2 inhibitors has been the subject of at least two lawsuits. Brigham Young University has sued Pfizer, alleging breach of contract from relations BYU had with the company at the time of Dr. Simmons work. A settlement was reached in April 2012 in which Pfizer agreed to pay $450 million. The other litigation is based on United States Pat. No. 6,048,850 owned by University of Rochester, which claimed a method to treat pain without causing gastro-intestinal distress by selectively inhibiting COX-2. When the patent issued, the university sued Searle (later Pfizer) in a case called, *University of Rochester v. G.D. Searle & Co.*, 358 F.3d 916 (Fed. Cir. 2004). The court ruled in favor of Searle in 2004, holding in essence that the university had claimed a method requiring, yet provided no written description of, a compound that could inhibit COX-2 and therefore the patent was invalid.

In the course of the search for a specific inhibitor of the negative effects of prostaglandins which spared the positive effects, it was discovered that prostaglandins could indeed be separated into two general classes which could loosely be regarded as "good prostaglandins" and "bad prostaglandins", according to the structure of a particular enzyme involved in their biosynthesis, cyclooxygenase.

Prostaglandins whose synthesis involves the cyclooxygenase-I enzyme, or COX-1, are responsible for maintenance and protection of the gastrointestinal tract, while prostaglandins whose synthesis involves the cyclooxygenase-II enzyme, or COX-2, are responsible for inflammation and pain.

The existing non-steroidal anti-inflammatory drugs (NSAIDs) differ in their relative specificities for COX-2 and COX-1; while aspirin and ibuprofen inhibit COX-2 and COX-1 enzymes, other NSAIDs appear to have partial COX-2 specificity, particularly meloxicam (Mobic). Aspirin is ≈170-fold more potent in inhibiting COX-1 than COX-2. Studies of meloxicam 7.5 mg per day for 23 days find a level of gastric injury similar to that of a placebo, and for meloxicam 15 mg per day a level of injury lower than that of other NSAIDs; however, in clinical practice meloxicam can still cause some ulcer complications.

Many COX-2-specific inhibitors have been removed from the U.S. market. As of December 2011, only Celebrex (generic name is celecoxib) is still available for purchase.

Valdecoxib and rofecoxib were about 300 times more potent at inhibiting COX-2 than COX-1, but too toxic for the heart, suggesting the possibility of relief from pain and inflammation without gastrointestinal irritation, and promising to be a boon for those who had previously experienced adverse effects or had comorbidities that could lead to such complications. Celecoxib is approximately 30 times more potent at inhibiting COX-2 than COX-1, with etoricoxib being 106 times more potent. Also, Tribulus terrestris was shown to have strong inhibitory activity on COX-2.

Research Fraud

Between 1996 and 2009, anesthesiologist Scott Reuben conducted clinical research on the use of COX-2 inhibitors, often in combination with gabapentin or pregabalin, for the prevention and treatment of post-surgical pain, research which was found in 2009 to have been faked. Reuben pleaded guilty, paid fines and served six months in jail, and lost his medical license. A 2009 review of meta-articles used in evidence-based medicine found that while some reviews were no longer valid when the Reuben studies were removed, the conclusions in the majority of them remained unchanged. The review found that the key Reuben claims that needed to be re-examined were "the absence of detrimental effects of coxibs on bone healing after spine surgery, the beneficial long-term outcome after preemptive administration of coxibs including an allegedly decreased incidence of chronic pain after surgery, and the analgesic efficacy of ketorolac or clonidine when added to local anesthetics for intravenous regional anesthesia."

Early COX-2-inhibiting Drugs

Celebrex (and other brand names for celecoxib) was introduced in 1999 and rapidly became the most frequently prescribed new drug in the United States. By October 2000, its US sales exceeded 100 million prescriptions per year for $3 billion, and was still rising. Sales of Celebrex alone reached $3.1 billion in 2001. A Spanish study found that between January 2000 and June 2001, 7% of NSAID prescriptions and 29% of NSAID expenditures were for COX-2 inhibitors. Over the period of the study, COX-2 inhibitors rose from 10.03% of total NSAIDs prescribed by specialty physicians to 29.79%, and from 1.52% to 10.78% of NSAIDs prescribed by primary care physicians (98.23% of NSAIDs and 94.61% of COX-2 inhibitors were prescribed by primary care physicians). For specialty physicians, rofecoxib and celecoxib were third and fifth most frequently prescribed NSAIDs but first and second in cost, respectively; for primary-care physicians they were ninth and twelfth most frequently prescribed NSAIDs and first and fourth in cost.

The cause of the rapid widespread acceptance of Celebrex and Vioxx by physicians was the publication of two large trials, the Celecoxib Long-term Arthritis Safety Study (CLASS) in *JAMA*, and the Vioxx Gastrointestinal Outcomes Research (VIGOR). The VIGOR trial was later proven to have been based on faulty data, and Vioxx was eventually withdrawn from the market.

VIGOR Study and Publishing Controversy

The VIGOR (Vioxx Gastrointestinal Outcomes Research) trial, "which was the making of Merck's drug rofecoxib (Vioxx)," was at the center of a dispute about the ethics of medical journals. VIGOR trial,1 was a trial in which over 8000 patients were randomized to receive either naproxen or rofecoxib (Vioxx), a Cox-2 inhibitor that Merck hoped would have fewer gastrointestinal side effects." Both publications concluded that COX-2 specific NSAIDs were associated with significantly fewer adverse gastrointestinal effects. In the CLASS trial comparing Celebrex 800 mg/day to ibuprofen 2400 mg/day and diclofenac 150 mg/day for osteoarthritis or rheumatoid arthritis for six months, Celebrex was associated with significantly fewer upper gastrointestinal complications (0.44% vs. 1.27%, P=0.04), with no significant difference in incidence of cardiovascular events in patients not taking aspirin for cardiovascular prophylaxis.

The VIGOR trial results were published in 2000 in the *New England Journal of Medicine* Bombardier and his research team claimed that there was "an increase in myocardial infarction in the patients given rofecoxib (0.4%) compared with those given naproxen (0.1%)" and "patients given naproxen experienced 121 side effects compared with 56 in the patients taking rofecoxib," a "marvellous result for Merck" which "contributed to huge sales of rofecoxib." Merck's scientists incorrectly interpreted the finding as a protective effect of naproxen, telling the FDA that the difference in heart attacks "is primarily due to" this protective effect. In September 2001, the United States Food and Drug Administration (FDA) sent a warning letter to the CEO of Merck, stating, "Your promotional campaign discounts the fact that in the VIGOR study, patients on Vioxx were observed to have a four to five fold increase in myocardial infarctions (MIs) compared to patients on the comparator non-steroidal anti-inflammatory drug (NSAID), Naprosyn (naproxen)." This led to the introduction, in April 2002, of warnings on Vioxx labeling concerning the increased risk of cardiovascular events (heart attack and stroke). By 2005 *The New England Journal of Medicine* published an editorial accusing the Bombardier et al. of deliberately withholding data.

Dr. Claire Bombardier, a University of Toronto rheumatologist, had claimed that the VIGOR trial testing resulted in Vioxx 50 mg/day versus naproxen for rheumatoid arthritis, Vioxx reduced the risk of symptomatic ulcers and clinical upper gastrointestinal events (perforations, obstructions and bleeding) by 54%, to 1.4% from 3%, the risk of complicated upper gastrointestinal events (complicated perforations, obstructions and bleeding in the upper gastrointestinal tract) by 57%, and the risk of bleeding from anywhere in the gastrointestinal tract by 62%. An enormous marketing effort capitalized on these publications; Vioxx was the most heavily advertised prescription drug in 2000, and Celebrex the seventh, according to IMS Health.

Neuroblastomas

Small tumors of the sympathetic nervous system (neuroblastoma) appear to have abnormal levels of COX-2 expressed. These studies report that overexpression of the COX-2 enzyme has an adverse effect on the tumor suppressor, p53. p53 is an apoptosis transcription factor normally found in the cytosol. When cellular DNA is damaged beyond repair, p53 is transported to the nucleus where it promotes p53 mediated apoptosis. Two of the metabolites of COX-2, prostaglandin A2 (PGA2) and A1 (PGA1), when present in high quantities bind to p53 in the cytosol and inhibit its ability to cross into the nucleus. This essentially sequesters p53 in the cytosol and prevents apoptosis. Coxibs such as Celebrex (celecoxib), by selectively inhibiting the overexpressed COX-2, allow p53 to work properly. Functional p53 allows DNA damaged neuroblastoma cells to commit suicide through apoptosis, halting tumor growth.

COX-2 up-regulation has also been linked to the phosphorylation and activation of the E3 ubiquitin ligase HDM2, a protein that mediates p53 ligation and tagged destruction, through ubiquitination. The mechanism for this neuroblastoma HDM2 hyperactivity is unknown. Studies have shown that COX-2 inhibitors block the phosphorylation of HDM2 preventing its activation. In vitro, the use of COX-2 inhibitors lowers the level of active HDM2 found in neuroblastoma cells. The exact process of how COX-2 inhibitors block HDM2 phosphorylation is unknown, but this mediated reduction in active HDM2 concentration level restores the cellular p53 levels. After treatment with a COX-2 inhibitor, the restored p53 function allows DNA damaged neuroblastoma cells to commit suicide through apoptosis reducing the size of growth of the tumor.

Patient-controlled Analgesia

Patient-controlled analgesia (PCA) is any method of allowing a person in pain to administer their own pain relief. The infusion is programmable by the prescriber. If it is programmed and functioning as intended, the machine is unlikely to deliver an overdose of medication. Providers must always observe the first administration of any PCA medication which has not already been administered by the provider to respond to allergic reactions.

Routes of Administration

Oral

The most common form of patient-controlled analgesia is self-administration of oral over-the-counter or prescription painkillers. For example, if a headache does not resolve with a small dose of an oral analgesic, more may be taken. As pain is a combination of tissue damage and emotional state, being in control means reducing the emotional component of pain.

Intravenous

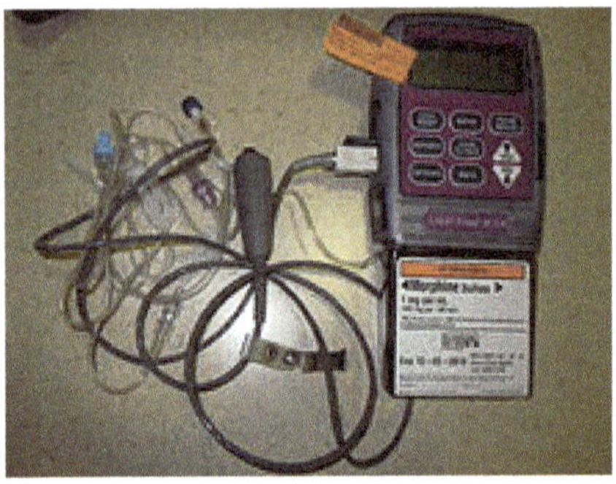

A patient-controlled analgesia infusion pump, configured for intravenous administration of morphine for postoperative analgesia

In a hospital setting, a PCA refers to an electronically controlled infusion pump that delivers an amount of intravenous analgesic when the patient presses a button. PCA can be used for both acute and chronic pain patients. It is commonly used for post-operative pain management, and for end-stage cancer patients.

Narcotics are the most common analgesics administered through PCAs. It is important for caregivers to monitor patients for the first two to twenty-four hours to ensure they are using the device properly.

With a PCA the patient is protected from overdose by the caregiver programming the PCA to deliver a dose at set intervals. If the patient presses the button sooner than the prescribed intake pressing the button does not operate the PCA. (The PCA can be set to emit a beep telling the patient a dose was NOT delivered). Dosage is also controlled when the patient is too sedated to press the button; preventing the patient from receiving needless doses and keeping the patient safe from overdosing.

Epidural

Patient-controlled epidural analgesia (PCEA) is a related term describing the patient-controlled administration of analgesic medicine in the epidural space, by way of intermittent boluses or infusion pumps. This can be used by women in labour, terminally ill cancer patients or to manage post-operative pain.

Inhaled

In 1968, Robert Wexler of Abbott Laboratories developed the Analgizer, a disposable inhaler that allowed the self-administration of methoxyflurane vapor in air for analgesia. The Analgizer consisted of a polyethylene cylinder 5 inches long and 1 inch in diameter with a 1 inch long mouthpiece. The device contained a rolled wick of polypropylene felt which held 15 milliliters of methoxyflurane. Because of the simplicity of the Analgizer and the pharmacological characteristics of methoxyflurane, it was easy for patients to self-administer the drug and rapidly achieve a level of conscious analgesia which could be maintained and adjusted as necessary over a period of time lasting from a few minutes to several hours. The 15 milliliter supply of methoxyflurane would typically last for two to three hours, during which time the user would often be partly amnesic to the sense of pain; the device could be refilled if necessary. The Analgizer was found to be safe, effective, and simple to administer in obstetric patients during childbirth, as well as for patients with bone fractures and joint dislocations, and for dressing changes on burn patients. When used for labor analgesia, the Analgizer allows labor to progress normally and with no apparent adverse effect on Apgar scores. All vital signs remain normal in obstetric patients, newborns, and injured patients. The Analgizer was widely utilized for analgesia and sedation until the early 1970s, in a manner that foreshadowed the patient-controlled analgesia infusion pumps of today. The Analgizer inhaler was withdrawn in 1974, but use of methoxyflurane as a sedative and analgesic continues in Australia and New Zealand in the form of the Penthrox inhaler.

Nasal

Patient Controlled Intranasal Analgesia (PCINA or Nasal PCA) refers to PCA devices in a Nasal spray form with inbuilt features to control the number of sprays that can be delivered in a fixed time period.

Transcutaneous

Transcutaneous delivery systems, including iontophoretic systems, are available. These are popular for administration of opioids such as fentanyl, or local anesthetics such as lidocaine. Iontocaine is one example of such a system.

Advantages and Disadvantages

Advantages of patient-controlled analgesia include self-delivery of pain medication, faster alleviation of pain because the patient can address pain with medication, and dosage monitoring by medical staff (dosage can be increased or decreased depending on need). With a PCA the patient spends less time in pain and as a corollary to this, patients tend to use less medication than in cases in which medication is given according to a set schedule or on a timer.

Disadvantages include the possibility that a patient will use the pain medication non-medically, self-administering the pain medication to get high. If a PCA device is not programmed properly for the patient this can result in an under-dose or overdose in a medicine. The system may also be inappropriate for certain individuals, for example patients with learning difficulties or confusion. Also, patients with poor manual dexterity may be unable to press the buttons as would those who are critically ill. PCA may not be appropriate for younger patients.

History

The PCA pump was developed and introduced by Philip H. Sechzer in the late 1960s and described in 1971.

Opioid

Opioids are substances that act on opioid receptors to produce morphine-like effects. Opioids are most often used medically to relieve pain, and by people addicted to opioids. Opioids include *opiates*, an older term that refers to such drugs derived from *opium*, including morphine itself. Other opioids are semi-synthetic and synthetic drugs such as hydrocodone, oxycodone and fentanyl; antagonist drugs such as naloxone and endogenous peptides such as the endorphins. The terms *opiate* and *narcotic* are sometimes encountered as synonyms for opioid. *Opiate* is properly limited to the natural alkaloids found in the resin of the opium poppy although some include semi-synthetic derivatives. *Narcotic*, derived from words meaning *numbness* or *sleep*, as an American legal term, refers to cocaine and opioids, and their source materials; it is also loosely applied to any illegal or controlled psychoactive drug. In some jurisdictions all controlled drugs are legally classified as *narcotics*. The term can have pejorative connotations and its use is generally discouraged where that is the case.

Primarily used for pain relief, including anesthesia they are also used to suppress cough, suppress diarrhea, treat addiction, reverse opioid overdose, and suppress opioid induced constipation. Extremely strong opioids are approved only for veterinary use such as immobilizing large mammals. Opioids act by binding to opioid receptors, which are found principally in the central and peripheral nervous system and the gastrointestinal tract. These receptors mediate both the psychoactive and the somatic effects of opioids. Opioid drugs include partial agonists, like the anti-diarrhea drug loperamide and antagonists like naloxegol for opioid-induced constipation, which do not cross the blood-brain barrier, but can displace other opioids from binding in those receptors.

The side effects of opioids may include itchiness, sedation, nausea, respiratory depression, constipation, and euphoria. Tolerance and dependence will develop with continuous use, requiring increasing doses and leading to a withdrawal syndrome upon abrupt discontinuation. The euphoria attracts recreational use, and frequent, escalating recreational use of opioids typically results in addiction. Accidental overdose or concurrent use with other depressant drugs commonly results in death from respiratory depression. Because of opioid drugs' reputation for addiction and fatal overdose, most are controlled substances.

Illicit production, smuggling, and addiction to opioids prompted treaties, laws and policing which have realized limited success. In 2013 between 28 and 38 million people used opioids illicitly (0.6% to 0.8% of the global population between the ages of 15 and 65). In 2011 an estimated 4 million people in the United States used opioids recreationally or were dependent on them. Current increased rates of recreational use and addiction are attributed to over-prescription of opioid medications and inexpensive illicit heroin. Conversely, fears about over-prescribing, exaggerated side effects and addiction from opioids are similarly blamed for under-treatment of pain.

Medical Uses

Pain

Opioids are indicated for the relief of mild to severe pain, but are usually reserved for moderate to severe pain. The weak opioid codeine, in low doses and combined with one or more other drugs, is commonly available without a prescription.

Acute Pain

Opioids are effective for the treatment of acute pain (such as pain following surgery). For immediate relief of moderate to severe acute pain opioids are frequently the treatment of choice due to their rapid onset, efficacy and reduced risk of dependence. They have also been found to be important in palliative care to help with the severe, chronic, disabling pain that may occur in some terminal conditions such as cancer, and degenerative conditions such as rheumatoid arthritis. In many cases opioids are a successful long-term care strategy for those with chronic cancer pain.

Chronic Non-cancer Pain

Guidelines have suggested that the risk of opioids is likely greater than their benefits when used for most non-cancer chronic conditions including headaches, back pain, and fibromyalgia. Thus they should be used cautiously in chronic non-cancer pain. If used the benefits and harms should be reassessed at least every three months.

In treating chronic pain, opioids are an option to be tried after other less risky pain relievers have been considered, including paracetamol/acetaminophen or NSAIDs like ibuprofen or naproxen. Some types of chronic pain, including the pain caused by fibromyalgia or migraine, are preferentially treated with drugs other than opioids. The efficacy of using opioids to lessen chronic neuropathic pain is uncertain.

Opioids are contraindicated as a first-line treatment for headache because they impair alertness, bring risk of dependence, and increase the risk that episodic headaches will become chronic. Opioids can also cause heightened sensitivity to headache pain. When other treatments fail or are unavailable, opioids may be appropriate for treating headache if the patient can be monitored to prevent the development of chronic headache.

Opioids are being used more frequently in the management of non-malignant chronic pain. This practice has now led to a new and growing problem with addiction and misuse of opioids. Because of various negative effects the use of opioids for long term management of chronic pain is not indicated unless other less risky pain relievers have been found ineffective. Chronic pain which occurs only periodically, such as that from nerve pain, migraines, and fibromyalgia, frequently is better treated with medications other than opioids. Paracetamol and non-steroidal anti-inflammatory drugs including ibuprofen and naproxen are considered safer alternatives. They are frequently used combined with opioids, such as paracetamol combined with oxycodone (Percocet) and ibuprofen combined with hydrocodone (Vicoprofen), which boosts the pain relief but is also intended to deter recreational use.

Other

Cough

Codeine was once viewed as the "gold standard" in cough suppressants, but this position is now questioned. Some recent placebo-controlled trials have found that it may be no better than a placebo for some causes including acute cough in children. Thus, it is not recommended for children. Additionally, there is no evidence that hydrocodone is useful in children. Similarly, a 2012 Dutch guideline regarding the treatment of acute cough does not recommend its use. (The opioid analogue dextromethorphan, long claimed to be as effective a cough suppressant as codeine, has similarly demonstrated little benefit in several recent studies).

Low dose morphine may help chronic cough but its use is limited by side effects.

Diarrhea and Constipation

In cases of diarrhea-predominate irritable bowel syndrome, opioids may be used to suppress diarrhea. Loperamide is a peripherally selective opioid available without a prescription used to suppress diarrhea.

The ability to suppress diarrhea also produces constipation when opioids are used beyond several weeks. Naloxegol, a peripherally-selective opioid antagonist is now available to treat opioid induced constipation.

Shortness of Breath

Opioids may help with shortness of breath particularly in advanced diseases such as cancer and COPD among others.

Adverse Effects

Adverse effects of opioids

Common and short term

- Itch
- Nausea
- Vomiting
- Constipation
- Drowsiness
- Dry mouth

Other

- Cognitive effects
- Opioid dependence
- Dizziness
- Decreased sex drive
- Impaired sexual function
- Decreased testosterone levels
- Depression
- Immunodeficiency
- Increased pain sensitivity
- Irregular menstruation
- Increased risk of falls
- Slowed breathing
- Coma

Studies have shown opioids to be safe when they are used correctly and in the ways that are well understood.

Carefully titrating the dose of opioids can provide for effective pain relief while minimizing adverse effects. Morphine and diamorphine have been shown to have a wider therapeutic range or "safety margin" than some other opioids. Because the required dose varies and cannot be predicted, titration usually starts at low doses, increasing until the desired effect or adverse effects occur.

Opioid analgesics do not cause any specific organ toxicity, unlike many other drugs, such as aspirin and paracetamol. They are not associated with upper gastrointestinal bleeding and kidney toxicity.

In older adults, opioid use is associated with increased adverse effects such as "sedation, nausea, vomiting, constipation, urinary retention, and falls". As a result, older adults taking opioids are at greater risk for injury.

Research suggests that when methadone is used long-term it can build up unpredictably in the body and lead to potentially deadly slowed breathing. Used medically, approaching toxicity goes unrecognized because the pain medication effect ends long before the drug's elimination half-life. According to the USCDC, methadone was involved in 31% of opioid related deaths in the US between 1999-2010 and 40% as the sole drug involved, far higher than other opioids. Regular physician monitoring reduces the likelihood of problems.

According to a cohort study, the rate of opioid related death was 0.017% per year amongst patients prescribed opioids for non-cancer pain from 1997 to 2005 in Washington State. Increasing dose and age were found to correlate with increased risk of overdose. While a cohort study is a higher level of evidence than case-control, a case-control study done in Canada correlates well as it had an opioid related death rate of 0.024% per year amongst patients prescribed opioids for non-cancer pain over a 10-year period.

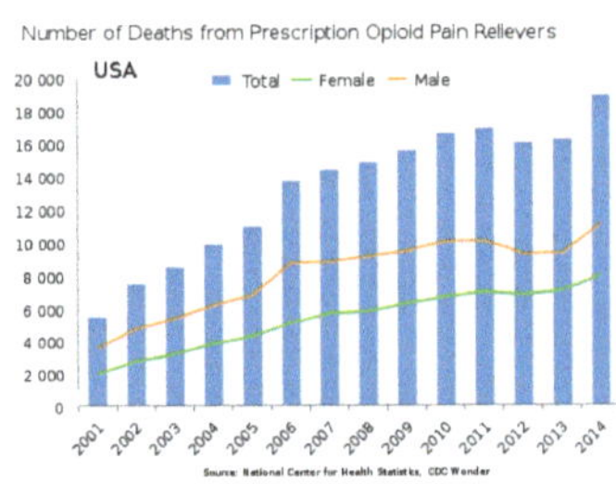

Timeline of number of yearly U.S. overdose deaths involving prescription opioid pain relievers.

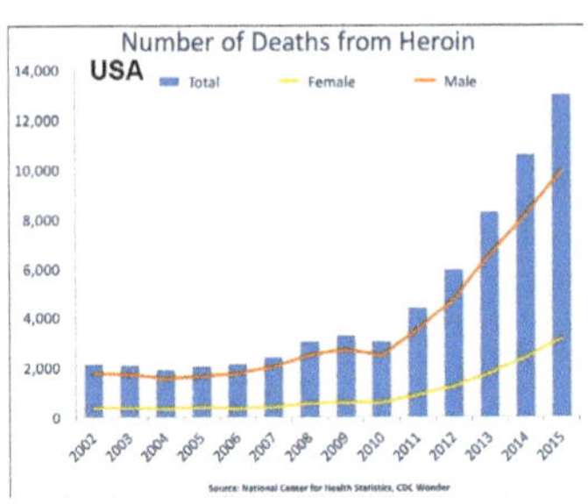

Timeline of number of yearly U.S. overdose deaths involving heroin.

Reinforcement Disorders

Tolerance

Tolerance is a process characterized by neuroadaptations that result in reduced drug effects. While receptor upregulation may often play an important role other mechanisms are also known. Tolerance is more pronounced for some effects than for others; tolerance occurs slowly to the effects on mood, itching, urinary retention, and respiratory depression, but occurs more quickly to the analgesia and other physical side effects. However, tolerance does not develop to constipation or miosis (the constriction of the pupil of the eye to less than or equal to two millimeters). This idea has been challenged, however, with some authors arguing that tolerance *does* develop to miosis.

Tolerance to opioids is attenuated by a number of substances, including:

- calcium channel blockers
- intrathecal magnesium and zinc
- NMDA antagonists, such as dextromethorphan, ketamine, and memantine.
- cholecystokinin antagonists, such as proglumide
- Newer agents such as the phosphodiesterase inhibitor ibudilast have also been researched for this application.

Tolerance is a physiologic process where the body adjusts to a medication that is frequently present, usually requiring higher doses of the same medication over time to achieve the same effect. It is a common occurrence in individuals taking high doses of opioids for extended periods, but does not predict any relationship to misuse or addiction.

Physical Dependence

Physical dependence is the physiological adaptation of the body to the presence of a substance, in this case opioid medication. It is defined by the development of withdrawal symptoms when the substance is discontinued, when the dose is reduced abruptly or, specifically in the case of opioids, when an antagonist (e.g., naloxone) or an agonist-antagonist (e.g., pentazocine) is administered. Physical dependence is a normal and expected aspect of certain medications and does not necessarily imply that the patient is addicted.

The withdrawal symptoms for opiates may include severe dysphoria, craving for another opiate dose, irritability, sweating, nausea, rhinorrea, tremor, vomiting and myalgia. Slowly reducing the intake of opioids over days and weeks can reduce or eliminate the withdrawal symptoms. The speed and severity of withdrawal depends on the half-life of the opioid; heroin and morphine withdrawal occur more quickly and are more severe than methadone withdrawal. The acute withdrawal phase is often followed by a protracted phase of depression and insomnia that can last for months. The symptoms of opioid withdrawal can be treated with other medications, such as clonidine. Physical dependence does not predict drug misuse or true addiction, and is closely related to the same mechanism as tolerance. While there is anecdotal claims of benefit with ibogaine, data to support its use in substance dependence is poor.

Addiction

Drug addiction is a complex set of behaviors typically associated with misuse of certain drugs, developing over time and with higher drug dosages. Addiction includes psychological compulsion, to the extent that the sufferer persists in actions leading to dangerous or unhealthy outcomes. Opioid addiction includes insufflation or injection, rather than taking opioids orally as prescribed for medical reasons.

In European nations such as Austria, Bulgaria, and Slovakia, slow release oral morphine formulations are used in opiate substitution therapy (OST) for patients who do not well tolerate the side effects of buprenorphine or methadone. In other European countries including the UK, this is also legally used for OST although on a varying scale of acceptance.

Tamper-release formulations of time-controlled preparations of medications are intended to curb abuse and addiction rates while trying to still provide legitimate pain relief and ease of use to pain patients. Questions remain, however, about the efficacy and safety of these types of preparations. Further tamper resistant medications are currently under consideration with trials for market approval by the FDA.

The amount of evidence available only permits making a weak conclusion, but it suggests that a physician properly managing opioid use in patients with no history of substance dependence or substance abuse can give long-term pain relief with little risk of developing addiction, abuse, or other serious side effects.

Problems with opioids include the following:

1. Some people find that opioids do not relieve all of their pain.
2. Some people find that opioids side effects cause problems which outweigh the therapy's benefit
3. Some people build tolerance to opioids over time. This requires them to increase their drug dosage to maintain the benefit, and that in turn also increases the unwanted side effects.
4. Long-term opioid use can cause opioid-induced hyperalgesia, which is a condition in which the patient has increased sensitivity to pain.

All of the opioids can cause side effects. Common adverse reactions in patients taking opioids for pain relief include nausea and vomiting, drowsiness, itching, dry mouth, dizziness, and constipation.

Nausea and Vomiting

Tolerance to nausea occurs within 7–10 days, during which antiemetics (e.g. low dose haloperidol once at night) are very effective. Due to severe side effects such as tardive dyskinesia, haloperidol is now rarely used. A related drug, prochlorperazine is more often used, although it has similar risks. Stronger antiemetics such as ondansetron or tropisetron are sometimes used when nausea is severe or continuous and disturbing, despite their greater cost. A less expensive alternative is dopamine antagonists such as domperidone and metoclopramide. Domperidone does not cross the blood–brain barrier and produce adverse central antidopaminergic effects, but blocks opioid emetic action in the chemoreceptor trigger zone. (The drug is not available in the U.S.) Some antihistamines with anticholinergic properties (e.g. orphenadrine or diphenhydramine) may also be effective. The first-generation antihistamine hydroxyzine is very commonly used, with the added advantages of not causing movement disorders, and also possessing analgesic-sparing properties. Δ^9-tetrahydrocannabinol relieves nausea and vomiting; it also produces analgesia that may allow lower doses of opioids with reduced nausea and vomiting.

- 5-HT_3 antagonists (e.g. ondansetron)
- Dopamine antagonists (e.g. domperidone)
- Anti-cholinergic antihistamines (e.g. diphenhydramine)
- Δ^9-tetrahydrocannabinol (e.g. dronabinol)

Vomiting is due to gastric stasis (large volume vomiting, brief nausea relieved by vomiting, oesophageal reflux, epigastric fullness, early satiation), besides direct action on the chemoreceptor trigger zone of the area postrema, the vomiting centre of the brain. Vomiting can thus be prevented by prokinetic agents (e.g. domperidone or metoclopramide). If vomiting has already started, these drugs need to be administered by a non-oral route (e.g. subcutaneous for metoclopramide, rectally for domperidone).

- Prokinetic agents (e.g. domperidone)
- Anti-cholinergic agents (e.g. orphenadrine)

Drowsiness

Tolerance to drowsiness usually develops over 5–7 days, but if troublesome, switching to an alternative opioid often helps. Certain opioids such as fentanyl, morphine and diamorphine (heroin) tend to be particularly sedating, while others such as oxycodone, tilidine and meperidine (pethidine) tend to produce comparatively less sedation, but individual patients responses can vary markedly and some degree of trial and error may be needed to find the most suitable drug for a particular patient. Otherwise, treatment with CNS stimulants is generally effective.

- Stimulants (e.g. caffeine, modafinil, amphetamine, methylphenidate)

Itching

Itching tends not to be a severe problem when opioids are used for pain relief, but antihistamines are useful for counteracting itching when it occurs. Non-sedating antihistamines such as fexofenadine are often preferred as they avoid increasing opioid induced drowsiness. However, some sedating antihistamines such as orphenadrine can produce a synergistic pain relieving effect permitting smaller doses of opioids be used. Consequently, several opioid/antihistamine combination products have been marketed, such as *Meprozine* (meperidine/promethazine) and *Diconal* (dipipanone/cyclizine), and these may also reduce opioid induced nausea.

- Antihistamines (e.g. fexofenadine)

Constipation

Opioid-induced constipation (OIC) develops in 90 to 95% of people taking opioids long-term. Since tolerance to this problem does not develop readily, most people on long-term opioids need to take a laxative or enemas.

Treatment

Treatment of OIC is successional and dependent on severity. The first mode of treatment is non-pharmacological, and includes lifestyle modifications like increasing dietary fiber, fluid intake (around 1.5 L (51 US fl oz) per day), and physical activity. If non-pharmacological measures are ineffective, laxatives, including stool softeners (e.g., docusate), bulk-forming laxatives (e.g., fiber supplements), stimulant laxatives (e.g., bisacodyl, senna), and/or enemas, may be used. A common laxative regimen for OIC is the combination of docusate and bisacodyl. Osmotic laxatives, including lactulose, polyethylene glycol, and milk of magnesia (magnesium hydroxide), as well as mineral oil (a lubricant laxative), are also commonly used for OIC.

If laxatives are insufficiently effective (which is often the case), opioid formulations or regimens that include a peripherally-selective opioid antagonist, such as methylnaltrexone bromide, naloxegol, alvimopan, or naloxone (as in oxycodone/naloxone), may be tried. A 2008 Cochrane review found that the evidence was tentative for alvimopan, naloxone, or methylnaltrexone bromide.

Respiratory Depression

Respiratory depression is the most serious adverse reaction associated with opioid use, but it usually is seen with the use of a single, intravenous dose in an opioid-naïve patient. In patients taking opioids regularly for pain relief, tolerance to respiratory depression occurs rapidly, so that it is not a clinical problem. Several drugs have been developed which can partially block respiratory depression, although the only respiratory stimulant currently approved for this purpose is doxapram, which has only limited efficacy in this application. Newer drugs such as BIMU-8 and CX-546 may be much more effective.

- Respiratory stimulants: carotid chemoreceptor agonists (e.g. doxapram), 5-HT_4 agonists (e.g. BIMU8), δ-opioid agonists (e.g. BW373U86) and AMPAkines (e.g. CX717) can all reduce respiratory depression caused by opioids without affecting analgesia, but most of these drugs are only moderately effective or have side effects which preclude use in humans. 5-HT_{1A} agonists such as 8-OH-DPAT and repinotan also counteract opioid-induced respiratory depression, but at the same time reduce analgesia, which limits their usefulness for this application.

- Opioid antagonists (e.g. naloxone, nalmefene, diprenorphine)

Opioid-induced Hyperalgesia

Opioid-induced hyperalgesia – where individuals using opioids to relieve pain paradoxically experience more pain as a result of that medication – has been observed in some people. This phenomenon, although uncommon, is seen in some people receiving palliative care, most often when dose is increased rapidly. If encountered, rotation between several different opioid pain medications may decrease the development of increased pain. Opioid induced hyperalgesia more commonly occurs with chronic use or brief high doses but some research suggests that it may also occur with very low doses.

Side effects such as hyperalgesia and allodynia, sometimes accompanied by a worsening of neuropathic pain, may be consequences of long-term treatment with opioid analgesics, especially when increasing tolerance has resulted in loss of efficacy and consequent progressive dose escalation over time. This appears to largely be a result of actions of opioid drugs at targets other than the three classic opioid receptors, including the nociceptin receptor, sigma receptor and Toll-like receptor 4, and can be counteracted in animal models by antagonists at these targets such as J-113,397, BD-1047 or (+)-naloxone respectively. No drugs are currently approved specifically for counteracting opioid-induced hyperalgesia in humans and in severe cases the only solution may be to discontinue use of opioid analgesics and replace them with non-opioid analgesic drugs. However, since individual sensitivity to the development of this side effect is highly dose dependent and may vary depending which opioid analgesic is used, many patients can avoid this side effect simply through dose reduction of the opioid drug (usually accompanied by the addition of a supplemental non-opioid analgesic), rotating between different opioid drugs, or by switching to a milder opioid with a mixed mode of action that also counteracts neuropathic pain, particularly tramadol or tapentadol.

- NMDA antagonists such as ketamine
- SNRIs such as milnacipran
- anticonvulsants such as gabapentin or pregabalin

Other Adverse Effects

Hormone Imbalance

Clinical studies have consistently associated medical and recreational opioid use with hypogonadism and hormone imbalance in different sexes. The effect is dose-dependent. Most studies suggest that the majority (perhaps as much as 90%) of chronic opioid users suffer hormone imbalances. Opioids can also interfere with menstruation in women by limiting the production of luteinizing hormone (LH). Opioid-induced endocrinopathy likely causes the strong association of opioid use with osteoporosis and bone fracture. It also may increase pain and thereby interfere with the intended clinical effect of opioid treatment. Opioid-induced endocrinopathy is likely caused their agonism of opioid receptors in the hypothalamus and the pituitary gland. One study found that the depressed testosterone levels of heroin addicts returned to normal within one month of abstinence, suggesting that the effect is not permanent. As of 2013, the effect of low-dose or acute opiate use on the endocrine system is unclear.

Disruption of Work

Use of opioids may be a risk factor for failing to return to work.

Persons performing any safety-sensitive task should not use opioids. Health care providers should not recommend that workers who drive or use heavy equipment including cranes or forklifts treat chronic or acute pain with opioids. Workplaces which manage workers who perform safety-sensitive operations should assign workers to less sensitive duties for so long as those workers are treated by their physician with opioids.

People who take opioids long term have increased likelihood of being unemployed. Taking opioids may further disrupt the patient's life and the adverse effects of opioids themselves can become a significant barrier to patients having an active life, gaining employment, and sustaining a career.

In addition, lack of employment may be a predictor of aberrant use of prescription opioids.

Increased Accident-proneness

Opioid use may increase accident-proneness. Opioids may increase risk of traffic accidents and accidental falls.

Rare Side Effects

Infrequent adverse reactions in patients taking opioids for pain relief include: dose-related respiratory depression (especially with more potent opioids), confusion, hallucinations, delirium, urticaria, hypothermia, bradycardia/tachycardia, orthostatic hypotension, dizziness, headache, urinary retention, ureteric or biliary spasm, muscle rigidity, myoclonus (with high doses), and flushing (due to histamine release, except fentanyl and remifentanil). Both therapeutic and chronic use of opioids can compromise the function of the immune system. Opioids decrease the proliferation of macrophage progenitor cells and lymphocytes, and affect cell differentiation (Roy & Loh, 1996). Opioids may also inhibit leukocyte migration. However the relevance of this in the context of pain relief is not known.

Interactions

Physicians treating patients using opioids in combination with other drugs keep continual documentation that further treatment is indicated and remain aware of opportunities to adjust treatment if the patient's condition changes to merit less risky therapy.

With Other Depressant Drugs

The concurrent use of opioids with other depressant drugs such as benzodiazepines or ethanol increases the rates of adverse events and overdose. As with an overdose of opioid alone, the combination of an opioid and another depressant may precipitate respiratory depression often leading to death. These risks are lessened with close monitoring by a physician, who may conduct ongoing screening for changes in patient behavior and treatment compliance.

Opioid Antagonist

Finally, opioid effects (adverse or otherwise) can be reversed with an opioid antagonist such as naloxone or naltrexone. These competitive antagonists bind to the opioid receptors with higher affinity than agonists but do not activate the receptors. This displaces the agonist, attenuating or reversing the agonist effects. However, the elimination half-life of naloxone can be shorter than that of the opioid itself, so repeat dosing or continuous infusion may be required, or a longer acting antagonist such as nalmefene may be used. In patients taking opioids regularly it is essential that the opioid is only partially reversed to avoid a severe and distressing reaction of waking in excruciating pain. This is achieved by not giving a full dose but giving this in small doses until the respiratory rate has improved. An infusion is then started to keep the reversal at that level, while maintaining pain relief. Opioid antagonists remain the standard treatment for respiratory depression following opioid overdose, with naloxone being by far the most commonly used, although the longer acting antagonist nalmefene may be used for treating overdoses of long-acting opioids such as methadone, and diprenorphine is used for reversing the effects of extremely potent opioids used in veterinary medicine such as etorphine and carfentanil. However, since opioid antagonists also block the beneficial effects of opioid analgesics, they are generally useful only for treating overdose, with use of opioid antagonists alongside opioid analgesics to reduce side effects, requiring careful dose titration and often being poorly effective at doses low enough to allow analgesia to be maintained.

Pharmacology

Opioid comparison				
Drug	**Relative Potency**	**Nonionized Fraction**	**Protein Binding**	**Lipid Solubility**
Morphine	1	++	++	++
Meperidine	0.1	+	+++	++
Hydromorphone	10		+	+++
Alfentanil	10–25	++++	++++	+++
Fentanyl	75–125	+	+++	++++
Remifentanil	250	+++	+++	++
Sufentanil	500–1000	++	++++	++++
Etorphine	1000–3000			

Opioids bind to specific opioid receptors in the nervous system and other tissues. There are three principal classes of opioid receptors, μ, κ, δ (mu, kappa, and delta), although up to seventeen have been reported, and include the ε, ι, λ, and ζ (Epsilon, Iota, Lambda and Zeta) receptors. Conversely, σ (Sigma) receptors are no longer considered to be opioid receptors because their activation is not reversed by the opioid inverse-agonist naloxone, they do not exhibit high-affinity binding for classical opioids, and they are stereoselective for dextro-rotatory isomers while the other opioid receptors are stereo-selective for levo-rotatory isomers. In addition, there are three subtypes of μ-receptor: μ_1 and μ_2, and the newly discovered μ_3. Another receptor of clinical importance is the opioid-receptor-like receptor 1 (ORL1), which is involved in pain responses as well as having a major role in the development of tolerance to μ-opioid agonists used as analgesics. These are all G-protein coupled receptors acting on GABAergic neurotransmission.

The pharmacodynamic response to an opioid depends upon the receptor to which it binds, its affinity for that receptor, and whether the opioid is an agonist or an antagonist. For example, the supraspinal analgesic properties of the opioid agonist morphine are mediated by activation of the μ_1 receptor; respiratory depression and physical dependence by the μ_2 receptor; and sedation and spinal analgesia by the κ receptor. Each group of opioid receptors elicits a distinct set of neurological responses, with the receptor subtypes (such as μ_1 and μ_2 for example) providing even more [measurably] specific responses. Unique to each opioid is its distinct binding affinity to the various classes of opioid receptors (e.g. the μ, κ, and δ opioid receptors are activated at different magnitudes according to the specific receptor binding affinities of the opioid). For example, the opiate alkaloid morphine exhibits high-affinity binding to the μ-opioid receptor, while ketazocine exhibits high affinity to κ receptors. It is this combinatorial mechanism that allows for such a wide class of opioids and molecular designs to exist, each with its own unique effect profile. Their individual molecular structure is also responsible for their different duration of action, whereby metabolic breakdown (such as *N*-dealkylation) is responsible for opioid metabolism.

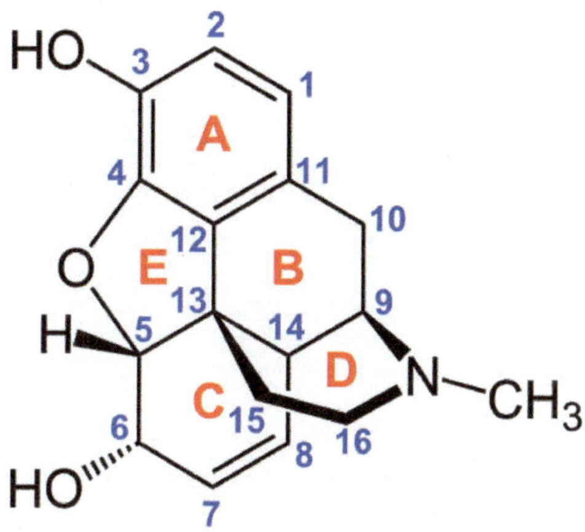

Locants of the morphine molecule

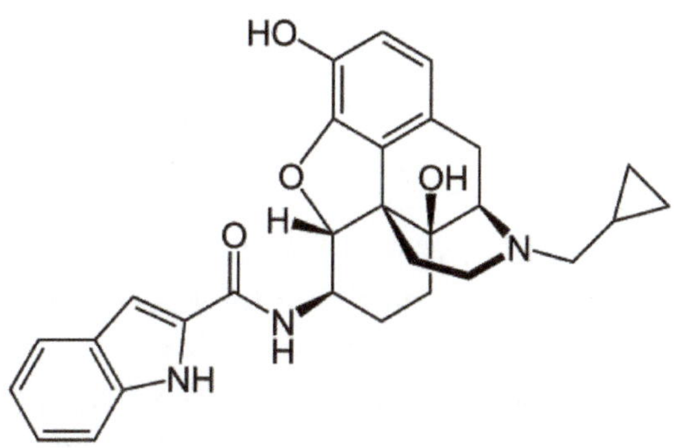

INTA: selective agonist of KOR-DOR and KOR-MOR heteromers.
Does not recruit β-arrestin II. Antinociceptive devoid of aversion, tolerance, and dependence in mice.

Functional Selectivity

A new strategy of drug development takes receptor signal transduction into consideration. This strategy strives to increase the activation of desirable signalling pathways while reducing the impact on undesirable pathways. This differential strategy has been given several names, including functional selectivity and biased agonism. The first opioid that was intentionally designed as a biased agonist and placed into clinical evaluation is the drug oliceridine. It displays analgesic activity and reduced adverse effects.

Opioid Comparison

Extensive research has been conducted to determine equivalence ratios comparing the relative potency of opioids. Given a dose of an opioid, an equianalgesic table is used to find the equivalent dosage of another. Such tables are used in opioid rotation practices, and to describe an opioid by comparison to morphine, the reference opioid. Equianalgesic tables typically list drug half-lives, and sometimes equianalgesic doses of the same drug by means of administration, such as morphine: oral and intravenous.

Usage

Global estimates of illegal drug users in 2014 (in millions of users)			
Substance	**Best estimate**	**Low estimate**	**High estimate**
Amphetamine-type stimulants	35.65	15.34	55.90
Cannabis	182.50	127.54	233.65
Cocaine	18.26	14.88	22.08
Ecstasy	19.40	9.89	29.01
Opiates	17.44	13.74	21.59
Opioids	33.12	28.57	38.52

Opioid prescriptions in the US increased from 76 million in 1991 to 207 million in 2013.

In the 1990s, opioid prescribing increased significantly. Once used almost exclusively for the treatment of acute pain or pain due to cancer, opioids are now prescribed liberally for people experiencing chronic pain. This has been accompanied by rising rates of accidental addiction and accidental overdoses leading to death. According to the International Narcotics Control Board, the United States and Canada lead the per capita consumption of prescription opioids. The number of opioid prescriptions in the United States and Canada is double the consumption in the European Union, Australia, and New Zealand. Certain populations have been affected by the opioid addiction crisis more than others, including First World communities and low-income populations. Public health specialists say that this may result from unavailability or high cost of alternative methods for addressing chronic pain.

History

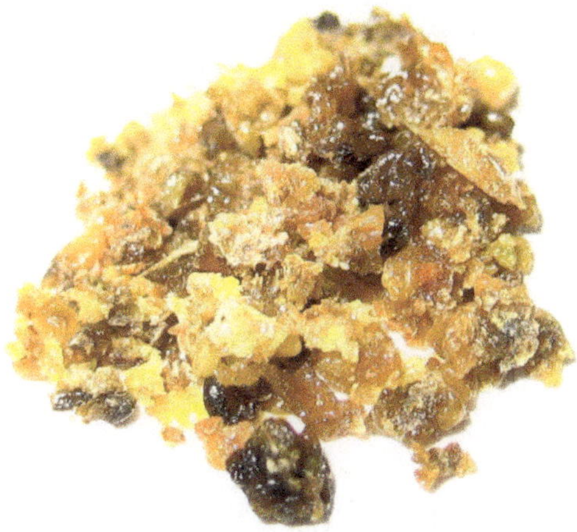

A sample of raw opium

Opioids are among the world's oldest known drugs. The medical, recreational, and religious use of the opium poppy predates the common era. In the 19th century morphine was isolated and marketed, and the hypodermic needle invented, introducing rapid, metered administration of the primary active compound. Synthetic opioids were invented, and biological mechanisms discovered in the 20th century.

Non-clinical use was criminalized in the United States by the Harrison Narcotics Tax Act of 1914, and by other laws worldwide. Since then, nearly all non-clinical use of opioids has been rated zero on the scale of approval of nearly every social institution. However, in United Kingdom the 1926 report of the Departmental Committee on Morphine and Heroin Addiction under the Chairmanship of the President of the Royal College of Physicians reasserted medical control and established the "British system" of control—which lasted until the 1960s; in the U.S. the Controlled Substances Act of 1970 markedly relaxed the harshness of the Harrison Act.

Before the twentieth century, institutional approval was often higher, even in Europe and America. In some cultures, approval of opioids was significantly higher than approval of alcohol. Opiates were used to treat depression and anxiety until the mid-1950s.

Society and Culture

Definition

The term "opioid" originated in the 1950s. It combines "opium" + "-oid" meaning "opiate-like" ("opiates" being morphine and similar drugs derived from opium). The first scientific publication to use it, in 1963, included a footnote stating, "In this paper, the term, 'opioid', is used in the sense originally proposed by George H. Acheson (personal communication) to refer to any chemical compound with morphine-like activities". By the late 1960s, research found that opiate effects are mediated by activation of specific molecular receptors in the nervous system, which were termed "opioid receptors". The definition of "opioid" was later refined to refer to substances that have morphine-like activities that are mediated by the activation of opioid receptors. One modern pharmacology textbook states: "the term opioid applies to all agonists and antagonists with morphine-like activity, and also the naturally occurring and synthetic opioid peptides". Another pharmacology reference eliminates the *morphine-like* requirement: "Opioid, a more modern term, is used to designate all substances, both natural and synthetic, that bind to opioid receptors (including antagonists)". Some sources define the term *opioid* to exclude *opiates*, and others use *opiate* comprehensively instead of *opioid*, but *opioid* used inclusively is considered modern, preferred and is in wide use.

Efforts to Reduce Abuse in the US

In 2011, the Obama administration released a white paper describing the administration's plan to deal with the opioid crisis. The administration's concerns about addiction and accidental overdosing have been echoed by numerous other medical and government advisory groups around the world.

As of 2015, prescription drug monitoring programs exist in every state but one. These programs allow pharmacists and prescribers to access patients' prescription histories in order to identify suspicious use. However, a survey of US physicians published in 2015 found that only 53% of doctors used these programs, while 22% were not aware that the programs were available to them. The Centers for Disease Control and Prevention was tasked with establishing and publishing a new guideline, and was heavily lobbied. In 2016, the United States Centers for Disease Control and Prevention published its Guideline for Prescribing Opioids for Chronic Pain, recommending that opioids only be used when benefits for pain and function are expected to outweigh risks, and then used at the lowest effective dosage, with avoidance of concurrent opioid and benzodiazepine use whenever possible.

Global Shortages

Morphine and other poppy-based medicines have been identified by the World Health Organization as essential in the treatment of severe pain. As of 2002, seven countries (USA, UK, Italy, Australia, France, Spain and Japan) use 77% of the world's morphine supplies, leaving many emerging countries lacking in pain relief medication. The current system of supply of raw poppy materials to make poppy-based medicines is regulated by the International Narcotics Control Board under the provision of the 1961 Single Convention on Narcotic Drugs. The amount of raw poppy materials that each country can demand annually based on these provisions must correspond to an estimate of the country's needs taken from the national consumption within the preceding two years. In many countries, underprescription of morphine is rampant because of the high prices and the lack of training in the prescription of poppy-based drugs. The World Health Organization is now working with administrations from various countries to train healthworkers and to develop national regulations regarding drug prescription to facilitate a greater prescription of poppy-based medicines.

Another idea to increase morphine availability is proposed by the Senlis Council, who suggest, through their proposal for Afghan Morphine, that Afghanistan could provide cheap pain relief solutions to emerging countries as part of a second-tier system of supply that would complement the current INCB regulated system by maintaining the balance and closed system that it establishes while providing finished product morphine to those suffering from severe pain and unable to access poppy-based drugs under the current system.

Recreational Use

Drug misuse is the use of drugs for reasons other than what the drug was prescribed for. Opioids are primarily misused due to their ability to produce strong euphoria. Misuse can also include giving drugs to people for whom it was not prescribed or selling the medication, both of which are crimes punishable by imprisonment in some, if not most, countries. In 2014, almost 2 million Americans abused or were dependent on prescription opioids.

Classification

There are a number of broad classes of opioids:

- Natural opiates: alkaloids contained in the resin of the opium poppy, primarily morphine, codeine, and thebaine, but not papaverine and noscapine which have a different mechanism of action; The following could be considered natural opiates: The leaves from Mitragyna speciosa (also known as kratom) contain a few naturally-occurring opioids, active via Mu- and Delta receptors. Salvinorin A, found naturally in the Salvia divinorum plant, is a kappa-opioid receptor agonist.
- Esters of morphine opiates: slightly chemically altered but more natural than the semi-synthetics, as most are morphine prodrugs, diacetylmorphine (morphine diacetate; heroin), nicomorphine (morphine dinicotinate), dipropanoylmorphine (morphine dipropionate), desomorphine, acetylpropionylmorphine, dibenzoylmorphine, diacetyldihydromorphine;
- Semi-synthetic opioids: created from either the natural opiates or morphine esters, such as hydromorphone, hydrocodone, oxycodone, oxymorphone, ethylmorphine and buprenorphine;
- Fully synthetic opioids: such as fentanyl, pethidine, levorphanol, methadone, tramadol, tapentadol, and dextropropoxyphene;
- Endogenous opioid peptides, produced naturally in the body, such as endor-

phins, enkephalins, dynorphins, and endomorphins. Morphine, and some other opioids, which are produced in small amounts in the body, are included in this category.

Tramadol and tapentadol, which act as monoamine uptake inhibitors also act as mild and potent agonists (respectively) of the μ-opioid receptor. Both drugs produce analgesia even when naloxone, an opioid antagonist, is administered.

Some minor opium alkaloids and various substances with opioid action are also found elsewhere, including molecules present in kratom, *Corydalis*, and *Salvia divinorum* plants and some species of poppy aside from *Papaver somniferum*. There are also strains which produce copious amounts of thebaine, an important raw material for making many semi-synthetic and synthetic opioids. Of all of the more than 120 poppy species, only two produce morphine.

Amongst analgesics there are a small number of agents which act on the central nervous system but not on the opioid receptor system and therefore have none of the other (narcotic) qualities of opioids although they may produce euphoria by relieving pain—a euphoria that, because of the way it is produced, does not form the basis of habituation, physical dependence, or addiction. Foremost amongst these are nefopam, orphenadrine, and perhaps phenyltoloxamine or some other antihistamines. Tricyclic antidepressants have painkilling effect as well, but they're thought to do so by indirectly activating the endogenous opioid system. Paracetamol is predominantly a centrally acting analgesic (non-narcotic) which mediates its effect by action on descending serotoninergic (5-hydroxy triptaminergic) pathways, to increase 5-HT release (which inhibits release of pain mediators). It also decreases cyclo-oxygenase activity. It has recently been discovered that most or all of the therapeutic efficacy of paracetamol is due to a metabolite (AM404, making paracetamol a prodrug) which enhances the release of serotonin and also interacts with the cannabinoid receptors by inhibiting the uptake of anandamide.

Other analgesics work peripherally (i.e., not on the brain or spinal cord). Research is starting to show that morphine and related drugs may indeed have peripheral effects as well, such as morphine gel working on burns. Recent investigations discovered opioid receptors on peripheral sensory neurons. A significant fraction (up to 60%) of opioid analgesia can be mediated by such peripheral opioid receptors, particularly in inflammatory conditions such as arthritis, traumatic or surgical pain. Inflammatory pain is also blunted by endogenous opioid peptides activating peripheral opioid receptors.

It has been discovered in 1953, that the human body, as well as those of some other animals, naturally produce minute amounts of morphine and codeine and possibly some of their simpler derivatives like heroin and dihydromorphine, in addition to the well known endogenous opioid peptides. Some bacteria are capable of producing some semi-synthetic opioids such as hydromorphone and hydrocodone when living in a solution containing morphine or codeine respectively.

Many of the alkaloids and other derivatives of the opium poppy are not opioids or narcotics; the best example is the smooth-muscle relaxant papaverine. Noscapine is a marginal case as it does have CNS effects but not necessarily similar to morphine, and it is probably in a category all its own.

Dextromethorphan (the stereoisomer of levomethorphan, a semi-synthetic opioid agonist) and its metabolite dextrorphan have no opioid analgesic effect at all despite their structural similarity to other opioids; instead they are potent NMDA antagonists and sigma 1 and 2-receptor agonists and are used in many over-the-counter cough suppressants. Salvinorin A is a unique selective, powerful κ-opioid receptor agonist. It is not properly considered an opioid nevertheless, because:

1. chemically, it is not an alkaloid; and
2. it has no typical opioid properties: absolutely no anxiolytic or cough-suppressant effects. It is instead a powerful hallucinogen.

Endogenous Opioids

Opioid-peptides that are produced in the body include:

- Endorphins
- Enkephalins
- Dynorphins
- Endomorphins

β-endorphin is expressed in Pro-opiomelanocortin (POMC) cells in the arcuate nucleus, in the brainstem and in immune cells, and acts through μ-opioid receptors. β-endorphin has many effects, including on sexual behavior and appetite. β-endorphin is also secreted into the circulation from pituitary corticotropes and melanotropes. α-neo-endorphin is also expressed in POMC cells in the arcuate nucleus.

met-enkephalin is widely distributed in the CNS and in immune cells; [met]-enkephalin is a product of the proenkephalin gene, and acts through μ and δ-opioid receptors. leu-enkephalin, also a product of the proenkephalin gene, acts through δ-opioid receptors.

Dynorphin acts through κ-opioid receptors, and is widely distributed in the CNS, including in the spinal cord and hypothalamus, including in particular the arcuate nucleus and in both oxytocin and vasopressin neurons in the supraoptic nucleus.

Endomorphin acts through μ-opioid receptors, and is more potent than other endogenous opioids at these receptors.

Opium Alkaloids and Derivatives

Opium Alkaloids

Phenanthrenes naturally occurring in (opium):

- Codeine
- Morphine
- Thebaine
- Oripavine

Preparations of mixed opium alkaloids, including papaveretum, are still occasionally used.

Esters of Morphine

- Diacetylmorphine (morphine diacetate; heroin)
- Nicomorphine (morphine dinicotinate)
- Dipropanoylmorphine (morphine dipropionate)
- Diacetyldihydromorphine
- Acetylpropionylmorphine
- Desomorphine
- Methyldesorphine
- Dibenzoylmorphine

Ethers of Morphine

- Dihydrocodeine
- Ethylmorphine
- Heterocodeine

Semi-synthetic Alkaloid Derivatives

- Buprenorphine
- Etorphine
- Hydrocodone

- Hydromorphone
- Oxycodone
- Oxymorphone

Synthetic Opioids

Anilidopiperidines

- Fentanyl
- Alphamethylfentanyl
- Alfentanil
- Sufentanil
- Remifentanil
- Carfentanyl
- Ohmefentanyl

Phenylpiperidines

- Pethidine (meperidine)
- Ketobemidone
- MPPP
- Allylprodine
- Prodine
- PEPAP
- Promedol

Diphenylpropylamine Derivatives

- Propoxyphene
- Dextropropoxyphene
- Dextromoramide
- Bezitramide
- Piritramide

- Methadone
- Dipipanone
- Levomethadyl Acetate (LAAM)
- Difenoxin
- Diphenoxylate
- Loperamide (does cross the blood-brain barrier but is quickly pumped into the non-central nervous system by P-Glycoprotein. Mild opiate withdrawal in animal models exhibits this action after sustained and prolonged use including rhesus monkeys, mice, and rats).

Benzomorphan Derivatives

- Dezocine—agonist/antagonist
- Pentazocine—agonist/antagonist
- Phenazocine

Oripavine Derivatives

- Buprenorphine—partial agonist
- Dihydroetorphine
- Etorphine

Morphinan Derivatives

- Butorphanol—agonist/antagonist
- Nalbuphine—agonist/antagonist
- Levorphanol
- Levomethorphan
- Racemethorphan

Others

- Lefetamine
- Menthol (Kappa-Opioid agonist)
- Meptazinol

- Mitragynine
- Tilidine
- Tramadol
- Tapentadol
- Eluxadoline
- AP-237
- 7-Hydroxymitragynine

Allosteric Modulators

Plain allosteric modulators do not belong to the opioids, instead they are classified as opioidergics.

Opioid Antagonists

- Nalmefene
- Naloxone
- Naltrexone
- Methylnaltrexone (Methylnaltrexone is only peripherally active as it does not cross the blood-brain barrier in sufficient quantities to be centrally active. As such, it can be considered the antithesis of loperamide).
- Naloxegol (Naloxegol is only peripherally active as it does not cross the blood-brain barrier in sufficient quantities to be centrally active. As such, it can be considered the antitheses of loperamide).

Morphine

Morphine is a pain medication of the opiate type which is found naturally in a number of plants and animals. It acts directly on the central nervous system (CNS) to decrease the feeling of pain. It can be taken for both acute pain and chronic pain. Morphine is frequently used for pain from myocardial infarction and during labour. It can be given by mouth, by injection into a muscle, by injecting under the skin, intravenously, into the space around the spinal cord, or rectally. Maximum effect is around 20 min when given intravenously and 60 min when given by mouth while duration of effect is between three and 7 h. Long-acting formulations also exist.

Potentially serious side effects include a decreased respiratory effort and low blood pressure. Morphine has a high potential for addiction and abuse. If the dose is reduced after long-term use, withdrawal may occur. Common side effects include drowsiness, vomiting, and constipation. Caution is advised when used during pregnancy or breast feeding, as morphine will affect the baby.

Morphine was first isolated between 1803 and 1805 by Friedrich Sertürner. This is generally believed to be the first isolation of an active ingredient from a plant. Merck began marketing it commercially in 1827. Morphine was more widely used after the invention of the hypodermic syringe in 1853–1855. Sertürner originally named the substance *morphium* after the Greek god of dreams, Morpheus, as it has a tendency to cause sleep.

The primary source of morphine is isolation from poppy straw of the opium poppy. In 2013, an estimated 523,000 kilograms of morphine were produced. About 45 000 kg were used directly for pain, an increase over the last twenty years of four times. Most use for this purpose was in the developed world. About 70% of morphine is used to make other opioids such as hydromorphone, oxymorphone, and heroin. It is a Schedule II drug in the United States, Class A in the United Kingdom, and Schedule I in Canada. It is on the World Health Organization's List of Essential Medicines, the most effective and safe medicines needed in a health system. Morphine is sold under many trade names.

Medical Uses

Pain

Morphine is used primarily to treat both acute and chronic severe pain. It is also used for pain due to myocardial infarction and for labor pains. Its duration of analgesia is about three to seven hours.

However, concerns exist that morphine may increase mortality in the setting of non ST elevation myocardial infarction. Morphine has also traditionally been used in the treatment of acute pulmonary edema. A 2006 review, though, found little evidence to support this practice. A 2016 Cochrane review concluded that morphine is effective in relieving cancer pain. Side-effects of nausea and constipation are rarely severe enough to warrant stopping treatment.

Shortness of Breath

Immediate-release morphine is beneficial in reducing the symptom of shortness of breath due to both cancer and noncancer causes. In the setting of breathlessness at rest or on minimal exertion from conditions such as advanced cancer or end-stage cardiorespiratory diseases, regular, low-dose sustained-release morphine significantly reduces breathlessness safely, with its benefits maintained over time.

Opioid Use Disorder

Morphine is also available as a slow-release formulation for opiate substitution therapy

(OST) in Austria, Bulgaria, and Slovenia, for addicts who cannot tolerate either methadone or buprenorphine.

Contraindications

Relative contraindications to morphine include:

- Respiratory depression when appropriate equipment is not available
- Although it has previously been thought that morphine was contraindicated in acute pancreatitis, a review of the literature shows no evidence for this.

Adverse Effects of Opioids

Common and short term

- Itch
- Nausea
- Vomiting
- Constipation
- Drowsiness
- Dry mouth

Other

- Opioid dependence
- Dizziness
- Decreased sex drive
- Impaired sexual function
- Decreased testosterone levels
- Depression
- Immunodeficiency
- Opioid-induced abnormal pain sensitivity
- Irregular menstruation
- Increased risk of falls
- Slowed breathing

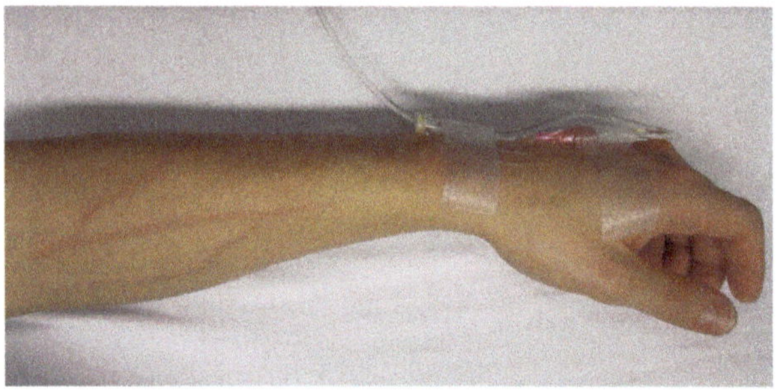

A localized reaction to intravenous morphine caused by histamine release in the veins

Constipation

Like loperamide and other opioids, morphine acts on the myenteric plexus in the intestinal tract, reducing gut motility, causing constipation. The gastrointestinal effects of morphine are mediated primarily by μ-opioid receptors in the bowel. By inhibiting gastric emptying and reducing propulsive peristalsis of the intestine, morphine decreases the rate of intestinal transit. Reduction in gut secretion and increased intestinal fluid absorption also contribute to the constipating effect. Opioids also may act on the gut indirectly through tonic gut spasms after inhibition of nitric oxide generation. This effect was shown in animals when a nitric oxide precursor, L-arginine, reversed morphine-induced changes in gut motility.

Hormone Imbalance

Clinical studies consistently conclude that morphine, like other opioids, often causes hypogonadism and hormone imbalances in chronic users of both sexes. This side effect is dose-dependent and occurs in both therapeutic and recreational users. Morphine can interfere with menstruation in women by suppressing levels of luteinizing hormone. Many studies suggest the majority (perhaps as much as 90%) of chronic opioid users have opioid-induced hypogonadism. This effect may cause the increased likelihood of osteoporosis and bone fracture observed in chronic morphine users. Studies suggest the effect is temporary. As of 2013, the effect of low-dose or acute use of morphine on the endocrine system is unclear.

Effects on Human Performance

Most reviews conclude that opioids produce minimal impairment of human performance on tests of sensory, motor, or attentional abilities. However, recent studies have been able to show some impairments caused by morphine, which is not surprising, given that morphine is a central nervous system depressant. Morphine has resulted in impaired functioning on critical flicker frequency (a measure of overall CNS arousal) and impaired performance on the Maddox wing test (a measure of deviation of the visual axes of the eyes). Few studies have investigated the effects of morphine on motor abilities; a high dose of morphine can impair finger tapping and the ability to maintain a low constant level of isometric force (i.e. fine motor control is impaired), though no studies have shown a correlation between morphine and gross motor abilities.

In terms of cognitive abilities, one study has shown that morphine may have a negative impact on anterograde and retrograde memory, but these effects are minimal and transient. Overall, it seems that acute doses of opioids in non-tolerant subjects produce minor effects in some sensory and motor abilities, and perhaps also in attention and cognition. It is likely that the effects of morphine will be more pronounced in opioid-naive subjects than chronic opioid users.

In chronic opioid users, such as those on Chronic Opioid Analgesic Therapy (COAT) for managing severe, chronic pain, behavioural testing has shown normal functioning on perception, cognition, coordination and behaviour in most cases. One 2000 study analysed COAT patients to determine whether they were able to safely operate a motor vehicle. The findings from this study suggest that stable opioid use does not significantly impair abilities inherent in driving (this includes physical, cognitive and perceptual skills). COAT patients showed rapid completion of tasks that require speed of responding for successful performance but made more errors than controls. COAT patients showed no deficits in visual-spatial perception and organization but did show impaired immediate and short-term visual memory. These patients showed no impairments in higher order cognitive abilities (i.e., planning). COAT patients appeared to have difficulty following instructions and showed a propensity toward impulsive behaviour, yet this did not reach statistical significance. It is important to note that this study reveals that COAT patients have no domain-specific deficits, which supports the notion that chronic opioid use has minor effects on psychomotor, cognitive, or neuropsychological functioning.

Reinforcement Disorders

Addiction

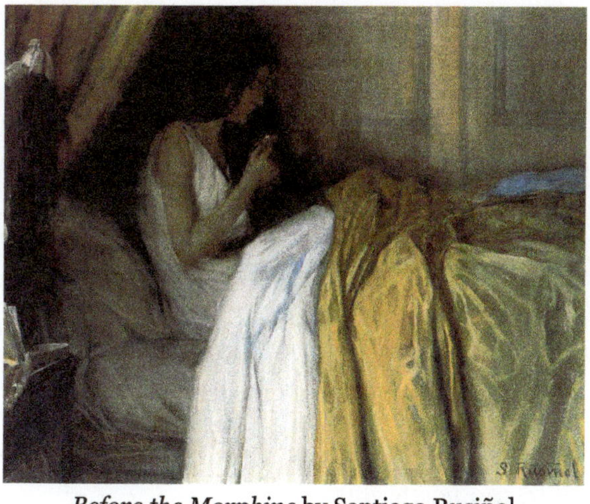

Before the Morphine by Santiago Rusiñol

Morphine is a highly addictive substance. In controlled studies comparing the physiological and subjective effects of heroin and morphine in individuals formerly addicted to opiates, subjects showed no preference for one drug over the other. Equipotent, injected doses had comparable action courses, with no difference in subjects' self-rated feelings of euphoria, ambition, nervousness, relaxation, drowsiness, or sleepiness. Short-term addiction studies by the same researchers demonstrated that tolerance developed at a similar rate to both heroin and morphine. When compared to the opioids hydromorphone, fentanyl, oxycodone, and pethidine/meperidine, former addicts showed a strong preference for heroin and morphine, suggesting that heroin and morphine are particularly susceptible to abuse and addiction. Morphine and heroin were also much more likely to produce euphoria and other positive subjective effects when compared to these other opioids. The choice of heroin and morphine over other opioids by former drug addicts may also be because heroin (also known as morphine diacetate, diamorphine, or diacetyl morphine) is an ester of morphine and a morphine prodrug, essentially meaning they are identical drugs *in vivo*. Heroin is converted to morphine before binding to the opioid receptors in the brain and spinal cord, where morphine causes the subjective effects, which is what the addicted individuals are seeking.

Tolerance

Several hypotheses are given about how tolerance develops, including opioid receptor phosphorylation (which would change the receptor conformation), functional decoupling of receptors from G-proteins (leading to receptor desensitization), μ-opioid receptor internalization or receptor down-regulation (reducing the number of available receptors for morphine to act on), and upregulation of the cAMP pathway (a counter-regulatory mechanism to opioid effects). CCK might mediate some counter-regulatory pathways responsible for opioid tolerance. CCK-antagonist drugs, specifically proglumide, have been shown to slow the development of tolerance to morphine.

Dependence and Withdrawal

Cessation of dosing with morphine creates the prototypical opioid withdrawal syndrome, which, unlike that of barbiturates, benzodiazepines, alcohol, or sedative-hypnotics, is not fatal by itself in neurologically healthy patients without heart or lung problems.

Acute morphine withdrawal, along with that of any other opioid, proceeds through a number of stages. Other opioids differ in the intensity and length of each, and weak opioids and mixed agonist-antagonists may have acute withdrawal syndromes that do not reach the highest level. As commonly cited, they are:

- Stage I, 6 to 14 hours after last dose: Drug craving, anxiety, irritability, perspiration, and mild to moderate dysphoria.

- Stage II, 14 to 18 hours after last dose: Yawning, heavy perspiration, mild depression, lacrimation, crying, headaches, runny nose, dysphoria, also intensification of the above symptoms, "yen sleep" (a waking trance-like state).
- Stage III, 16 to 24 hours after last dose: Rhinorrhea (runny nose) and increase in other of the above, dilated pupils, piloerection (goose bumps – a purported origin of the phrase, 'cold turkey,' but in fact the phrase originated outside of drug treatment), muscle twitches, hot flashes, cold flashes, aching bones and muscles, loss of appetite, and the beginning of intestinal cramping.
- Stage IV, 24 to 36 hours after last dose: Increase in all of the above including severe cramping and involuntary leg movements ("kicking the habit" also called restless leg syndrome), loose stool, insomnia, elevation of blood pressure, moderate elevation in body temperature, increase in frequency of breathing and tidal volume, tachycardia (elevated pulse), restlessness, nausea.
- Stage V, 36 to 72 hours after last dose: Increase in the above, fetal position, vomiting, free and frequent liquid diarrhea, which sometimes can accelerate the time of passage of food from mouth to out of system, weight loss of 2 to 5 kg per 24 hours, increased white cell count, and other blood changes.
- Stage VI, after completion of above: Recovery of appetite and normal bowel function, beginning of transition to postacute and chronic symptoms that are mainly psychological, but may also include increased sensitivity to pain, hypertension, colitis or other gastrointestinal afflictions related to motility, and problems with weight control in either direction.

In advanced stages of withdrawal, ultrasonographic evidence of pancreatitis has been demonstrated in some patients and is presumably attributed to spasm of the pancreatic sphincter of Oddi.

The withdrawal symptoms associated with morphine addiction are usually experienced shortly before the time of the next scheduled dose, sometimes within as early as a few hours (usually 6–12 hours) after the last administration. Early symptoms include watery eyes, insomnia, diarrhea, runny nose, yawning, dysphoria, sweating, and in some cases a strong drug craving. Severe headache, restlessness, irritability, loss of appetite, body aches, severe abdominal pain, nausea and vomiting, tremors, and even stronger and more intense drug craving appear as the syndrome progresses. Severe depression and vomiting are very common. During the acute withdrawal period, systolic and diastolic blood pressures increase, usually beyond premorphine levels, and heart rate increases, which have potential to cause a heart attack, blood clot, or stroke.

Chills or cold flashes with goose bumps ("cold turkey") alternating with flushing (hot flashes), kicking movements of the legs ("kicking the habit") and excessive sweating are also characteristic symptoms. Severe pains in the bones and muscles of the back and extremities occur, as do muscle spasms. At any point during this process, a suitable narcotic can be administered that will dramatically reverse the withdrawal symptoms. Major withdrawal symptoms peak between 48 and 96 hours after the last dose and subside after about 8 to 12 days. Sudden withdrawal by heavily dependent users who are in poor health is very rarely fatal. Morphine withdrawal is considered less dangerous than alcohol, barbiturate, or benzodiazepine withdrawal.

The psychological dependence associated with morphine addiction is complex and protracted. Long after the physical need for morphine has passed, the addict will usually continue to think and talk about the use of morphine (or other drugs) and feel strange or overwhelmed coping with daily activities without being under the influence of morphine. Psychological withdrawal from morphine is usually a very long and painful process. Addicts often suffer severe depression, anxiety, insomnia, mood swings, amnesia (forgetfulness), low self-esteem, confusion, paranoia, and other psychological disorders. Without intervention, the syndrome will run its course, and most of the overt physical symptoms will disappear within 7 to 10 days including psychological dependence. A high probability of relapse exists after morphine withdrawal when neither the physical environment nor the behavioral motivators that contributed to the abuse have been altered. Testimony to morphine's addictive and reinforcing nature is its relapse rate. Abusers of morphine (and heroin) have one of the highest relapse rates among all drug users, ranging up to 98% in the estimation of some medical experts.

Overdose

A large overdose can cause asphyxia and death by respiratory depression if the person does not receive medical attention immediately. Overdose treatment includes the administration of naloxone. The latter completely reverses morphine's effects, but may result in immediate onset of withdrawal in opiate-addicted subjects. Multiple doses may be needed.

The minimum lethal dose is 200 mg, but in case of hypersensitivity, 60 mg can bring sudden death. In serious drug dependency (high tolerance), 2000–3000 mg per day can be tolerated.

Pharmacology

Pharmacodynamics

Endogenous opioids include endorphins, enkephalins, dynorphins, and even morphine itself. Morphine appears to mimic endorphins. Endorphins, a contraction of the term endogenous morphines, are responsible for analgesia (reducing pain), causing sleepiness, and feelings of pleasure. They can be released in response to pain, strenuous exercise, orgasm, or excitement.

Morphine is the prototype narcotic drug and is the standard against which all other opioids are tested. It interacts predominantly with the μ–δ-opioid (Mu-Delta) receptor heteromer. The μ-binding sites are discretely distributed in the human brain, with high densities in the posterior amygdala, hypothalamus, thalamus, nucleus caudatus, putamen, and certain cortical areas. They are also found on the terminal axons of primary afferents within laminae I and II (substantia gelatinosa) of the spinal cord and in the spinal nucleus of the trigeminal nerve.

Morphine is a phenanthrene opioid receptor agonist – its main effect is binding to and activating the μ-opioid receptors in the central nervous system. In clinical settings, morphine exerts its principal pharmacological effect on the central nervous system and gastrointestinal tract. Its primary actions of therapeutic value are analgesia and sedation. Activation of the μ-opioid receptors is associated with analgesia, sedation, euphoria, physical dependence, and respiratory depression. Morphine is a rapid-acting narcotic, and it is known to bind very strongly to the μ-opioid receptors, and for this reason, it often has a higher incidence of euphoria/dysphoria, respiratory depression, sedation, pruritus, tolerance, and physical and psychological dependence when compared to other opioids at equianalgesic doses. Morphine is also a κ-opioid and δ-opioid receptor agonist, κ-opioid's action is associated with spinal analgesia, miosis (pinpoint pupils) and psychotomimetic effects. δ-Opioid is thought to play a role in analgesia. Although morphine does not bind to the σ-receptor, it has been shown that σ-agonists, such as (+)-pentazocine, inhibit morphine analgesia, and σ-antagonists enhance morphine analgesia, suggesting downstream involvement of the σ-receptor in the actions of morphine.

The effects of morphine can be countered with opioid antagonists such as naloxone and naltrexone; the development of tolerance to morphine may be inhibited by NMDA antagonists such as ketamine or dextromethorphan. The rotation of morphine with chemically dissimilar opioids in the long-term treatment of pain will slow down the growth of tolerance in the longer run, particularly agents known to have significantly incomplete cross-tolerance with morphine such as levorphanol, ketobemidone, piritramide, and methadone and its derivatives; all of these drugs also have NMDA antagonist properties. It is believed that the strong opioid with the most incomplete cross-tolerance with morphine is either methadone or dextromoramide.

Gene Expression

Studies have shown that morphine can alter the expression of a number of genes. A single injection of morphine has been shown to alter the expression of two major groups of genes, for proteins involved in mitochondrial respiration and for cytoskeleton-related proteins.

Effects on the Immune System

Morphine has long been known to act on receptors expressed on cells of the central nervous system resulting in pain relief and analgesia. In the 1970s and '80s, evidence suggesting that opioid drug addicts show increased risk of infection (such as increased pneumonia, tuberculosis, and HIV/AIDS) led scientists to believe that morphine may also affect the immune system. This possibility increased interest in the effect of chronic morphine use on the immune system.

The first step of determining that morphine may affect the immune system was to establish that the opiate receptors known to be expressed on cells of the central nervous system are also expressed on cells of the immune system. One study successfully showed that dendritic cells, part of the innate immune system, display opiate receptors. Dendritic cells are responsible for producing cytokines, which are the tools for communication in the immune system. This same study showed that dendritic cells chronically treated with morphine during their differentiation produce more interleukin-12 (IL-12), a cytokine responsible for promoting the proliferation, growth, and differentiation of T-cells (another cell of the adaptive immune system) and less interleukin-10 (IL-10), a cytokine responsible for promoting a B-cell immune response (B cells produce antibodies to fight off infection).

This regulation of cytokines appear to occur via the p38 MAPKs (mitogen-activated protein kinase)-dependent pathway. Usually, the p38 within the dendritic cell expresses TLR 4 (toll-like receptor 4), which is activated through the ligand LPS (lipopolysaccharide). This causes the p38 MAPK to be phosphorylated. This phosphorylation activates the p38 MAPK to begin producing IL-10 and IL-12. When the dendritic cells are chronically exposed to morphine during their differentiation process then treated with LPS, the production of cytokines is different. Once treated with morphine, the p38 MAPK does not produce IL-10, instead favoring production of IL-12. The exact mechanism through which the production of one cytokine is increased in favor over another is not known. Most likely, the morphine causes increased phosphorylation of the p38 MAPK. Transcriptional level interactions between IL-10 and IL-12 may further increase the production of IL-12 once IL-10 is not being produced. This increased production of IL-12 causes increased T-cell immune response.

Further studies on the effects of morphine on the immune system have shown that morphine influences the production of neutrophils and other cytokines. Since cytokines are produced as part of the immediate immunological response (inflammation), it has been suggested that they may also influence pain. In this way, cytokines may be a logical target for analgesic development. Recently, one study has used an animal model (hind-paw incision) to observe the effects of morphine administration on the acute immunological response. Following hind-paw incision, pain thresholds and cytokine production were measured. Normally, cytokine production in and around the wounded area increases in order to fight infection and control healing (and, possibly, to control pain), but pre-incisional morphine administration (0.1–10.0 mg/kg) reduced the number of cytokines found around the wound in a dose-dependent manner. The authors suggest that morphine administration in the acute post-injury period may reduce resistance to infection and may impair the healing of the wound.

Pharmacokinetics

Absorption and Metabolism

Morphine can be taken orally, sublingually, bucally, rectally, subcutaneously, intranasally, intravenously, intrathecally or epidurally and inhaled via a nebulizer. As a recreational drug, it is becoming more common to inhale ("Chasing the Dragon"), but, for medical purposes, intravenous (IV) injection is the most common method of administration. Morphine is subject to extensive first-pass metabolism (a large proportion is broken down in the liver), so, if taken orally, only 40% to 50% of the dose reaches the central nervous system. Resultant plasma levels after subcutaneous (SC), intramuscular (IM), and IV injection are all comparable. After IM or SC injections, morphine plasma levels peak in approximately 20 min, and, after oral administration, levels peak in approximately 30 min. Morphine is metabolised primarily in the liver and approximately 87% of a dose of morphine is excreted in the urine within 72 h of administration. Morphine is metabolized primarily into morphine-3-glucuronide (M3G) and morphine-6-glucuronide (M6G) via glucuronidation by phase II metabolism enzyme UDP-glucuronosyl transferase-2B7 (UGT2B7). About 60% of morphine is converted to M3G, and 6% to 10% is converted to M6G. Not only does the metabolism occur in the liver but it may also take place in the brain and the kidneys. M3G does not undergo opioid receptor binding and has no analgesic effect. M6G binds to μ-receptors and is half as potent an analgesic as morphine in humans. Morphine may also be metabolized into small amounts of normorphine, codeine, and hydromorphone. Metabolism rate is determined by gender, age, diet, genetic makeup, disease state (if any), and use of other medications. The elimination half-life of morphine is approximately 120 min, though there may be slight differences between men and women. Morphine can be stored in fat, and, thus, can be detectable even after death. Morphine can cross the blood–brain barrier, but, because of poor lipid solubility, protein binding, rapid conjugation with glucuronic acid and ionization, it does not cross easily. Diacetylmorphine, which is derived from morphine, crosses the blood–brain barrier more easily, making it more potent.

Extended-release

There are extended-release formulations of orally administered morphine whose effect last longer, which can be given once per day. Brand names for this formulation of morphine include Avinza, Kadian, MS Contin and Dolcontin. For constant pain, the relieving effect of extended-release morphine given once (for Kadian) or twice (for MS Contin) every 24 hours is roughly the same as multiple administrations of *immediate release* (or "regular") morphine. Extended-release morphine can be administered together with "rescue doses" of immediate-release morphine as needed in case of breakthrough pain, each generally consisting of 5% to 15% of the 24-hour extended-release dosage.

Detection in Body Fluids

Morphine and its major metabolites, morphine-3-glucuronide and morphine-6-glucuronide, can be detected in blood, plasma, hair, and urine using an immunoassay. Chromatography can be used to test for each of these substances individually. Some testing procedures hydrolyze metabolic products into morphine before the immunoassay, which must be considered when comparing morphine levels in separately published results. Morphine can also be isolated from whole blood samples by solid phase extraction (SPE) and detected using liquid chromatography-mass spectrometry (LC-MS).

Ingestion of codeine or food containing poppy seeds can cause false positives.

A 1999 review estimated that relatively low doses of heroin (which metabolizes immediately into morphine) are detectable by standard urine tests for 1-1.5 days after use. A 2009 review determined that, when the analyte is morphine and the limit of detection is 1 ng/ml, a 20 mg intravenous (IV) dose of morphine is detectable for 12–24 hours. A limit of detection of 0.6 ng/ml had similar results.

Natural Occurrence

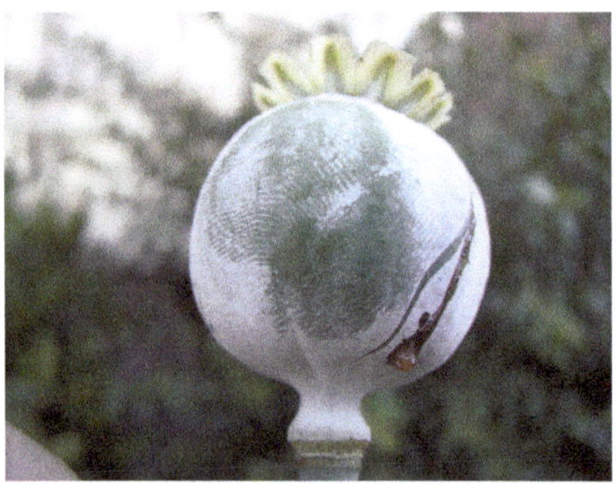

A freshly-scored opium poppy seedpod bleeding latex.

Morphine is the most abundant opiate found in opium, the dried latex extracted by shallowly scoring the unripe seedpods of the *Papaver somniferum* poppy. Morphine is generally 8–14% of the dry weight of opium, although specially bred cultivars reach 26% or produce little morphine at all (under 1%, perhaps down to 0.04%). The latter varieties, including the 'Przemko' and 'Norman' cultivars of the opium poppy, are used to produce two other alkaloids, thebaine and oripavine, which are used in the manufacture of semi-synthetic and synthetic opioids like oxycodone and etorphine and some other types of drugs. *P. bracteatum* does not contain morphine or codeine, or other narcotic phenanthrene-type, alkaloids. This species is rather a source of thebaine. Occurrence of morphine in other Papaverales and Papaveraceae, as well as in some species of hops and mulberry trees has not been confirmed. Morphine is produced most predominantly early in the life cycle of the plant. Past the optimum point for extraction, various processes in the plant produce codeine, thebaine, and in some cases negligible amounts of hydromorphone, dihydromorphine, dihydrocodeine, tetrahydro-thebaine, and hydrocodone (these compounds are rather synthesized from thebaine and oripavine).

In the brain of mammals, morphine is detectable in trace steady-state concentrations. The human body also produces endorphins, which are chemically related endogenous opioid peptides that function as neuropeptides and have similar effects as morphine.

Human Biosynthesis

Morphine is an endogenous opioid in humans that can be synthesized and released by white blood cells. CYP2D6, a cytochrome P450 isoenzyme, catalyzes the biosynthesis of morphine from codeine and dopamine from tyramine along the biosynthetic pathway of morphine in humans. The morphine biosynthetic pathway in humans occurs as follows:

L-tyrosine → *para*-tyramine or L-DOPA → dopamine → (*S*)-norlaudanosoline → (*S*)-reticuline → 1,2-dehydroretinulinium → (*R*)-reticuline → salutaridine → salutaridinol → thebaine → neopinone → codeinone → codeine → morphine

(*S*)-Norlaudanosoline (also known as tetrahydropapaveroline) can also be synthesized from 3,4-dihydroxyphenylacetaldehyde (DOPAL), a metabolite of L-DOPA and dopamine. Urinary concentrations of endogenous codeine and morphine have been found to significantly increase in individuals taking L-DOPA for the treatment of Parkinson's disease.

Biosynthesis in the Opium Poppy

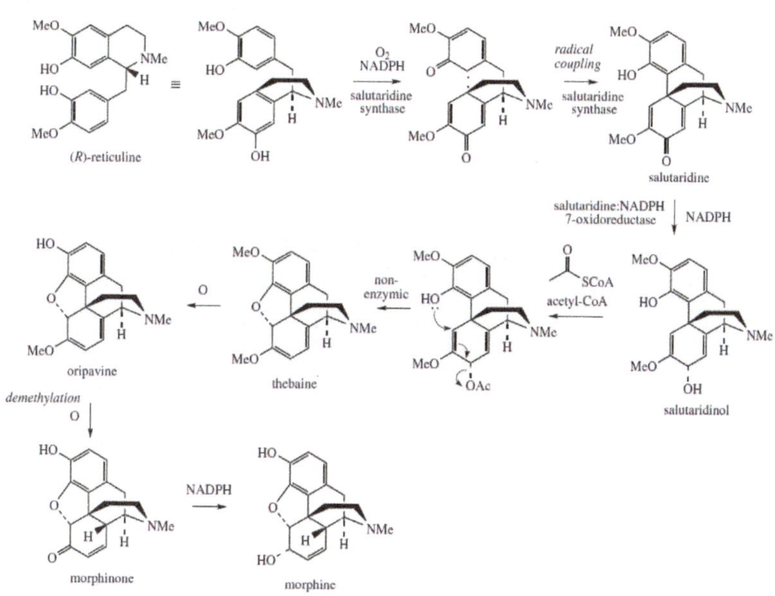

Morphine biosynthesis in the opium poppy

Morphine is biosynthesized in the opium poppy from the tetrahydroisoquinoline reticuline. It is converted into salutaridine, thebaine, and oripavine. The enzymes involved in this process are the salutaridine synthase, salutaridine:NADPH 7-oxidoreductase and the codeinone reductase. Researchers are attempting to reproduce the biosynthetic pathway that produces morphine in genetically engineered yeast. In June 2015 the *S*-reticuline could be produced from sugar and *R*-reticuline could be converted to morphine, but the intermediate reaction could not be performed. In August 2015 the first complete synthesis of thebaine and hydrocodone in yeast were reported, but the process would need to be 100,000 times more productive to be suitable for commercial use.

Chemistry

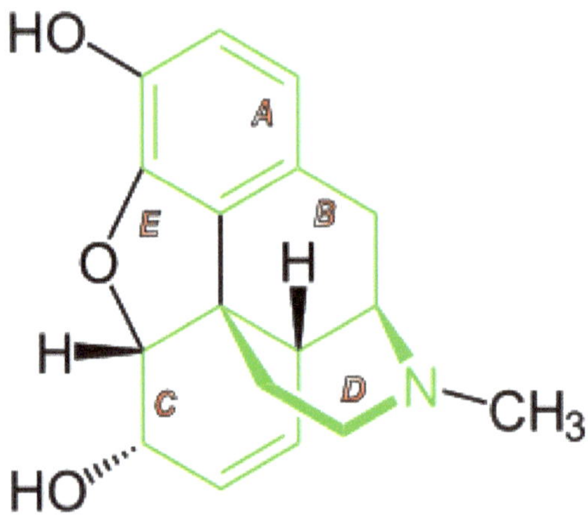

Chemical structure of morphine. The benzylisoquinoline backbone is shown in green.

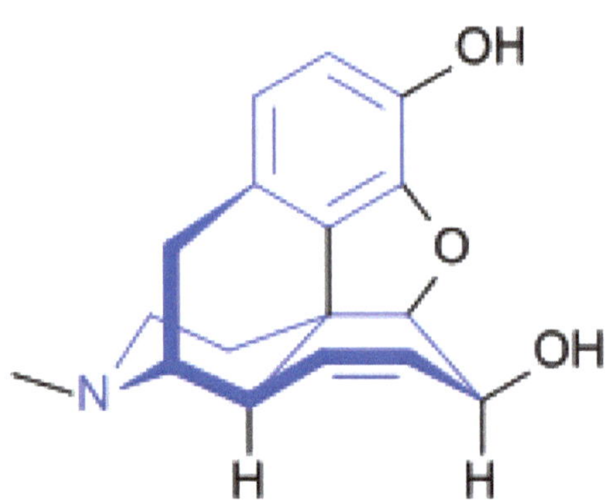

Same structure with correct 3D configuration; backbone in blue.

Morphine is a benzylisoquinoline alkaloid with two additional ring closures. It has:

- A rigid pentacyclic structure consisting of a benzene ring (A), two partially unsaturated cyclohexane rings (B and C), a piperidine ring (D) and a tetrahydrofuran ring (E). Rings A, B and C are the phenanthrene ring system. This ring system has little conformational flexibility.

- Two hydroxyl functional groups: a C3-phenolic OH (pK_a 9.9) and a C6-allylic OH,
- An ether linkage between C4 and C5,
- Unsaturation between C7 and C8,
- A basic, tertiary amine function at position 17,
- 5 centers of chirality (C5, C6, C9, C13 and C14) with morphine exhibiting a high degree of stereoselectivity of analgesic action.

Most of the licit morphine produced is used to make codeine by methylation. It is also a precursor for many drugs including heroin (3,6-diacetylmorphine), hydromorphone (dihydromorphinone), and oxymorphone (14-hydroxydihydromorphinone); many morphine derivatives can also be manufactured using thebaine or codeine as a starting material. Replacement of the *N*-methyl group of morphine with an *N*-phenylethyl group results in a product that is 18 times more powerful than morphine in its opiate agonist potency. Combining this modification with the replacement of the 6-hydroxyl with a 6-methylene group produces a compound some 1,443 times more potent than morphine, stronger than the Bentley compounds such as etorphine (M99, the Immobilon tranquilliser dart) by some measures.

The structure-activity relationship of morphine has been extensively studied. As a result of the extensive study and use of this molecule, more than 250 morphine derivatives (also counting codeine and related drugs) have been developed since the last quarter of the 19th century. These drugs range from 25% the analgesic strength of codeine (or slightly more than 2% of the strength of morphine) to several thousand times the strength of morphine, to powerful opioid antagonists, including naloxone (Narcan), naltrexone (Trexan), diprenorphine (M5050, the reversing agent for the Immobilon dart) and nalorphine (Nalline). Some opioid agonist-antagonists, partial agonists, and inverse agonists are also derived from morphine. The receptor-activation profile of the semi-synthetic morphine derivatives varies widely and some, like apomorphine are devoid of narcotic effects.

Morphine and most of its derivatives do not exhibit optical isomerism, although some more distant relatives like the morphinan series (levorphanol, dextorphan and the racemic parent chemical dromoran) do, and as noted above stereoselectivity in vivo is an important issue.

Morphine-derived agonist–antagonist drugs have also been developed. Elements of the morphine structure have been used to create completely synthetic drugs such as the morphinan family (levorphanol, dextromethorphan and others) and other groups that have many members with morphine-like qualities. The modification of morphine and the aforementioned synthetics has also given rise to non-narcotic drugs with other uses such as emetics, stimulants, antitussives, anticholinergics, muscle relaxants, local anaesthetics, general anaesthetics, and others.

Most semi-synthetic opioids, both of the morphine and codeine subgroups, are created by modifying one or more of the following:

- Halogenating or making other modifications at positions 1 or 2 on the morphine carbon skeleton.
- The methyl group that makes morphine into codeine can be removed or added back, or replaced with another functional group like ethyl and others to make codeine analogues of morphine-derived drugs and vice versa. Codeine analogues of morphine-based drugs often serve as prodrugs of the stronger drug, as in codeine and morphine, hydrocodone and hydromorphone, oxycodone and oxymorphone, nicocodeine and nicomorphine, dihydrocodeine and dihydromorphine, etc.
- Saturating, opening, or other changes to the bond between positions 7 and 8, as well as adding, removing, or modifying functional groups to these positions; saturating, reducing, eliminating, or otherwise modifying the 7–8 bond and attaching a functional group at 14 yields hydromorphinol; the oxidation of the hydroxyl group to a carbonyl and changing the 7–8 bond to single from double changes codeine into oxycodone.
- Attachment, removal or modification of functional groups to positions 3 or 6 (dihydrocodeine and related, hydrocodone, nicomorphine); in the case of moving the methyl functional group from position 3 to 6, codeine becomes heterocodeine, which is 72 times stronger, and therefore six times stronger than morphine.
- Attachment of functional groups or other modification at position 14 (oxymorphone, oxycodone, naloxone).
- Modifications at positions 2, 4, 5 or 17, usually along with other changes to the molecule elsewhere on the morphine skeleton. Often this is done with drugs produced by catalytic reduction, hydrogenation, oxidation, or the like, producing strong derivatives of morphine and codeine.

Both morphine and its hydrated form, $C_{17}H_{19}NO_3H_2O$, are sparingly soluble in water. In five liters of water, only one gram of the hydrate will dissolve. For this reason, pharmaceutical companies produce sulfate and hydrochloride salts of the drug, both of which are over 300 times more water-soluble than their parent molecule. Whereas the pH of a saturated morphine hydrate solution is 8.5, the salts are acidic. Since they derive from a strong acid but weak base, they are both at about pH = 5; as a consequence, the morphine salts are mixed with small amounts of NaOH to make them suitable for injection.

A number of salts of morphine are used, with the most common in current clinical use being the hydrochloride, sulfate, tartrate, and citrate; less commonly methobromide, hydrobromide, hydroiodide, lactate, chloride, and bitartrate and the others listed below. Morphine diacetate, which is another name for heroin, is a Schedule I controlled substance, so it is not used clinically in the United States; it is a sanctioned medication in the United Kingdom and in Canada and some countries in Continental Europe, its use being particularly common (nearly to the degree of the hydrochloride salt) in the United Kingdom. Morphine meconate is a major form of the alkaloid in the poppy, as is morphine pectinate, nitrate, sulphate, and some others. Like codeine, dihydrocodeine and other (especially older) opiates, morphine has been used as the salicylate salt by some suppliers and can be easily compounded, imparting the therapeutic advantage of both the opioid and the NSAID; multiple barbiturate salts of morphine were also used in the past, as was/is morphine valerate, the salt of the acid being the active principle of valerian. Calcium morphenate is the intermediate in various latex and poppy-straw methods of morphine production, more rarely sodium morphenate takes its place. Morphine ascorbate and other salts such as the tannate, citrate, and acetate, phosphate, valerate and others may be present in poppy tea depending on the method of preparation. Morphine valerate produced industrially was one ingredient of a medication available for both oral and parenteral administration popular many years ago in Europe and elsewhere called Trivalin, which also included the valerates of caffeine and cocaine, with a version containing codeine valerate as a fourth ingredient being distributed under the name Tetravalin.

Closely related to morphine are the opioids morphine-*N*-oxide (genomorphine), which is a pharmaceutical that is no longer in common use; and pseudomorphine, an alkaloid that exists in opium, form as degradation products of morphine.

The salts listed by the United States Drug Enforcement Administration for reporting purposes, in addition to a few others, are as follows:

Synthesis

The first morphine total synthesis, devised by Marshall D. Gates, Jr. in 1952, remains a widely used example of total synthesis. Several other syntheses were reported, notably by the research groups of Rice, Evans, Fuchs, Parker, Overman, Mulzer-Trauner, White, Taber, Trost, Fukuyama, Guillou, and Stork. It is "highly unlikely" that a chemical synthesis will ever be able to compete with the cost of producing morphine from the opium poppy.

Production

In the opium poppy, the alkaloids are bound to meconic acid. The method is to extract from the crushed plant with diluted sulfuric acid, which is a stronger acid than meconic acid, but not so strong to react with alkaloid molecules. The extraction is performed in many steps (one amount of crushed plant is extracted at least six to ten times, so practically every alkaloid goes into the solution). From the solution obtained at the last extraction step, the alkaloids are precipitated by either ammonium hydroxide or sodium carbonate. The last step is purifying and separating morphine from other opium alkaloids. The somewhat similar Gregory process was developed in the United Kingdom during the Second World War, which begins with stewing the entire plant, in most cases save the roots and leaves, in plain or mildly acidified water, then proceeding through steps of concentration, extraction, and purification of alkaloids. Other methods of processing "poppy straw" (i.e., dried pods and stalks) use steam, one or more of several types of alcohol, or other organic solvents.

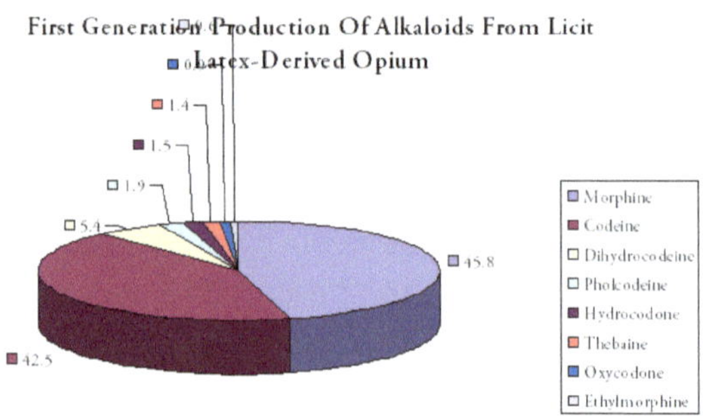

First generation production of Alkaloids from licit latex-derived opium

The poppy straw methods predominate in Continental Europe and the British Commonwealth, with the latex method in most common use in India. The latex method can involve either vertical or horizontal slicing of the unripe pods with a two-to five-bladed knife with a guard developed specifically for this purpose to the depth of a fraction of a millimetre and scoring of the pods can be done up to five times. An alternative latex method sometimes used in China in the past is to cut off the poppy heads, run a large needle through them, and collect the dried latex 24 to 48 hours later.

In India, opium harvested by licensed poppy farmers is dehydrated to uniform levels of hydration at government processing centers, and then sold to pharmaceutical companies that extract morphine from the opium. However, in Turkey and Tasmania, morphine is obtained by harvesting and processing the fully mature dry seed pods with attached stalks, called *poppy straw*. In Turkey, a water extraction process is used, while in Tasmania, a solvent extraction process is used.

Opium poppy contains at least 50 different alkaloids, but most of them are of very low concentration. Morphine is the principal alkaloid in raw opium and constitutes roughly 8–19% of opium by dry weight (depending on growing conditions). Some purpose-developed strains of poppy now produce opium that is up to 26% morphine by weight. A rough rule of thumb to determine the morphine content of pulverised dried poppy straw is to divide the percentage expected for the strain or crop via the latex method by eight or an empirically determined factor, which is often in the range of 5 to 15. The Norman strain of *P. Somniferum*, also developed in Tasmania, produces down to 0.04% morphine but with much higher amounts of thebaine and oripavine, which can be used to synthesise semi-synthetic opioids as well as other drugs like stimulants, emetics, opioid antagonists, anticholinergics, and smooth-muscle agents.

In the 1950s and 1960s, Hungary supplied nearly 60% of Europe's total medication-purpose morphine production. To this day, poppy farming is legal in Hungary, but poppy farms are limited by law to 2 acres (8,100 m^2). It is also legal to sell dried poppy in flower shops for use in floral arrangements.

It was announced in 1973 that a team at the National Institutes of Health in the United States had developed a method for total synthesis of morphine, codeine, and thebaine using coal tar as a starting material. A shortage in codeine-hydrocodone class cough suppressants (all of which can be made from morphine in one or more steps, as well as from codeine or thebaine) was the initial reason for the research.

Most morphine produced for pharmaceutical use around the world is actually converted into codeine as the concentration of the latter in both raw opium and poppy straw is much lower than that of morphine; in most countries, the usage of codeine (both as end-product and precursor) is at least equal or greater than that of morphine on a weight basis.

Precursor to Other Opioids

Pharmaceutical

Morphine is a precursor in the manufacture in a large number of opioids such as dihydromorphine, hydromorphone, hydrocodone, and oxycodone as well as codeine, which itself has a large family of semi-synthetic derivatives. Morphine is commonly treated with acetic anhydride and ignited to yield heroin. Throughout Europe there is growing acceptance within the medical community of the use of slow release oral morphine as a substitution treatment alternative to methadone and buprenorphine for patients not able to tolerate the side-effects of buprenorphine and methadone. Slow-release oral morphine has been in widespread use for opiate maintenance therapy in Austria, Bulgaria, and Slovakia for many years and it is available on a small scale in many other countries including the UK. The long-acting nature of slow-release morphine mimics that of buprenorphine because the sustained blood levels are relatively flat so there is no "high" per se that a patient would feel but rather a sustained feeling of wellness and avoidance of withdrawal symptoms. For patients sensitive to the side-effects that in part may be a result of the unnatural pharmacological actions of buprenorphine and methadone, slow-release oral morphine formulations offer a promising future for use managing opiate addiction. The pharmacology of heroin and morphine is identical except the two acetyl groups increase the lipid solubility of the heroin molecule, causing heroin to cross the blood–brain barrier and enter the brain more rapidly in injection. Once in the brain, these acetyl groups are removed to yield morphine, which causes the subjective effects of heroin. Thus, heroin may be thought of as a more rapidly acting form of morphine.

Illicit

Illicit morphine is rarely produced from codeine found in over-the-counter cough and pain medicines. This demethylation reaction is often performed using pyridine and hydrochloric acid.

Another source of illicit morphine comes from the extraction of morphine from extended-release morphine products, such as MS-Contin. Morphine can be extracted from these products with simple extraction techniques to yield a morphine solution that can be injected. As an alternative, the tablets can be crushed and snorted, injected or swallowed, although this provides much less euphoria but retains some of the extended-release effect, and the extended-release property is why MS-Contin is used in some countries alongside methadone, dihydrocodeine, buprenorphine, dihydroetorphine, piritramide, levo-alpha-acetylmethadol (LAAM), and special 24-hour formulations of hydromorphone for maintenance and detoxification of those physically dependent on opioids.

Another means of using or misusing morphine is to use chemical reactions to turn it into heroin or another stronger opioid. Morphine can, using a technique reported in New Zealand (where the initial precursor is codeine) and elsewhere known as home-bake, be turned into what is usually a mixture of morphine, heroin, 3-monoacetylmorphine, 6-monoacetylmorphine, and codeine derivatives like acetylcodeine if the process is using morphine made from demethylating codeine.

Since heroin is one of a series of 3,6 diesters of morphine, it is possible to convert morphine to nicomorphine (Vilan) using nicotinic anhydride, dipropanoylmorphine with propionic anhydride, dibutanoylmorphine and disalicyloylmorphine with the respective acid anhydrides. Glacial acetic acid can be used to obtain a mixture high in 6-monoacetylmorphine, niacin (vitamin B_3) in some form would be precursor to 6-nicotinylmorphine, salicylic acid may yield the salicyoyl analogue of 6-MAM, and so on.

The clandestine conversion of morphine to ketones of the hydromorphone class or other derivatives like dihydromorphine (Paramorfan), desomorphine (Permonid), metopon, etc. and codeine to hydrocodone (Dicodid), dihydrocodeine (Paracodin), etc. is more involved, time-consuming, requires lab equipment of various types, and usually requires expensive catalysts and large amounts of morphine at the outset and is less common but still has been discovered by authorities in various ways during the last 20 years or so. Dihydromorphine can be acetylated into another 3,6 morphine diester, namely diacetyldihydromorphine (Paralaudin), and hydrocodone into thebacon.

History

An opium-based elixir has been ascribed to alchemists of Byzantine times, but the specific formula was lost during the Ottoman conquest of Constantinople (Istanbul). Around 1522, Paracelsus made reference to an opium-based elixir that he called *lau-*

danum from the Latin word *laudare*, meaning "to praise" He described it as a potent painkiller, but recommended that it be used sparingly. In the late eighteenth century, when the East India Company gained a direct interest in the opium trade through India, another opiate recipe called laudanum became very popular among physicians and their patients.

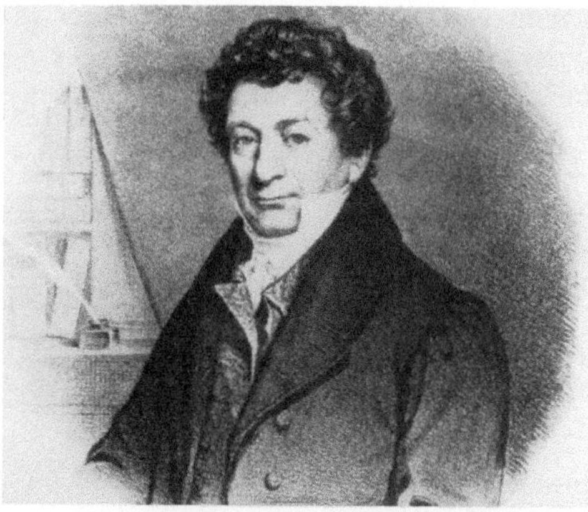

Friedrich Sertürner

Morphine was discovered as the first active alkaloid extracted from the opium poppy plant in December 1804 in Paderborn, Germany, by Friedrich Sertürner. In 1817 Sertürner reported experiments in which he administered morphine to himself, three young boys, three dogs, and a mouse; all four people almost died. Sertürner originally named the substance *morphium* after the Greek god of dreams, Morpheus as it has a tendency to cause sleep.

The drug was first marketed to the general public by Sertürner and Company in 1817 as a pain medication, and also as a treatment for opium and alcohol addiction. It was first used as a poison in 1822 when Dr. Edme Castaing of France was convicted of murdering a patient. Commercial production began in Darmstadt, Germany in 1827 by the pharmacy that became the pharmaceutical company Merck, with morphine sales being a large part of their early growth. In the 1850s Alexander Wood reported that he had injected morphine into his wife as an experiment; his wife died from respiratory depression.

Later it was found that morphine was more addictive than either alcohol or opium, and its extensive use during the American Civil War allegedly resulted in over 400,000 sufferers from the "soldier's disease" of morphine addiction. This idea has been a subject of controversy, as there have been suggestions that such a disease was in fact a fabrication; the first documented use of the phrase "soldier's disease" was in 1915.

Diacetylmorphine (better known as heroin) was synthesized from morphine in 1874 and brought to market by Bayer in 1898. Heroin is approximately 1.5 to 2 times more potent than morphine weight for weight. Due to the lipid solubility of diacetylmorphine, it can cross the blood–brain barrier faster than morphine, subsequently increasing the reinforcing component of addiction. Using a variety of subjective and objective measures, one study estimated the relative potency of heroin to morphine administered intravenously to post-addicts to be 1.80–2.66 mg of morphine sulfate to 1 mg of diamorphine hydrochloride (heroin).

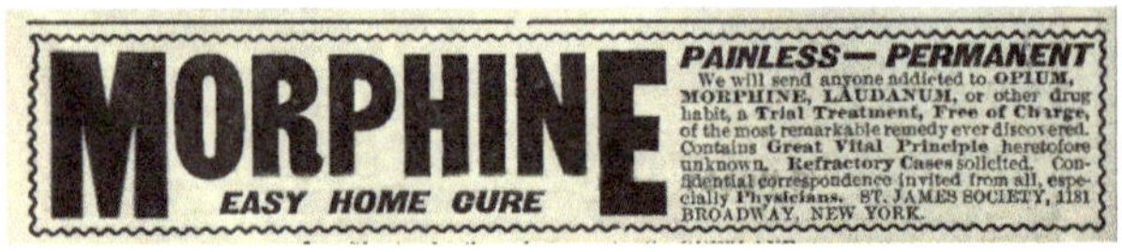

Advertisement for curing morphine addiction, ca. 1900

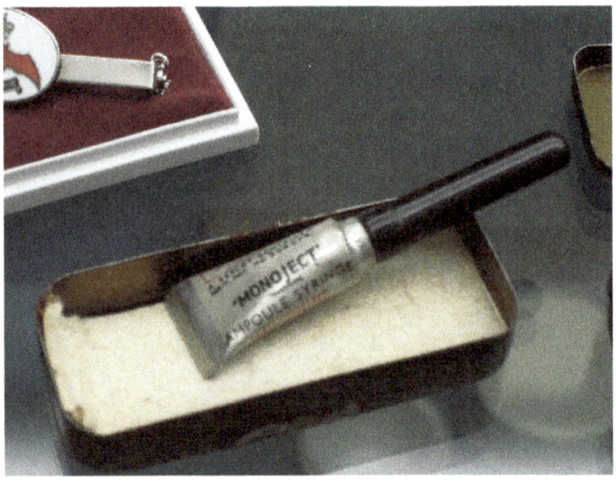

An ampoule of morphine with integral needle for immediate use. Also known as a "syrette". From WWII. On display at the Army Medical Services Museum.

Morphine became a controlled substance in the US under the Harrison Narcotics Tax Act of 1914, and possession without a prescription in the US is a criminal offense. Morphine was the most commonly abused narcotic analgesic in the world until heroin was synthesized and came into use. In general, until the synthesis of dihydromorphine (ca. 1900), the dihydromorphinone class of opioids (1920s), and oxycodone (1916) and similar drugs, there were no other drugs in the same efficacy range as opium, morphine, and heroin, with synthetics still several years away (pethidine was invented in Germany in 1937) and opioid agonists among the semi-synthetics were analogues and derivatives of codeine such as dihydrocodeine (Paracodin), ethylmorphine (Dionine), and benzylmorphine (Peronine). Even today, morphine is the most sought after prescription narcotic by heroin addicts when heroin is scarce, all other things being equal; local conditions and user preference may cause hydromorphone, oxymorphone, high-dose oxycodone, or methadone as well as dextromoramide in specific instances such as 1970s Australia, to top that particular list. The stop-gap drugs used by the largest absolute number of heroin addicts is probably codeine, with significant use also of dihydrocodeine, poppy straw derivatives like poppy pod and poppy seed tea, propoxyphene, and tramadol.

The structural formula of morphine was determined by 1925 by Robert Robinson. At least three methods of total synthesis of morphine from starting materials such as coal tar and petroleum distillates have been patented, the first of which was announced in 1952, by Dr. Marshall D. Gates, Jr. at the University of Rochester. Still, the vast majority of morphine is derived from the opium poppy by either the traditional method of gathering latex from the scored, unripe pods of the poppy, or processes using poppy straw, the dried pods and stems of the plant, the most widespread of which was invented in Hungary in 1925 and announced in 1930 by the chemist János Kabay.

In 2003, there was discovery of endogenous morphine occurring naturally in the human body. Thirty years of speculation were made on this subject because there was a receptor that, it appeared, reacted only to morphine: the μ_3-opioid receptor in human tissue. Human cells that form in reaction to cancerous neuroblastoma cells have been found to contain trace amounts of endogenous morphine.

Society and Culture

Legal Status

- In Australia, morphine is classified as a Schedule 8 drug under the variously titled State and Territory Poisons Acts.
- In Canada, morphine is classified as a Schedule I drug under the Controlled Drugs and Substances Act.
- In France, morphine is in the strictest schedule of controlled substances, based upon the December 1970 French controlled substances law.
- In Germany, morphine is a *verkehrsfähiges und verschreibungsfähiges Betäubungsmittel* listed under *Anlage III* (the equivalent of CSA Schedule II) of the Betäubungsmittelgesetz.
- In Switzerland, morphine is similarly scheduled to Germany's legal classification of the drug.
- In Japan, morphine is classified as a narcotic under the Narcotics and Psychotropics Control Act.
- In the Netherlands, morphine is classified as a List 1 drug under the Opium Law.
- In the United Kingdom, morphine is listed as a Class A drug under the Misuse of Drugs Act 1971 and a Schedule 2 Controlled Drug under the Misuse of Drugs Regulations 2001.
- In the United States, morphine is classified as a Schedule II controlled substance under the Controlled Substances Act with a main Administrative Con-

trolled Substances Code Number (ACSCN) of ACSCN 9300. Morphine pharmaceuticals in the US are subject to annual manufacturing quotas; morphine production for use in extremely dilute formulations and its production as an intermediate, or chemical precursor, for conversion into other drugs is excluded from the US manufacturing quota.

- Internationally (UN), morphine is a Schedule I drug under the Single Convention on Narcotic Drugs.

Non-medical Use

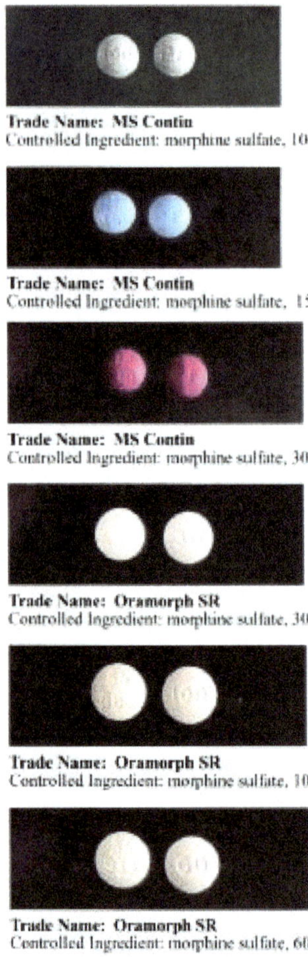

Example of different morphine tablets

The euphoria, comprehensive alleviation of distress and therefore all aspects of suffering, promotion of sociability and empathy, “body high”, and anxiolysis provided by narcotic drugs including the opioids can cause the use of high doses in the absence of pain for a protracted period, which can impart a morbid craving for the drug in the user. Being the prototype of the entire opioid class of drugs means that morphine has properties that may lend it to misuse. Morphine addiction is the model upon which the current perception of addiction is based.

Animal and human studies and clinical experience back up the contention that morphine is one of the most euphoric drugs known, and via all but the IV route heroin and morphine cannot be distinguished according to studies because heroin is a prodrug for the delivery of systemic morphine. Chemical changes to the morphine molecule yield other euphorigenics such as dihydromorphine, hydromorphone (Dilaudid, Hydal), and oxymorphone (Numorphan, Opana), as well as the latter three's methylated equivalents dihydrocodeine, hydrocodone, and oxycodone, respectively; in addition to heroin, there are dipropanoylmorphine, diacetyldihydromorphine, and other members of the 3,6 morphine diester category like nicomorphine and other similar semi-synthetic opiates like desomorphine, hydromorphinol, etc. used clinically in many countries of the world but in many cases also produced illicitly in rare instances.

In general, non-medical use of morphine entails taking more than prescribed or outside of medical supervision, injecting oral formulations, mixing it with unapproved potentiators such as alcohol, cocaine, and the like, or defeating the extended-release mechanism by chewing the tablets or turning into a powder for snorting or preparing injectables. The latter method can be as time-consuming and involved as traditional methods of smoking opium. This and the fact that the liver destroys a large percentage of the drug on the first pass impacts the demand side of the equation for clandestine re-sellers, as many customers are not needle users and may have been disappointed with ingesting the drug orally. As morphine is generally as hard or harder to divert than oxycodone in a lot of cases, morphine in any form is uncommon on the street, although ampoules and phials of morphine injection, pure pharmaceutical morphine powder, and soluble multi-purpose tablets are very popular where available.

Morphine is also available in a paste that is used in the production of heroin, which can be smoked by itself or turned to a soluble salt and injected; the same goes for the penultimate products of the Kompot (Polish Heroin) and black tar processes. Poppy straw as well as opium can yield morphine of purity levels ranging from poppy tea to near-pharmaceutical-grade morphine by itself or with all of the more than 50 other alkaloids. It also is the active narcotic ingredient in opium and all of its forms, derivatives, and analogues as well as forming from breakdown of heroin and otherwise present in many batches of illicit heroin as the result of incomplete acetylation.

Slang Terms

Informal names for morphine include: Cube Juice, Dope, Dreamer, Emsel, First Line, God's Drug, Hard Stuff, Hocus, Hows, Lydia, Lydic, M, Miss Emma, Mister Blue, Monkey, Morf, Morph, Morphide, Morphie, Morpho, Mother, MS, Ms. Emma, Mud, New Jack Swing (if mixed with heroin), Sister, Tab, Unkie, Unkie White, and Stuff.

MS Contin tablets are known as misties, and the 100 mg extended-release tablets as greys and blockbusters. The "speedball" can use morphine as the opioid component, which is combined with cocaine, amphetamines, methylphenidate, or similar drugs. "Blue Velvet" is a combination of morphine with the antihistamine tripelennamine (Pyrabenzamine, PBZ, Pelamine) taken by injection, or less commonly the mixture when swallowed or used as a retention enema; the name is also known to refer to a combination of tripelennamine and dihydrocodeine or codeine tablets or syrups taken by mouth. "Morphia" is an older official term for morphine also used as a slang term. "Driving Miss Emma" is intravenous administration of morphine. Multi-purpose tablets (readily soluble hypodermic tablets that can also be swallowed or dissolved under the tongue or betwixt the cheek and jaw) are known, as are some brands of hydromorphone, as Shake & Bake or Shake & Shoot.

Morphine can be smoked, especially diacetylmorphine (heroin), the most common method being the "Chasing The Dragon" method. To perform a relatively crude acetylation to turn the morphine into heroin and related drugs immediately prior to use is known as AAing (for Acetic Anhydride) or home-bake, and the output of the procedure also known as home-bake or, Blue Heroin.

Trade Names

Morphine is marketed under many different brand names in various parts of the world.

Access in Developing Countries

Although morphine is cheap, people in poorer countries often do not have access to it. According to a 2005 estimate by the International Narcotics Control Board, six countries (Australia, Canada, France, Germany, the United Kingdom, and the United States) consume 79% of the world's morphine. The less affluent countries, accounting for 80% of the world's population, consumed only about 6% of the global morphine supply. Some countries import virtually no morphine, and in others the drug is rarely available even for relieving severe pain while dying.

Experts in pain management attribute the under-distribution of morphine to an unwarranted fear of the drug's potential for addiction and abuse. While morphine is clearly addictive, Western doctors believe it is worthwhile to use the drug and then wean the patient off when the treatment is over.

References

- Satoskar, R. S.; Rege, Nirmala; Bhandarkar, S. D. (2015). Pharmacology and Pharmacotherapeutics. Elsevier Health Sciences. ISBN 9788131243718
- Simone Rossi, ed. (2006). Australian medicines handbook 2006. Adelaide: Australian Medicines Handbook Pty Ltd. ISBN 0-9757919-2-3
- Clive P. Page, Michael J. Curtis, Morley Sutter, Michael Walker, Brian Hoffman. Farmacología integrada (in Spanish). Published by Elsevier España, 1998. ISBN 84-8174-340-2

- Bayer HealthCare Pharmaceuticals Inc (September 2008). "CIPRO (ciprofloxacin hydrochloride) TABLETS CIPRO,(ciprofloxacin*) ORAL SUSPENSION" (PDF). USA: FDA. Retrieved 31 August 2009
- Thomas MC (February 2000). "Diuretics, ACE inhibitors and NSAIDs—the triple whammy". The Medical journal of Australia. 172 (4): 184–5. ISSN 0025-729X. PMID 10772593
- Staff (9 July 2015). "FDA Strengthens Warning of Heart Attack and Stroke Risk for Non-Steroidal Anti-Inflammatory Drugs". FDA. Retrieved 9 July 2015
- Royal Pharmaceutical Society of Great Britain (2009). "5 Infections". British National Formulary (BNF 57). BMJ Group and RPS Publishing. ISBN 978-0-85369-845-6
- Reza Nakhai-Pour, Hamid. "Use of nonaspirin nonsteroidal anti-inflammatory drugs during pregnancy and the risk of spontaneous abortion" (PDF). Canadian Medical Association Journal. Retrieved 7 September 2011
- "Non-Steroidal Anti-Inflammatory Drugs (NSAIDs) in Metal Complexes and Their Effect at the Cellular Level". European Journal of Inorganic Chemistry. 2016: 3048–3071. doi:10.1002/ejic.201501480
- Cathy S. Jewell; Chambers, James Q.; Chearney, Lee Ann; Romaine, Deborah S.; Candace B. Levy (2007). The Facts on File encyclopedia of health and medicine. New York: Facts on File. ISBN 0-8160-6063-0
- Shionoiri H (July 1993). "Pharmacokinetic drug interactions with ACE inhibitors". Clinical pharmacokinetics. 25 (1): 20–58. doi:10.2165/00003088-199325010-00003. PMID 8354016. Retrieved 30 November 2012
- Glanze, Walter D.; Anderson, Kenneth; Anderson, Lois E. (1998). Mosby's medical, nursing, & allied health dictionary. St. Louis: Mosby. ISBN 0-8151-4800-3
- Knights, Kathleen. "Defining the COX Inhibitor Selectivity of NSAIDs: Implications for Understanding Toxicity". Web MD LLC. Retrieved 17 February 2013
- Loeser, John David; Bonica, John J.; Butler, Stephen H.; Chapman, C. Richard (2001). Bonica's Management of Pain (3 ed.). Philadelphia, PA: Lippincott Williams & Wilkins. p. 772. ISBN 0-683-30462-3
- Wexler RE (1968). "Analgizer: Inhaler for supervised self-administration of inhalation anesthesia". Abbott Park, Illinois: Abbott Laboratories. Retrieved 2010-11-21
- Benzon, Honorio; Raja, Srinivasa N.; Fishman, Scott E.; Liu, Spencer; Cohen, Steven P. (2011). Essentials of Pain Medicine. Elsevier Health Sciences. p. 85. ISBN 1437735932

5

Anesthesia: An Overview

Anesthesia is given to a patient to temporarily make them unconscious. It can be of various types like general anesthesia, local anesthesia and spinal anesthesia. This chapter is an overview of the subject matter incorporating all the major aspects of anesthesia.

Anesthesia

In the practice of medicine (especially surgery and dentistry), anesthesia or anaesthesia is a state of temporary induced loss of sensation or awareness. It may include analgesia (relief from or prevention of pain), paralysis (muscle relaxation), amnesia (loss of memory), or unconsciousness. A patient under the effects of anesthetic drugs is referred to as being anesthetized.

Anesthesia enables the painless performance of medical procedures that would cause severe or intolerable pain to an unanesthetized patient. Three broad categories of anaesthesia exist:

- General anesthesia suppresses central nervous system activity and results in unconsciousness and total lack of sensation.
- Sedation suppresses the central nervous system to a lesser degree, inhibiting both anxiety and creation of long-term memories without resulting in unconsciousness.
- Regional anesthesia and local anesthesia, which block transmission of nerve impulses between a targeted part of the body and the central nervous system, causing loss of sensation in the targeted body part. A patient under regional or local anesthesia remains conscious, unless general anaesthesia or sedation is administered at the same time. Two broad classes exist:
    - Peripheral blockade inhibits sensory perception in an isolated part of the body, such as numbing a tooth for dental work or administering a nerve block to inhibit sensation in an entire limb.
    - Central, or neuraxial, blockade administers the anesthetic in the region of the central nervous system itself, suppressing incoming sensation from out-

side the area of the block. Examples include epidural anaesthesia and spinal anaesthesia.

In preparing for a medical procedure, the health care provider giving anesthesia chooses and determines the doses of one or more drugs to achieve the types and degree of anesthesia characteristics appropriate for the type of procedure and the particular patient. The types of drugs used include general anesthetics, hypnotics, sedatives, neuromuscular-blocking drugs, narcotic, and analgesics.

There are both major and minor risks of anesthesia. Examples of major risks include death, heart attack and pulmonary embolism whereas minor risks can include postoperative nausea and vomiting and hospital readmission. The likelihood of a complication occurring is proportional to the relative risk of a variety of factors related to the patient's health, the complexity of the surgery being performed and the type of anesthetic used. Of these factors, the person's health prior to surgery (stratified by the ASA physical status classification system) has the greatest bearing on the probability of a complication occurring. Patients typically wake within minutes of an anesthetic being terminated and regain their senses within hours. One exception is a condition called long-term post-operative cognitive dysfunction, characterized by persistent confusion lasting weeks or months, which is more common in those undergoing cardiac surgery and in the elderly.

Medical uses

The purpose of anesthesia can be distilled down to three basic goals or end points:

- hypnosis (a temporary loss of consciousness and with it a loss of memory. In a pharmacological context, the word hypnosis usually has this technical meaning, in contrast to its more familiar lay or psychological meaning of an altered state of consciousness not necessarily caused by drugs).
- analgesia (lack of sensation which also blunts autonomic reflexes).
- muscle relaxation.

Different types of anesthesia affect the endpoints differently. Regional anesthesia, for instance, affects analgesia; benzodiazepine-type sedatives (used in twilight sleep) favor amnesia; and general anesthetics can affect all of the endpoints. The goal of anesthesia is to achieve the endpoints required for the given surgical procedure with the least risk to the patient.

To achieve the goals of anesthesia, drugs act on different but interconnected parts of the nervous system. Hypnosis, for instance, is generated through actions on the nuclei in the brain and is similar to the activation of sleep. The effect is to make people less aware and less reactive to noxious stimuli.

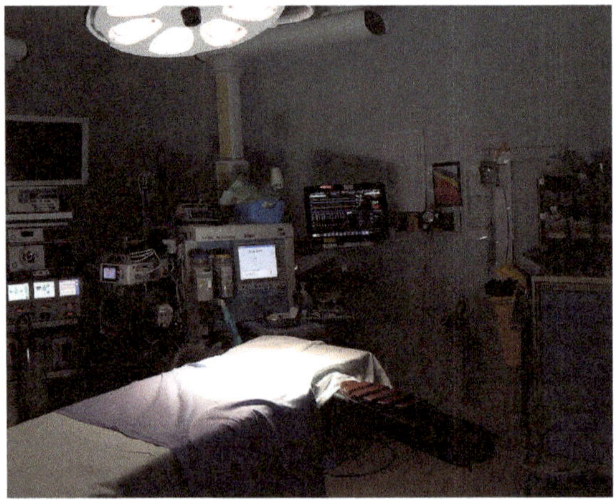

The anesthetic area of an operating room

Loss of memory (amnesia) is created by action of drugs on multiple (but specific) regions of the brain. Memories are created as either declarative or non-declarative memories in several stages (short-term, long-term, long-lasting) the strength of which is determined by the strength of connections between neurons termed synaptic plasticity. Each anesthetic produces amnesia through unique effects on memory formation at variable doses. Inhalational anesthetics will reliably produce amnesia through general suppression of the nuclei at doses below those required for loss of consciousness. Drugs like midazolam produce amnesia through different pathways by blocking the formation of long-term memories.

Tied closely to the concepts of amnesia and hypnosis is the concept of consciousness. Consciousness is the higher order process that synthesizes information. For instance, the "sun" conjures up feelings, memories and a sensation of warmth rather than a description of a round, orange warm ball seen in the sky for part of a 24hour cycle. Likewise, a person can have dreams (a state of subjective consciousness) during anesthetic or have consciousness of the procedure despite having no indication of it under anesthetic. It is estimated that 22% of people dream during general anesthesia and 1 or 2 cases per 1000 have some consciousness termed "awareness during general anesthesia".

Techniques

Anesthesia is unique, in that it is not a direct means of treatment, rather it allows others to do things that may treat, diagnose, or cure an ailment which would otherwise be painful or complicated. The best anesthetic, therefore is the one with the lowest risk to the patient that still achieves the endpoints required to complete the procedure. The first stage of an anesthetic is the pre-operative risk assessment made up of the medical history, physical examination and lab tests. Diagnosing a person's pre-operative physical status allows the clinician to minimize anesthetic risks. A well completed medical history will arrive at the correct diagnosis 56% of the time which increases to 73% with a physical examination. Lab tests help in diagnosis but only in 3% of cases, underscoring the need for a full history and physical examination prior to anesthetics. Incorrect pre-operative assessments or preparations are the root cause of 11% of all adverse anesthetic events.

One part of the risk assessment is based on the patients' health. The American Society of Anesthesiologists have developed a six-tier scale which stratifies the pre-operative physical state of the patient called the ASA physical status. The scale assesses a high-order of risk as the patient's general health relates to an anesthetic.

The more detailed pre-operative medical history aims to discover genetic disorders (such as malignant hyperthermia or pseudocholinesterase deficiency), habits (tobacco, drug and alcohol use), physical attributes (such as obesity or a difficult airway) and any coexisting diseases (especially cardiac and respiratory diseases) that might impact the anesthetic. The physical examination helps quantify the impact of anything found in the medical history in addition to lab tests.

Aside from the generalities of the patients health assessment, an evaluation of the specific factors as they relate to the surgery also need to be considered for anesthesia. For instance, anesthesia during childbirth must consider not only the mother but the baby. Cancers and tumors that occupy the lungs or throat create special challenges to general anesthesia. After determining the health of the person undergoing anesthetic and the endpoints that are required to complete the procedure, the type of anesthetic can be selected. Choice of surgical method and anaesthetic technique aims to reduce risk of complications, shorten time needed for recovery and minimise the surgical stress response.

Equipment

The core instrument in an inhalational anesthetic delivery system is an anesthetic machine. It has vaporizers, ventilators, an anesthetic breathing circuit, waste gas scavenging system and pressure gauges. The purpose of the anesthetic machine is to provide anesthetic gas at a constant pressure, oxygen for breathing and to remove carbon dioxide or other waste anesthetic gases. Since inhalational anaesthetics are flammable, various checklists have been developed to confirm that the machine is ready for use, that the safety features are active and the electrical hazards are removed. Intravenous anesthetic is delivered either by bolus doses or an infusion pump. There are also many smaller instruments used in airway management and monitoring the patient. The common thread to modern machinery in this field is the use of fail-safe systems that decrease the odds of catastrophic misuse of the machine.

Monitoring

Patients under general anesthesia must undergo continuous physiological monitoring to ensure safety. In the US, the American Society of Anesthesiologists (ASA) have established minimum monitoring guidelines for patients receiving general anesthesia, regional anesthesia, or sedation. This includes electrocardiography (ECG), heart rate, blood pressure, inspired and expired gases, oxygen saturation of the blood (pulse oximetry), and temperature. In the UK the Association of Anaesthetists (AAGBI) have set minimum monitoring guidelines for general and regional anesthesia. For minor surgery, this generally includes monitoring of heart rate, oxygen saturation, blood pressure, and inspired and expired concentrations for oxygen, carbon dioxide, and inhalational anesthetic agents. For more invasive surgery, monitoring may also include temperature, urine output, blood pressure, central venous pressure, pulmonary artery pressure and pulmonary artery occlusion pressure, cardiac output, cerebral activity, and neuromuscular function. In addition, the operating room environment must be monitored for ambient temperature and humidity, as well as for accumulation of exhaled inhalational anesthetic agents, which might be deleterious to the health of operating room personnel.

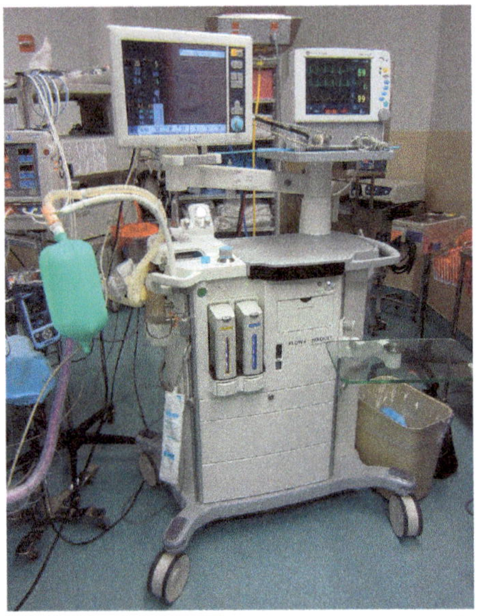

An anesthetic machine with integrated systems for monitoring of several vital parameters.

Sedation

Sedation (also referred to as *dissociative anesthesia* or *twilight anesthesia*) creates hypnotic, sedative, anxiolytic, amnesic, anticonvulsant, and centrally produced muscle-relaxing properties. From the perspective of the person giving the sedation, the patient will appear sleepy, relaxed and forgetful, allowing unpleasant procedures to be more easily completed. Sedatives such as benzodiazepines are usually given with pain relievers (such as narcotics, or local anesthetics or both) because they don't, by themselves, provide significant pain relief.

From the perspective of the person receiving sedative, the effect is a feeling of general relaxation, amnesia (loss of memory) and time passing quickly. Many drugs can produce a sedative effect including benzodiazepines, propofol, thiopental, ketamine and inhaled general anesthetics. The advantage of sedation over a general anesthetic is that it generally does not require support of the airway or breathing (no tracheal intubation or mechanical ventilation) and can have less of an effect on the cardiovascular system which may add to a greater margin of safety in some patients.

Regional Anesthesia

When pain is blocked from a part of the body using local anesthetics, it is generally referred to as regional anesthesia. There are many types of regional anesthesia either by injecting into the tissue itself, a vein that feeds the area or around a nerve trunk that supplies sensation to the area. The latter are called nerve blocks and are divided into peripheral or central nerve blocks.

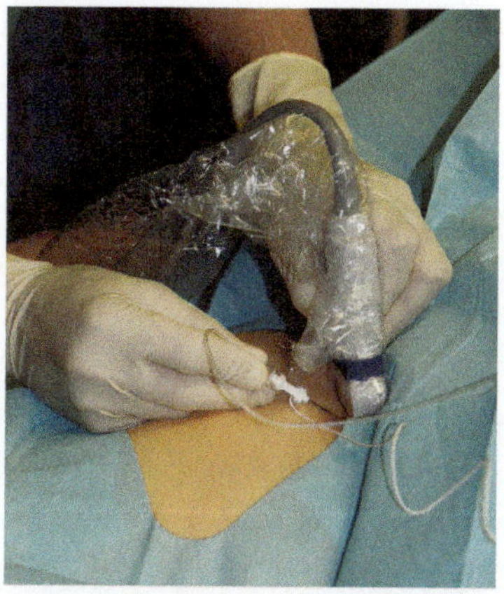

Sonography guided femoral nerve block

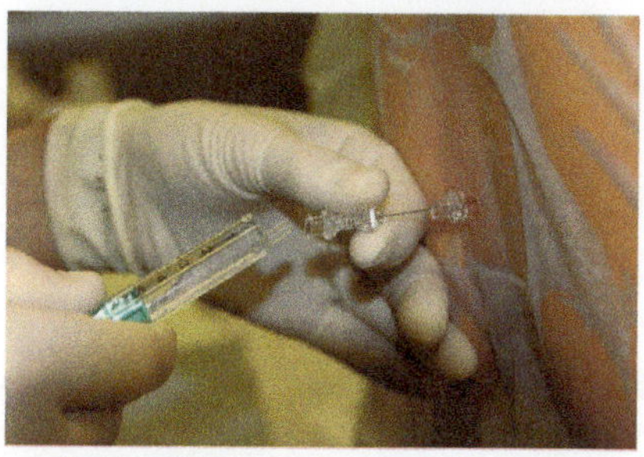

Backflow of cerebrospinal fluid through a spinal needle after puncture of the arachnoid mater during spinal anaesthesia

The following are the types of regional anesthesia:

- *Infiltrative anesthesia*: a small amount of local anesthetic is injected in a small area to stop any sensation (such as during the closure of a laceration, as a continuous infusion or "freezing" a tooth). The effect is almost immediate.
- *Peripheral nerve block*: local anesthetic is injected near a nerve that provides sensation to particular portion of the body. There is significant variation in the speed of onset and duration of anesthesia depending on the potency of the drug (e.g. Mandibular block).

- *Intravenous regional anesthesia* (also called a Bier block): dilute local anesthetic is infused to a limb through a vein with a tourniquet placed to prevent the drug from diffusing out of the limb.
- *Central nerve blockade*: Local anesthetic is injected or infused in or around a portion of the central nervous system (discussed in more detail below in Spinal, epidural and caudal anesthesia).
- *Topical anesthesia*: local anesthetics that are specially formulated to diffuse through the mucous membranes or skin to give a thin layer of analgesia to an area (e.g. EMLA patches).
- *Tumescent anesthesia*: a large amount of very dilute local anesthetics are injected into the subcutaneous tissues during liposuction.
- *Systemic local anesthetics*: local anesthetics are given systemically (orally or intravenous) to relieve neuropathic pain.

Nerve Blocks

When local anesthetic is injected around a larger diameter nerve that transmits sensation from an entire region it is referred to as a nerve block. Nerve blocks are commonly used in dentistry, when the mandibular nerve is blocked for procedures on the lower teeth. With larger diameter nerves (such as the interscalene block for upper limbs or psoas compartment block for lower limbs) the nerve and position of the needle is localized with ultrasound or electrical stimulation. The use of ultrasound may reduce complication rates and improve quality, performance time, and time to onset of blocks. Because of the large amount of local anesthetic required to affect the nerve, the maximum dose of local anesethetic has to be considered. Nerve blocks are also used as a continuous infusion, following major surgery such as knee, hip and shoulder replacement surgery, and may be associated with lower complications. Nerve blocks are also associated with a lower risk of neurologic complications when compared to neuraxial blocks.

Spinal, Epidural and Caudal Anesthesia

Central neuraxial anesthesia is the injection of local anesthetic around the spinal cord to provide analgesia in the abdomen, pelvis or lower extremities. It is divided into either spinal (injection into the subarachnoid space), epidural (injection outside of the subarachnoid space into the epidural space) and caudal (injection into the cauda equina or tail end of the spinal cord). Spinal and epidural are the most commonly used forms of central neuraxial blockade.

Spinal anesthesia is a "one-shot" injection that provides rapid onset and profound sensory anesthesia with lower doses of anesethetic, and is usually associated with neuromuscular blockade (loss of muscle control). Epidural anesthesia uses larger doses of anesthetic infused through an indwelling catheter which allows the anesthetic to be augmented should the effects begin to dissipate. Epidural anesthesia does not typically affect muscle control.

Because central neuraxial blockade causes arterial and vasodilation, a drop in blood pressure is common. This drop is largely dictated by the venous side of the circulatory system which holds 75% of the circulating blood volume. The physiologic effects are much greater when the block is placed above the 5th thoracic vertebra. An ineffective block is most often due to inadequate anxiolysis or sedation rather than a failure of the block itself.

Acute Pain Management

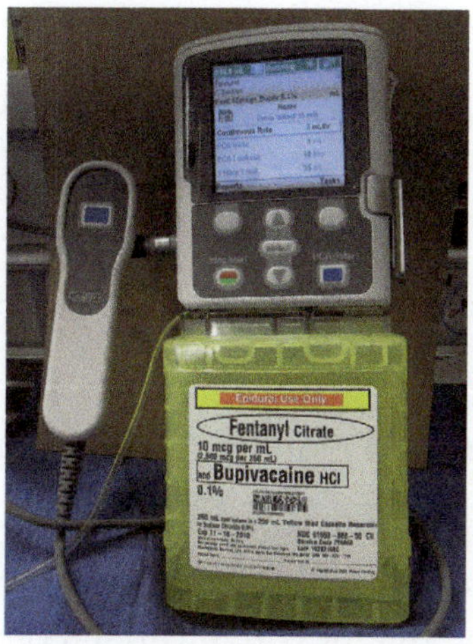

Pain that is well managed during and immediately after surgery improves the health of patients (by decreasing physiologic stress) and the potential for chronic pain. Nociception (pain sensation) is not hard-wired into the body. Instead, it is a dynamic process wherein persistent painful stimuli can sensitize the system and either make pain management difficult or promote the development of chronic pain. For this reason, preemptive acute pain management may reduce both acute and chronic pain and is tailored to the surgery, the environment in which it is given (in-patient/out-patient) and the individual patient.

Pain management is classified into either pre-emptive or on-demand. On-demand pain medications typically include either opioid or non-steroidal anti-inflammatory drugs but can also make use of novel approaches such as inhaled nitrous oxide or ketamine. On demand drugs can be administered by a clinician ("as needed drug orders") or by the patient using patient-controlled analgesia (PCA). PCA has been shown to provide slightly better pain control and increased patient satisfaction when compared with conventional methods. Common preemptive approaches include epidural neuraxial blockade or nerve blocks. One review which looked at pain control after abdominal aortic surgery found that epidural blockade provides better pain relief (especially during movement) in the period up to three postoperative days. It reduces the duration of postoperative tracheal intubation by roughly half. The occurrence of prolonged postoperative mechanical ventilation and myocardial infarction is also reduced by epidural analgesia.

Risks and Complications

Risks and complications as they relate to anesthesia are classified as either morbidity (a disease or disorder that results from anesthesia) or mortality (death that results from anesthesia). Attempting to quantify how anesthesia contributes to morbidity and mortality can be difficult because a person's health prior to surgery and the complexity of the surgical procedure can also contribute to the risks.

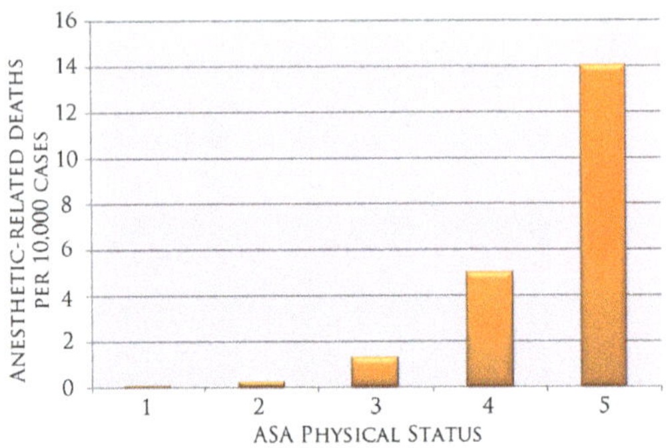

Anesthesia-related deaths by ASA status

Prior to the introduction of anesthesia in the early 19th century, the physiologic stress from surgery caused significant complications and many deaths from shock. The faster the surgery was, the lower the rate of complications (leading to reports of very quick amputations). The advent of anesthesia allowed more complicated and life-saving surgery to be completed, decreased the physiologic stress of the surgery, but added an element of risk. It was two years after the introduction of ether anesthetics that the first death directly related to the use of anesthesia was reported.

Morbidity can be major (myocardial infarction, pneumonia, pulmonary embolism, renal failure/insufficiency, postoperative cognitive dysfunction and allergy) or minor (minor nausea, vomiting, readmission). There is usually overlap in the contributing factors that lead to morbidity and mortality between the health of the patient, the surgery being performed and the anesthetic. To understand the relative risk of each contributing factor, consider that the rate of deaths totally attributed to the patient's health is 1:870. Compare that to the rate of deaths totally attributed to surgical factors (1:2860) or anesthesia alone (1:185,056) illustrating that the single greatest factor in anesthetic mortality is the health of the patient. These statistics can also be compared to the first such study on mortality in anesthesia from 1954, which reported a rate of death from all causes at 1:75 and a rate attributed to anesthesia alone at 1:2680. Direct comparisons between mortality statistics cannot reliably be made over time and across countries because of differences in the stratification of risk factors, however, there is evidence that anesthetics have made a significant improvement in safety but to what degree is uncertain.

Rather than stating a flat rate of morbidity or mortality, many factors are reported as contributing to the relative risk of the procedure and anesthetic combined. For instance, an operation on a person who is between the ages of 60–79 years old places the patient at 2.32 times greater risk than someone less than 60 years old. Having an ASA score of 3, 4 or 5 places the person at 10.65 times greater risk than someone with an ASA score of 1 or 2. Other variables include age greater than 80 (3.29 times risk compared to those under 60), gender (females have a lower risk of 0.77), urgency of the procedure (emergencies have a 4.44 times greater risk), experience of the person completing the procedure (less than 8 years experience and/or less than 600 cases have a 1.06 times greater risk) and the type of anesthetic (regional anesthetics are lower risk than general anesthetics). Obstetrical, the very young and the very old are all at greater risk of complication so extra precautions may need to be taken.

On 14 December 2016 the Food and Drug Administration issued a Public Safety Communication warning that "repeated or lengthy use of general anesthetic and sedation drugs during surgeries or procedures in children younger than 3 years or in pregnant women during their third trimester may affect the development of children's brains." The warning was criticized by the American College of Obstetricians and Gynecologists, which pointed out the absence of direct evidence regarding use in pregnant women and the possibility that "this warning could inappropriately dissuade providers from providing medically indicated care during pregnancy." Patient advocates noted that a randomized clinical trial would be unethical, that the mechanism of injury is well-established in animals, and that studies had shown exposure to multiple uses of anesthetic significantly increased the risk of developing learning disabilities in young children, with a hazard ratio of 2.12 (95% confidence interval, 1.26–3.54).

Recovery

The immediate time after anesthesia is called emergence. Emergence from general anesthesia or sedation requires careful monitoring because there is still a risk of complication. Nausea and vomiting are reported at 9.8% but will vary with the type of anesthetic and procedure. There is a need for airway support in 6.8%, there can be urinary retention (more common in those over 50 years of age) and hypotension in 2.7%. Hypothermia, shivering and confusion are also common in the immediate post-operative period because of the lack of muscle movement (and subsequent lack of heat production) during the procedure.

Postoperative cognitive dysfunction (also known as *POCD* and post-anesthetic confusion) is a disturbance in cognition after surgery. It may also be variably used to describe emergence delirium (immediate post-operative confusion) and early cognitive dysfunction (diminished cognitive function in the first post-operative week). Although the three entities (delirium, early POCD and long-term POCD) are separate, the presence of delirium post-operatively predicts the presence of early POCD. There does not appear to be an association between delirium or early POCD and long-term POCD. According to a recent study conducted at the David Geffen School of Medicine at UCLA, the brain navigates its way through a series of activity clusters, or "hubs" on its way back to consciousness. Dr. Andrew Hudson, an assistant professor in anesthesiology states, "Recovery from anesthesia is not simply the result of the anesthetic 'wearing off,' but also of the brain finding its way back through a maze of possible activity states to those that allow conscious experience. Put simply, the brain reboots itself."

Long-term postoperative cognitive dysfunction is a subtle deterioration in cognitive function, that can last for weeks, months, or longer. Most commonly, relatives of the person report a lack of attention, memory and loss of interest in activities previously dear to the person (such as crosswords). In a similar way, people in the workforce may report an inability to complete tasks at the same speed they could previously. There is good evidence that POCD occurs after cardiac surgery and the major reason for its occurrence is the formation of microemboli. POCD also appears to occur in non-cardiac surgery. Its causes in non-cardiac surgery are less clear but older age is a risk factor for its occurrence.

History

The first attempts at general anesthesia were probably herbal remedies administered in prehistory. Alcohol is one of the oldest known sedatives and it was used in ancient Mesopotamia thousands of years ago. The Sumerians are said to have cultivated and harvested the opium poppy (*Papaver somniferum*) in lower Mesopotamia as early as 3400 BC.

The ancient Egyptians had some surgical instruments, as well as crude analgesics and sedatives, including possibly an extract prepared from the mandrake fruit. Bian Que (Chinese: 扁鵲, Wade–Giles: *Pien Ch'iao*, c. 300 BC) was a legendary Chinese internist and surgeon who reportedly used general anesthesia for surgical procedures.

Throughout Europe, Asia, and the Americas a variety of *Solanum* species containing potent tropane alkaloids were used for anesthesia. In 13th century Italy, Theodoric Borgognoni used similar mixtures along with opiates to induce unconsciousness, and treatment with the combined alkaloids proved a mainstay of anesthesia until the nineteenth century. Local anesthetics were used in Inca civilization where shamans chewed coca leaves and performed operations on the skull while spitting into the wounds they had inflicted to anesthetize. Cocaine was later isolated and became the first effective local anesthetic. It was first used in 1859 by Karl Koller, at the suggestion of Sigmund Freud, in eye surgery in 1884. German surgeon August Bier (1861–1949) was the first to use cocaine for intrathecal anesthesia in 1898. Romanian surgeon Nicolae Racoviceanu-Piteşti (1860–1942) was the first to use opioids for intrathecal analgesia; he presented his experience in Paris in 1901.

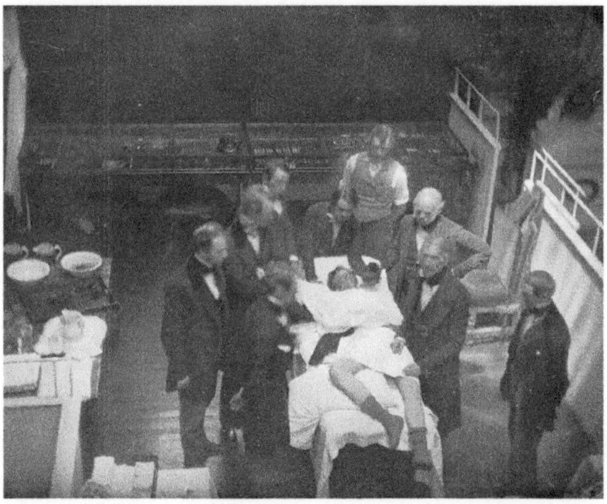

Contemporary re-enactment of Morton's 16 October 1846, ether operation; daguerrotype by Southworth & Hawes

Early Arab writings mention anesthesia by inhalation. This idea was the basis of the "soporific sponge" ("sleep sponge"), introduced by the Salerno school of medicine in the late twelfth century and by Ugo Borgognoni (1180–1258) in the thirteenth century. The sponge was promoted and described by Ugo's son and fellow surgeon, Theodoric Borgognoni (1205–1298). In this anesthetic method, a sponge was soaked in a dissolved solution of opium, mandragora, hemlock juice, and other substances. The sponge was then dried and stored; just before surgery the sponge was moistened and then held under the patient's nose. When all went well, the fumes rendered the patient unconscious.

The most famous anesthetic, ether, may have been synthesized as early as the 8th century, but it took many centuries for its anesthetic importance to be appreciated, even though the 16th century physician and polymath Paracelsus noted that chickens made to breathe it not only fell asleep but also felt no pain. By the early 19th century, ether was being used by humans, but only as a recreational drug.

Meanwhile, in 1772, English scientist Joseph Priestley discovered the gas nitrous oxide. Initially, people thought this gas to be lethal, even in small doses, like some other nitrogen oxides. However, in 1799, British chemist and inventor Humphry Davy decided to find out by experimenting on himself. To his astonishment he found that nitrous oxide made him laugh, so he nicknamed it laughing gas. Davy wrote about the potential anesthetic properties of nitrous oxide, but nobody at that time pursued the matter any further.

American physician Crawford W. Long noticed that his friends felt no pain when they injured themselves while staggering around under the influence of ether. He immediately thought of its potential in surgery. Conveniently, a participant in one of those "ether frolics", a student named James Venable, had two small tumors he wanted excised. But fearing the pain of surgery, Venable kept putting the operation off. Hence, Long suggested that he have his operation while under the influence of ether. Venable agreed, and on 30 March 1842 he underwent a painless operation. However, Long did not announce his discovery until 1849.

Horace Wells conducted the first public demonstration of the inhalational anesthetic at the Massachusetts General Hospital in Boston in 1845. However, the nitrous oxide was improperly administered and the patient cried out in pain. On 16 October 1846, Boston dentist William Thomas Green Morton gave a successful demonstration using diethyl ether to medical students at the same venue. Morton, who was unaware of Long's previous work, was invited to the Massachusetts General Hospital to demonstrate his new technique for painless surgery. After Morton had induced anesthesia, surgeon John Collins Warren removed a tumor from the neck of Edward Gilbert Abbott. This occurred in the surgical amphitheater now called the Ether Dome. The previously skeptical Warren was impressed and stated, "Gentlemen, this is no humbug." In a letter to Morton shortly thereafter, physician and writer Oliver Wendell Holmes, Sr. proposed naming the state produced "anesthesia", and the procedure an "anesthetic".

Morton at first attempted to hide the actual nature of his anesthetic substance, referring to it as Letheon. He received a US patent for his substance, but news of the successful anesthetic spread quickly by late 1846. Respected surgeons in Europe including Liston, Dieffenbach, Pirogov, and Syme quickly undertook numerous operations with ether. An American-born physician, Boott, encouraged London dentist James Robinson to perform a dental procedure on a Miss Lonsdale. This was the first case of an operator-anesthetist. On the same day, 19 December 1846, in Dumfries Royal Infirmary, Scotland, a Dr. Scott used ether for a surgical procedure. The first use of anesthesia in the Southern Hemisphere took place in Launceston, Tasmania, that same year. Drawbacks with ether such as excessive vomiting and its explosive flammability led to its replacement in England with chloroform.

Discovered in 1831 by an American physician Samuel Guthrie (1782–1848), and independently a few months later by Frenchman Eugène Soubeiran (1797–1859) and Justus von Liebig (1803–73) in Germany, chloroform was named and chemically characterised in 1834 by Jean-Baptiste Dumas (1800–84). Its anaesthetic properties were noted early in 1847 by Marie-Jean-Pierre Flourens (1794–1867). The use of chloroform in anesthesia is linked to James Young Simpson, who, in a wide-ranging study of organic compounds, found chloroform's efficacy on 4 November 1847. Its use spread quickly and gained royal approval in 1853 when John Snow gave it to Queen Victoria during the birth of Prince Leopold. Unfortunately, though free of ether's flammability and consequent explosion hazard, chloroform is not as safe pharmacologically, especially when administered by an untrained practitioner (medical students, nurses, and occasionally members of the public were often pressed into giving anesthetics at this time). This led to many deaths from the use of chloroform that (with hindsight) might have been preventable. The first fatality directly attributed to chloroform anesthesia was recorded on 28 January 1848 after the death of Hannah Greener.

John Snow of London published articles from May 1848 onwards "On Narcotism by the

Inhalation of Vapours" in the London Medical Gazette. Snow also involved himself in the production of equipment needed for the administration of inhalational anesthetics, the forerunner of today's anesthesia machines.

Of these first famous anesthetics, only nitrous oxide is still widely used today, with chloroform and ether having been replaced by safer but sometimes more expensive general anesthetics, and cocaine by more effective local anesthetics with less abuse potential.

Society and Culture

Almost all healthcare providers use anesthesia to some degree, however most health professions have their own field of specialists in the field including medicine, nursing and dentistry.

Doctors specializing in perioperative care, development of an anesthetic plan, and the administration of anesthetics are known in the US as *anesthesiologists* and in the UK, Canada, Australia, and NZ as *anaesthetists* or *anaesthesiologists*. All anesthetics in the UK, Australia, New Zealand, Hong Kong and Japan are administered by doctors. Nurse anesthetists also administer anesthesia in 109 nations. In the US, 35% of anesthetics are provided by physicians in solo practice, about 55% are provided by anesthesia care teams (ACTs) with anesthesiologists medically directing anesthesiologist assistants or certified registered nurse anesthetists (CRNAs), and about 10% are provided by CRNAs in solo practice. There can also be anesthesiologist assistants (US) or physician assistant (anaesthesia) (UK) who assist with anesthesia.

Special Populations

There are many circumstances when anesthesia needs to be altered for special circumstances due to the procedure (such as in cardiac surgery, cardiothoracic anesthesiology or neurosurgery), the patient (such as in pediatric anesthesia, geriatric, bariatric or obstetrical anesthesia) or special circumstances (such as in trauma, prehospital care, robotic surgery or extreme environments).

General Anaesthetic

A general anaesthetic is a drug that can bring about a reversible loss of consciousness. Anaesthetists, physician assistants or nurse anaesthetists administer these drugs to induce or maintain general anaesthesia to facilitate surgery. Some of these drugs are also used in lower dosages for pain management. The biological mechanisms of the action of general anaesthetics are not well understood.

Mode of Administration

Drugs given to induce general anaesthesia can be either as gases or vapours (inhalational anaesthetics), or as injections (intravenous anaesthetics or even intramuscular).

It is possible to deliver anaesthesia solely by inhalation or injection, but most commonly the two forms are combined, with an injection given to induce anaesthesia and a gas used to maintain it.

Inhalation

Inhalational anaesthetic substances are either volatile liquids or gases, and are usually delivered using an anaesthesia machine. An anaesthesia machine allows composing a mixture of oxygen, anaesthetics and ambient air, delivering it to the patient and monitoring patient and machine parameters. Liquid anaesthetics are vapourised in the machine. All of these agents share the property of being quite hydrophobic (i.e., as liquids, they are not freely miscible—or mixable—in water, and as gases they dissolve in oils better than in water).

Many compounds have been used for inhalation anaesthesia, but only a few are still in widespread use. Desflurane, isoflurane and sevoflurane are the most widely used volatile anaesthetics today. They are often combined with nitrous oxide. Older, less popular, volatile anaesthetics, include halothane, enflurane, and methoxyflurane. Researchers are also actively exploring the use of xenon as an anaesthetic.

Injection

Injectable anaesthetics are used for the induction and maintenance of a state of unconsciousness. Anaesthetists prefer to use intravenous injections, as they are faster, generally less painful and more reliable than intramuscular or subcutaneous injections. Among the most widely used drugs are:

- Propofol
- Etomidate
- Barbiturates such as methohexital and thiopentone/thiopental
- Benzodiazepines such as midazolam
- Ketamine is used in the UK as "field anaesthesia", for instance at a road traffic incidents or similar situations where an operation must be conducted at the scene or when there is not enough time to move to an operating room, while preferring other anaesthetics where conditions allow their use. It is more frequently used in the operative setting in the US.

Benzodiazepines are sedatives and are used in combinations with other general anaesthetics.

Method of Action

General anaesthetics are often defined as compounds that induce a reversible loss of consciousness in humans or loss of righting reflex in animals. Clinical definitions are also extended to include the lack of awareness to painful stimuli, sufficient to facilitate surgical applications in clinical and veterinary practice. General anaesthetics do not act as analgesics and should also not be confused with sedatives. General anaesthetics are a structurally diverse group of compounds whose mechanisms encompasses multiple biological targets involved in the control of neuronal pathways. The precise workings are the subject of some debate and ongoing research.

Lipid Theory

At the start of the 20th century, it was postulated by Overton and Meyer that general anaesthetics exert their action by acting on the plasma membrane. This was supported by evidence that the potency of the drug has a direct, positive correlation with the lipid solubility of the blood. The mechanism of action was proposed to be increased fluidity of the membrane. The interpretation of the Overton and Meyer finding has been challenged and discredited.

Ion Channels

It is postulated that general anaesthetics exert their action by the activation of inhibitory central nervous system (CNS) receptors, and the inactivation of CNS excitatory receptors. The relative roles of different receptors is still under much debate, but evidence has emerged for some targets being involved with particular anaesthetics.

Multiple anaesthetics have been found to affect the inhibitory $GABA_A$ receptor, including propofol, thiopental and isoflurane. However, xenon and nitrous oxide are thought to have no effect here. Glycine receptors have been suggested as putative target for at least the analgesic effect of inhalational anaesthetics.

2-pore-domain potassium channels, with the subfamilies TREK and TASK, have recently emerged as a potential target. These channels regulate membrane excitability, and halothane has been found to reduce neuronal firing by hyperpolarising neurons by a current similar to TASK. Knockout mouse models have provided support for TREK-1. NMDA receptors, HCN channels and some sodium channels.

Pharmacokinetics

Induction

Induction is a term that refers to the first stage of anaesthesia, Stage 1, prior to reaching a depth suitable for surgery, i.e. Stage 3. The speed of induction depends on the time taken for the drug to reach an effective concentration in the brain. Different compounds partition to different compartments of the body, such as fatty tissue, at different rates. Hence, different compounds have different rates of induction. Intravenous anaesthetics like Thiopental have been used for induction and it is common for anaesthesia to be maintained by inhalational anaesthetics such as Isoflurane. Propofol is now the most widely used intravenous general anaesthetic.

Elimination

Volatile anaesthetics are eliminated in the terminal phase via the lungs. A low blood:-gas partition coefficient is therefore necessary for quick removal of the anaesthetic. When the oil:water coefficient is high, there will be little anaesthetic in the blood, so elimination will be slow, giving a prolonged hangover effect.

Intravenous and intramuscular drugs are eliminated by metabolic pathways in the liver. It is not uncommon to produce toxic metabolites (e.g. chloroform).

General Anaesthesia

General anaesthesia or general anesthesia is a medically induced state of unconsciousness with loss of protective reflexes, resulting from the administration of one or more general anaesthetic agents. It is carried out to allow medical procedures that would otherwise be intolerably painful for the patient; or where the nature of the procedure itself precludes the patient being awake.

A variety of medications may be administered, with the overall aim of ensuring unconsciousness, amnesia, analgesia, loss of reflexes of the autonomic nervous system, and in some cases paralysis of skeletal muscles. The optimal combination of drugs for any given patient and procedure is typically selected by an anaesthetist, or another provider such as an Operating Department Practitioner, Anaesthetist Practitioner, physician assistant or nurse anaesthetist (depending on local practice), in consultation with the patient and the surgeon, dentist, or other practitioner performing the operative procedure.

History

Attempts at producing a state of general anaesthesia can be traced throughout recorded history in the writings of the ancient Sumerians, Babylonians, Assyrians, Egyptians, Greeks, Romans, Indians, and Chinese. During the Middle Ages, scientists and other scholars made significant advances in the Eastern world, while their European counterparts also made important advances.

The European Renaissance saw significant advances in anatomy and surgical technique. However, despite all this progress, surgery remained a treatment of last resort. Largely because of the associated pain, many patients chose certain death rather than undergo surgery. Although there has been a great deal of debate as to who deserves the most credit for the discovery of general anaesthesia, it is generally agreed that certain scientific discoveries in the late 18th and early 19th centuries were critical to the eventual introduction and development of modern anaesthetic techniques.

Two enormous leaps occurred in the late 19th century, which together allowed the transition to modern surgery. An appreciation of the germ theory of disease led rapidly to the development and application of antiseptic techniques in surgery. Antisepsis, which soon gave way to asepsis, reduced the overall morbidity and mortality of surgery to a far more acceptable rate than in previous eras. Concurrent with these developments were the significant advances in pharmacology and physiology which led to the development of general anaesthesia and the control of pain. On the 14 November 1804, Hanaoka Seishū, a Japanese doctor, became the first person to successfully perform surgery using general anesthesia.

In the 20th century, the safety and efficacy of general anaesthesia was improved by the routine use of tracheal intubation and other advanced airway management techniques. Significant advances in monitoring and new anaesthetic agents with improved pharmacokinetic and pharmacodynamic characteristics also contributed to this trend. Finally, standardized training programs for anaesthesiologists and nurse anaesthetists emerged during this period.

Purpose

General anaesthesia has many purposes, including:

1. Analgesia (loss of response to pain)
2. Amnesia (loss of memory)
3. Immobility (loss of motor reflexes)
4. Hypnosis (unconsciousness)
5. Paralysis (skeletal muscle relaxation)

Biochemical Mechanism of Action

The biochemical mechanism of action of general anaesthetics is not well understood. To induce unconsciousness, anaesthetics have myriad sites of action and affect the central nervous system (CNS) at multiple levels. Common areas of the central nervous system whose functions are interrupted or changed during general anesthesia include the cerebral cortex, thalamus, reticular activating system, and spinal cord. Current theories on the anaesthetized state identify not only target sites in the CNS but also neural networks and loops whose interruption is linked with unconsciousness. Potential pharmacologic targets of general anaesthetics are GABA, glutamate-activated ion channels, NMDA receptor families, voltage-gated ion channels, and glycine and serotonin receptors.

Halothane has been found to be a GABA agonist, and ketamine is an NMDA receptor antagonist.

Preanaesthetic Evaluation

Prior to a planned procedure, the anaesthetist reviews medical records and/or interviews the patient to determine the best combination of drugs and dosages and the degree to which monitoring will be required to ensure a safe and effective procedure. Key factors in this evaluation are the patient's age, body mass index, medical and surgical history, current medications, and fasting time. Thorough and accurate answering of the questions is important so that the anaesthetist can select the proper drugs and procedures. For example, a patient who consumes significant quantities of alcohol or illicit drugs could be undermedicated if s/he fails to disclose this fact, and this could lead to anaesthesia awareness or intraoperative hypertension. Commonly used medications can interact with anaesthetics, and failure to disclose such usage can increase the risk to the patient.

An important aspect of pre-anaesthetic evaluation is an assessment of the patient's airway, involving inspection of the mouth opening and visualisation of the soft tissues of the pharynx. The condition of teeth and location of dental crowns are checked, and neck flexibility and head extension are observed.

Premedication

Prior to administration of a general anaesthetic, the anaesthetist may administer one or more drugs that complement or improve the quality or safety of the anaesthetic.

One commonly used premedication is clonidine, an alpha-2 adrenergic agonist. Clonidine premedication reduces the need for anaesthetic induction agents, for volatile agents to maintain general anaesthesia, and for postoperative analgesics. It also reduces postoperative shivering, postoperative nausea and vomiting, and emergence delirium. In children, clonidine premedication is at least as effective as benzodiazepines and has less serious side effects. However, oral clonidine can take up to 45 minutes to take full effect, and drawbacks include hypotension and bradycardia.

Midazolam, a benzodiazepine characterized by a rapid onset and short duration, is effective in reducing preoperative anxiety, including separation anxiety in children. Dexmedetomidine and certain atypical antipsychotic agents may be used in uncooperative children.

Melatonin has been found to be effective as an anaesthetic premedication in both adults and children because of its hypnotic, anxiolytic, sedative, antinociceptive, and anticonvulsant properties. Unlike midazolam, melatonin does not impair psychomotor skills or hinder recovery. Recovery is more rapid after premedication with melatonin than with midazolam, and there is also a reduced incidence of post-operative agitation and delirium. Melatonin premedication also reduces the required induction dose of propofol and sodium thiopental.

Another example of anaesthetic premedication is the preoperative administration of beta adrenergic antagonists to reduce the incidence of postoperative hypertension, cardiac dysrhythmia, or myocardial infarction. Anaesthesiologists may administer an antiemetic agent such as ondansetron, droperidol, or dexamethasone to prevent post-operative nausea and vomiting, or subcutaneous heparin or enoxaparin to reduce the incidence of deep vein thrombosis. Other commonly used premedication agents include opioids such as fentanyl or sufentanil, gastrokinetic agents such as metoclopramide, and histamine antagonists such as famotidine.

Non-pharmacologic preanaesthetic interventions include playing relaxing music, massage, and reducing ambient light and noise levels in order to maintain the sleep-wake cycle. These techniques are particularly useful for children and patients with intellectual disabilities. Other options for children who refuse or cannot tolerate pharmacologic premedication include interventions by clowns and child life specialists. Minimizing sensory stimulation or distraction by video games may also help to reduce anxiety prior to or during induction of general anaesthesia.

Stages of Anaesthesia

Guedel's classification, introduced by Arthur Ernest Guedel in 1937, describes four stages of anaesthesia. Despite newer anaesthetic agents and delivery techniques, which have led to more rapid onset of—and recovery from—anaesthesia (in some cases bypassing some of the stages entirely), the principles remain.

Stage 1

> Stage 1, also known as *induction*, is the period between the administration of induction agents and loss of consciousness. During this stage, the patient progresses from analgesia without amnesia to analgesia with amnesia. Patients can carry on a conversation at this time.

Stage 2

> Stage 2, also known as the *excitement stage*, is the period following loss of consciousness and marked by excited and delirious activity. During this stage, the patient's respiration and heart rate may become irregular. In addition, there may be uncontrolled movements, vomiting, suspension of breathing, and pupillary dilation. Because the combination of spastic movements, vomiting, and irregular respiration may compromise the patient's airway, rapidly acting drugs are used to minimize time in this stage and reach Stage 3 as fast as possible.

Stage 3

In Stage 3, also known as *surgical anaesthesia*, the skeletal muscles relax, vomiting stops, respiratory depression occurs, and eye movements slow and then stop. The patient is unconscious and ready for surgery. This stage is divided into four planes:

1. The eyes roll, then become fixed;
2. Corneal and laryngeal reflexes are lost;
3. The pupils dilate and light reflex is lost;
4. Intercostal paralysis and shallow abdominal respiration occur.

Stage 4

Stage 4, also known as *overdose*, occurs when too much anaesthetic medication is given relative to the amount of surgical stimulation and the patient has severe brainstem or medullary depression, resulting in a cessation of respiration and potential cardiovascular collapse. This stage is lethal without cardiovascular and respiratory support.

Induction

General anaesthesia is usually induced in a medical facility, most commonly in an operating theatre or in a dedicated anaesthetic room adjacent to the theatre. However, it may also be conducted in other locations, such as an endoscopy suite, radiology or cardiology department, emergency department, or ambulance, or at the site of a disaster where extrication of the patient may be impossible or impractical.

Anaesthetic agents may be administered by various routes, including inhalation, injection (intravenous, intramuscular, or subcutaneous), oral, and rectal. Once they enter the circulatory system, the agents are transported to their biochemical sites of action in the central and autonomic nervous systems.

Most general anaesthetics are induced either intravenously or by inhalation. Intravenous injection works faster than inhalation, taking about 10–20 seconds to induce total unconsciousness. This minimizes the excitatory phase (Stage 2) and thus reduces complications related to the induction of anaesthesia. Commonly used intravenous induction agents include propofol, sodium thiopental, etomidate, and ketamine. Inhalational anaesthesia may be chosen when intravenous access is difficult to obtain (e.g., children), when difficulty maintaining the airway is anticipated, or when the patient prefers it. Sevoflurane is the most commonly used agent for inhalational induction, because it is less irritating to the tracheobronchial tree than other agents.

As an example sequence of induction drugs:

1. Pre-oxygenation to fill lungs with oxygen to permit a longer period of apnea during intubation without affecting blood oxygen levels
2. Lidocaine for sedation and systemic analgesia for intubation
3. Fentanyl for systemic analgesia for intubation
4. Propofol for sedation for intubation
5. Switching from oxygen to a mixture of oxygen and inhalational anesthetic

Laryngoscopy and intubation are both very stimulating and induction blunts the response to these maneuvers while simultaneously inducing a near-coma state to prevent awareness.

Physiologic Monitoring

Several monitoring technologies allow for a controlled induction of, maintenance of, and emergence from general anaesthesia.

1. Continuous electrocardiography (ECG or EKG): Electrodes are placed on the patient's skin to monitor heart rate and rhythm. This may also help the anaesthesiologist to identify early signs of heart ischaemia. Typically lead II and V5 are monitored for arrhythmias and ischemia, respectively.
2. Continuous pulse oximetry (SpO2): A device is placed, usually on a finger, to allow for early detection of a fall in a patient's haemoglobin saturation with oxygen (hypoxaemia).
3. Blood pressure monitoring: There are two methods of measuring the patient's blood pressure. The first, and most common, is non-invasive blood pressure (NIBP) monitoring. This involves placing a blood pressure cuff around the patient's arm, forearm, or leg. A machine takes blood pressure readings at regular, preset intervals throughout the surgery. The second method is invasive blood pressure (IBP) monitoring. This method is reserved for patients with significant heart or lung disease, the critically ill, and those undergoing major procedures such as cardiac or transplant surgery, or when large blood loss is expected. It involves placing a special type of plastic cannula in an artery, usually in the wrist (radial artery) or groin (femoral artery).
4. Agent concentration measurement: anaesthetic machines typically have monitors to measure the percentage of inhalational anaesthetic agents used as well as exhalation concentrations. These monitors include measuring oxygen, carbon dioxide, and inhalational anaesthetics (e.g., nitrous oxide, isoflurane).

5. Oxygen measurement: Almost all circuits have an alarm in case oxygen delivery to the patient is compromised. The alarm goes off if the fraction of inspired oxygen drops below a set threshold.

6. A circuit disconnect alarm or low pressure alarm indicates failure of the circuit to achieve a given pressure during mechanical ventilation.

7. Capnography measures the amount of carbon dioxide exhaled by the patient in percent or mmHg, allowing the anaesthesiologist to assess the adequacy of ventilation. MmHg is usually used to allow the provider to see more subtle changes.

8. Temperature measurement to discern hypothermia or fever, and to allow early detection of malignant hyperthermia.

9. Electroencephalography, entropy monitoring, or other systems may be used to verify the depth of anaesthesia. This reduces the likelihood of anesthesia awareness and of overdose.

Airway Management

Anaesthetized patients lose protective airway reflexes (such as coughing), airway patency, and sometimes a regular breathing pattern due to the effects of anaesthetics, opioids, or muscle relaxants. To maintain an open airway and regulate breathing, some form of breathing tube is inserted after the patient is unconscious. To enable mechanical ventilation, an endotracheal tube is often used, although there are alternative devices that can assist respiration, such as face masks or laryngeal mask airways. Generally, full mechanical ventilation is only used if a very deep state of general anesthesia is to be induced for a major procedure, and/or with a profoundly ill or injured patient. That said, induction of general anaesthesia usually results in apnea and requires ventillation until the drugs wear off and spontaneous breathing starts. In other words, ventilation may be required for both induction and maintenance of general anesthesia or just during the induction. However, mechanical ventilation can provide ventilatory support during spontaneous breathing to ensure adequate gas exchange.

General anaesthesia can also be induced with the patient spontaneously breathing and therefore maintaining their own oxygenation which can be beneficial in certain scenarios (e.g. difficult airway or tubeless surgery). Spontaneous ventilation has been traditionally maintained with inhalational agents (i.e. halothane or sevoflurane) which is called a gas or inhalational induction. Spontaneous ventilation can also be maintained using intravenous anaesthesia (e.g. propofol). Intravenous anaesthesia to maintain spontaneous respiration has certain advantages over inhalational agents (i.e. suppressed laryngeal reflexes) however it requires careful titration. SponTaneous Respiration using IntraVEnous anaesthesia and High-flow nasal oxygen (STRIVE Hi) is a technique that has been used in difficult and obstructed airways.

Eye Management

General anaesthesia reduces the tonic contraction of the orbicularis oculi muscle, causing lagophthalmos, or incomplete eye closure, in 59% of patients. In addition, tear production and tear-film stability are reduced, resulting in corneal epithelial drying and reduced lysosomal protection. The protection afforded by Bell's phenomenon (in which the eyeball turns upward during sleep, protecting the cornea) is also lost. Careful management is required to reduce the likelihood of eye injuries during general anaesthesia.

Neuromuscular Blockade

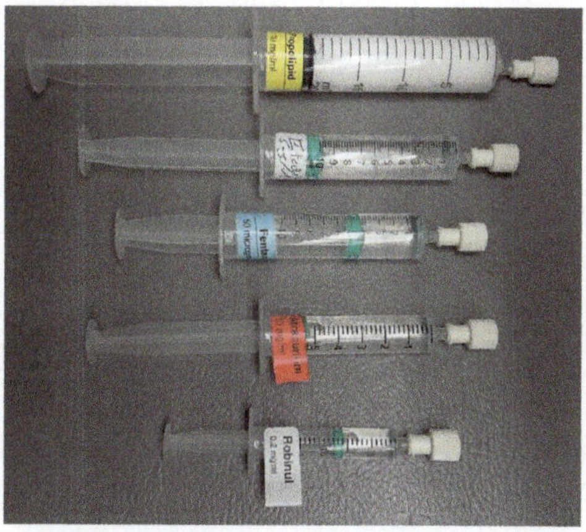

Syringes prepared with medications that are expected to be used during an operation under general anesthesia maintained by sevoflurane gas:

- Propofol, a hypnotic

- Ephedrine, in case of hypotension

- Fentanyl, for analgesia

- Atracurium, for neuromuscular block

- Glycopyrronium bromide (here under trade name Robinul), reducing secretions

Paralysis, or temporary muscle relaxation with a neuromuscular blocker, is an integral part of modern anaesthesia. The first drug used for this purpose was curare, introduced in the 1940s, which has now been superseded by drugs with fewer side effects and, generally, shorter duration of action. Muscle relaxation allows surgery within major body cavities, such as the abdomen and thorax, without the need for very deep anaesthesia, and also facilitates endotracheal intubation.

Acetylcholine, the natural neurotransmitter at the neuromuscular junction, causes muscles to contract when it is released from nerve endings. Muscle relaxants work by preventing acetylcholine from attaching to its receptor. Paralysis of the muscles of respiration—the diaphragm and intercostal muscles of the chest—requires that some form of artificial respiration be implemented. Because the muscles of the larynx are also paralysed, the airway usually needs to be protected by means of an endotracheal tube.

Paralysis is most easily monitored by means of a peripheral nerve stimulator. This device intermittently sends short electrical pulses through the skin over a peripheral nerve while the contraction of a muscle supplied by that nerve is observed. The effects of muscle relaxants are commonly reversed at the end of surgery by anticholinesterase drugs. Examples of skeletal muscle relaxants in use today are pancuronium, rocuronium, vecuronium, atracurium, mivacurium, and succinylcholine.

Maintenance

The duration of action of intravenous induction agents is generally 5 to 10 minutes, after which spontaneous recovery of consciousness will occur. In order to prolong unconsciousness for the required duration (usually the duration of surgery), anaesthesia must be maintained. This is achieved by allowing the patient to breathe a carefully controlled mixture of oxygen, nitrous oxide, and a volatile anaesthetic agent, or by administering medication (usually propofol) through an intravenous catheter. Inhaled agents are frequently supplemented by intravenous anaesthetics, such as opioids (usually fentanyl or a fentanyl derivative) and sedatives (usually propofol or midazolam). With propofol-based anaesthetics, however, supplementation by inhalation agents is not required.

At the end of surgery, administration of anaesthetic agents is discontinued. Recovery of consciousness occurs when the concentration of anaesthetic in the brain drops below a certain level (usually within 1 to 30 minutes, depending on the duration of surgery). In the 1990s, a novel method of maintaining anaesthesia was developed in Glasgow, Scotland. Called TCI (target controlled infusion), it involves using a computer-controlled syringe driver (pump) to infuse propofol throughout the duration of surgery, removing the need for a volatile anaesthetic and allowing pharmacologic principles to more precisely guide the amount of the drug used by setting the desired drug concentration. Advantages include faster recovery from anaesthesia, reduced incidence of postoperative nausea and vomiting, and absence of a trigger for malignant hyperthermia. At present, TCI is not permitted in the United States, but a syringe pump delivering a specific rate of medication is commonly used instead.

Other medications are occasionally used to treat side effects or prevent complications. They include antihypertensives to treat high blood pressure; ephedrine or phenylephrine to treat low blood pressure; salbutamol to treat asthma, laryngospasm, or bronchospasm; and epinephrine or diphenhydramine to treat allergic reactions. Glucocorticoids or antibiotics are sometimes given to prevent inflammation and infection, respectively.

Emergence

Emergence is the return to baseline physiologic function of all organ systems after the cessation of general anaesthetics. This stage may be accompanied by temporary neurologic phenomena, such as agitated emergence (acute mental confusion), aphasia (impaired production or comprehension of speech), or focal impairment in sensory or motor function. Shivering is also fairly common and can be clinically significant because it causes an increase in oxygen consumption, carbon dioxide production, cardiac output, heart rate, and systemic blood pressure. The proposed mechanism is based on the observation that the spinal cord recovers at a faster rate than the brain. This results in uninhibited spinal reflexes manifested as clonic activity (shivering). This theory is supported by the fact that doxapram, a CNS stimulant, is somewhat effective in abolishing postoperative shivering. Cardiovascular events such as increased or decreased blood pressure, rapid heart rate, or other cardiac dysrhythmias are also common during emergence from general anaesthesia, as are respiratory symptoms such as dyspnoea.

Postoperative Care

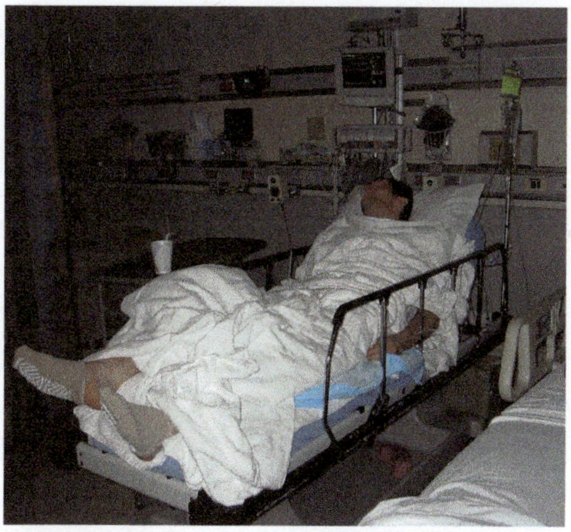

Anaesthetized patient in postoperative recovery.

Anaesthesia should conclude with a pain-free awakening and a management plan for postoperative pain relief. This may be in the form of regional analgesia or oral, transdermal, or parenteral medication. Minor surgical procedures are amenable to oral pain relief medications such as paracetamol and NSAIDs (e.g., ibuprofen). Moderate levels of pain require the addition of mild opiates such as tramadol. Major surgical procedures may require a combination of modalities to confer adequate pain relief. Parenteral methods include patient-controlled analgesia (PCA) involving a strong opiate such as morphine, fentanyl, or oxycodone. The patient presses a button to activate a syringe device and receive a preset dose or "bolus" of the drug (e.g., one milligram of morphine). The PCA device then "locks out" for a preset period to allow the drug to take effect. If the patient becomes too sleepy or sedated, he or she makes no more requests. This confers a fail-safe aspect that is lacking in continuous-infusion techniques.

Postanesthetic shivering is common. Apart from causing discomfort and exacerbating pain, shivering has been shown to increase oxygen consumption, catecholamine release, cardiac output, heart rate, blood pressure, and intraocular pressure. A number of techniques are used to reduce shivering, such as increased ambient temperature, conventional or forced warm air blankets, and warmed intravenous fluids.

In many cases, opioids used in general anaesthesia can cause postoperative ileus, even after non-abdominal surgery. Administration of a μ-opioid antagonist such as alvimopan immediately after surgery can help reduce the severity and duration of ileus.

Perioperative Mortality

Most perioperative mortality is attributable to complications from the operation, such as haemorrhage, sepsis, and failure of vital organs. Current estimates of perioperative mortality in procedures involving general anaesthesia range from one in 53 to one in 5,417. However, a 1997 Canadian retrospective review of 2,830,000 oral surgical procedures in Ontario between 1973 and 1995 reported only four deaths in cases in which an oral and maxillofacial surgeon or a dentist with specialized training in anaesthesia administered the general anaesthetic or deep sedation. The authors calculated an overall mortality rate of 1.4 per 1,000,000.

Mortality directly related to anaesthetic management is very uncommon but may be caused by pulmonary aspiration of gastric contents, asphyxiation, or anaphylaxis. These in turn may result from malfunction of anaesthesia-related equipment or, more commonly, human error. A 1978 study found that 82% of preventable anaesthesia mishaps were the result of human error. In a 1954 review of 599,548 surgical procedures at 10 hospitals in the United States between 1948 and 1952, 384 deaths were attributed to anaesthesia, for an overall mortality rate of 0.064%. In 1984, after a television programme highlighting anaesthesia mishaps aired in the United States, American anaesthesiologist Ellison C. Pierce appointed the Anesthesia Patient Safety and Risk Management Committee within the American Society of Anesthesiologists. This committee was tasked with determining and reducing the causes of anaesthesia-related morbidity and mortality. An outgrowth of this committee, the Anesthesia Patient Safety Foundation, was created in 1985 as an independent, nonprofit corporation with the goal "that no patient shall be harmed by anesthesia".

As with perioperative mortality rates in general, mortality attributable to the management of general anaesthesia is controversial. Estimates of the incidence of perioperative mortality directly attributable to anaesthesia range from one in 6,795 to one in 200,200.

Inhalational Anaesthetic

An inhalational anaesthetic is a chemical compound possessing general anaesthetic properties that can be delivered via inhalation. They are administered by anaesthetists (a term which includes anaesthesiologists, nurse anaesthetists, and anaesthesiologist assistants) through an anaesthesia mask, laryngeal mask airway or tracheal tube connected to an anaesthetic vaporiser and an anaesthetic delivery system. Agents of significant contemporary clinical interest include volatile anaesthetic agents such as isoflurane, sevoflurane and desflurane, as well as certain anaesthetic gases such as nitrous oxide and xenon.

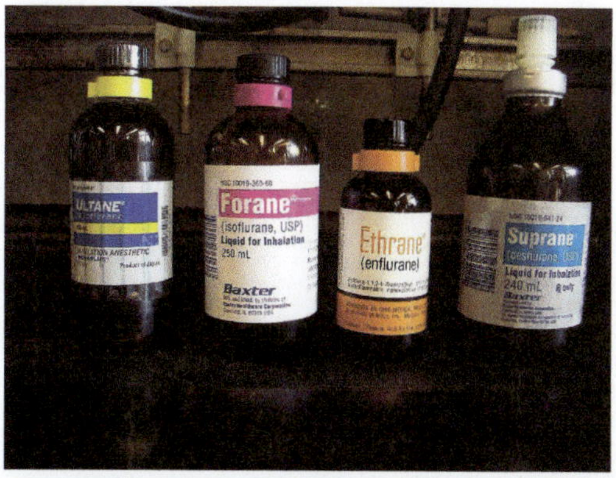

Bottles of sevoflurane, isoflurane, enflurane, and desflurane, the common fluorinated ether anaesthetics used in clinical practice. These agents are colour-coded for safety purposes. Note the special fitting for desflurane, which boils at room temperature.

List of Inhalational Anaesthetic Agents

Currently-used Agents

- Desflurane
- Isoflurane
- Nitrous oxide
- Sevoflurane
- Xenon

Previously-used Agents

Although some of these are still used in clinical practice and in research, the following anaesthetic agents are primarily of historical interest in developed countries:

- Chloroethane (ethyl chloride)
- Chloroform
- Cryofluorane
- Cyclopropane
- Diethyl ether

- Enflurane
- Ethylene
- Fluroxene
- Halothane
- Methoxyflurane (still used currently as an analgesic)
- Methoxypropane
- Trichloroethylene
- Vinyl ether

Never-marketed Agents

- Aliflurane
- Halopropane
- Norflurane
- Roflurane
- Synthane
- Teflurane

Volatile Anaesthetics

Volatile anaesthetic agents share the property of being liquid at room temperature, but evaporating easily for administration by inhalation. All of these agents share the property of being quite hydrophobic (i.e., as liquids, they are not freely miscible with water, and as gases they dissolve in oils better than in water). The ideal volatile anaesthetic agent offers smooth and reliable induction and maintenance of general anaesthesia with minimal effects on other organ systems. In addition it is odourless or pleasant to inhale; safe for all ages and in pregnancy; not metabolised; rapid in onset and offset; potent; and safe for exposure to operating room staff. It is also cheap to manufacture; easy to transport and store, with a long shelf life; easy to administer and monitor with existing equipment; stable to light, plastics, metals, rubber and soda lime; non-flammable and environmentally safe. None of the agents currently in use are ideal, although many have some of the desirable characteristics. For example, sevoflurane is pleasant to inhale and is rapid in onset and offset. It is also safe for all ages. However, it is expensive (approximately 3 to 5 times more expensive than isoflurane), and approximately half as potent as isoflurane.

Gases

Other gases or vapors which produce general anaesthesia by inhalation include nitrous oxide, cyclopropane and xenon. These are stored in gas cylinders and administered using flowmeters, rather than vaporisers. Cyclopropane is explosive and is no longer used for safety reasons, although otherwise it was found to be an excellent anaesthetic. Xenon is odourless and rapid in onset, but is expensive and requires specialized equipment to administer and monitor. Nitrous oxide, even at 80% concentration, does not quite produce surgical level anaesthesia in most persons at standard atmospheric pressure, so it must be used as an adjunct anaesthetic, along with other agents.

Hyperbaric Anaesthesia

Under hyperbaric conditions (pressures above normal atmospheric pressure), other gases such as nitrogen, and noble gases such as argon, krypton, and xenon become anaesthetics. When inhaled at high partial pressures (more than about 4 bar, encountered at depths below about 30 metres in scuba diving), nitrogen begins to act as an anaesthetic agent, causing nitrogen narcosis. However, the minimum alveolar concentration (MAC) for nitrogen is not achieved until pressures of about 20 to 30 atm (bar) are attained. Argon is slightly more than twice as anaesthetic as nitrogen per unit of partial pressure. Xenon however is a usable anaesthetic at 80% concentration and normal atmospheric pressure.

Neurological Theories of Action

The full mechanism of action of volatile anaesthetic agents is unknown and has been the subject of intense debate. "Anesthetics have been used for 160 years, and how they work is one of the great mysteries of neuroscience," says anaesthesiologist James Sonner of the University of California, San Francisco. Anaesthesia research "has been for a long time a science of untestable hypotheses," notes Neil L. Harrison of Cornell University.

"Most of the injectable anesthetics appear to act on a single molecular target," says Sonner. "It looks like inhaled anesthetics act on multiple molecular targets. That makes it a more difficult problem to pick apart."

The possibility of anaesthesia by the inert gas argon in particular (even at 10 to 15 bar) suggests that the mechanism of action of volatile anaesthetics is an effect best described by physical chemistry, and not a chemical bonding action. However, the agent may bind to a receptor with a weak interaction. A physical interaction such as swelling of nerve cell membranes from gas solution in the lipid bilayer may be operative. Notably, the gases hydrogen, helium, and neon have not been found to have anaesthetic properties at any pressure. Helium at high pressures produces nervous irritation ("anti-anaesthesia"), suggesting that the anaesthetic mechanism(s) may be operated in reverse by this gas (i.e., nerve membrane compression). Also, some halogenated ethers (such as flurothyl) also possess this "anti-anaesthetic" effect, providing further evidence for this theory.

History

The concept was first used by Paracelsus in 1540. He used sweet oil of vitriol (prepared by Valerius Cordus and named *Aether* by Frobenius): used to feed fowl: "it was taken even by chickens and they fall asleep from it for a while but awaken later without harm". Subsequently, about 40 years later, in 1581, Giambattista Delia Porta demonstrated the use of ether on humans although it was not employed for any type of surgical anesthesia.

Local Anesthesia

Local anesthesia is any technique to induce the absence of sensation in a specific part of the body, generally for the aim of inducing local analgesia, that is, local insensitivity to pain, although other local senses may be affected as well. It allows patients to undergo surgical and dental procedures with reduced pain and distress. In many situations, such as cesarean section, it is safer and therefore superior to general anesthesia. It is also used for relief of non-surgical pain and to enable diagnosis of the cause of some chronic pain conditions. Anesthetists sometimes combine both general and local anesthesia techniques.

The following terms are often used interchangeably:

- *Local anesthesia*, in a strict sense, is anesthesia of a small part of the body such as a tooth or an area of skin.
- *Regional anesthesia* is aimed at anesthetizing a larger part of the body such as a leg or arm.
- *Conduction anesthesia* encompasses a great variety of local and regional anesthetic techniques.

Medical

A local anesthetic is a drug that causes reversible local anesthesia and a loss of nociception. When it is used on specific nerve pathways (nerve block), effects such as analgesia (loss of pain sensation) and paralysis (loss of muscle power) can be achieved. Clinical local anesthetics belong to one of two classes: aminoamide and aminoester local anesthetics. Synthetic local anesthetics are structurally related to cocaine. They differ from cocaine mainly in that they have no abuse potential and do not act on the sympathoadrenergic system, i.e. they do not produce hypertension or local vasoconstriction, with the exception of Ropivacaine and Mepivacaine that do produce weak vasoconstriction.

Local anesthetics vary in their pharmacological properties and they are used in various techniques of local anesthesia such as:

- Topical anesthesia (surface)
- Infiltration
- Plexus block
- Epidural (extradural) block
- Spinal anesthesia (subarachnoid block)

Adverse effects depend on the local anesthetic agent, method, and site of administration and is discussed in depth in the local anesthetic sub-article, but overall, adverse effects can be:

1. localized prolonged anesthesia or paresthesia due to infection, hematoma, excessive fluid pressure in a confined cavity, and severing of nerves & support tissue during injection.
2. systemic reactions such as depressed CNS syndrome, allergic reaction, vasovagal episode, and cyanosis due to local anesthetic toxicity.
3. lack of anesthetic effect due to infectious pus such as an abscess.

Non-medical Local Anesthetic Techniques

Local pain management that uses other techniques than analgesic medication include:

- Transcutaneous electrical nerve stimulation, which has been found to be ineffective for lower back pain, however, it might help with diabetic neuropathy.
- Pulsed radiofrequency, neuromodulation, direct introduction of medication and nerve ablation may be used to target either the tissue structures and organ/systems responsible for persistent nociception or the nociceptors from the structures implicated as the source of chronic pain.

Local Anesthetic

A local anesthetic (LA) is a medication that causes reversible absence of pain sensation, although other senses are often affected, as well. Also, when it is used on specific nerve pathways (local anesthetic nerve block), paralysis (loss of muscle power) also can be achieved.

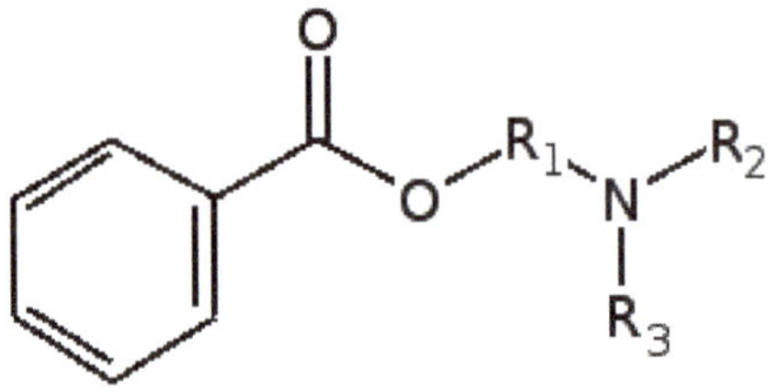

Aminoester

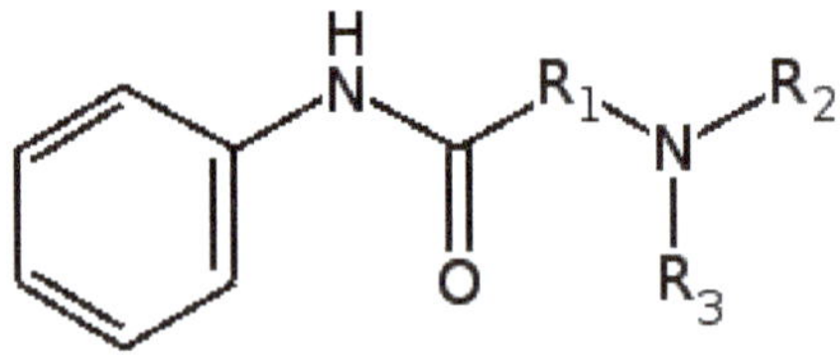

Aminoamide

Structure

Clinical LAs belong to one of two classes: aminoamide and aminoester local anesthetics. Synthetic LAs are structurally related to cocaine. They differ from cocaine mainly in that they have a very low abuse potential and do not produce hypertension or (with few exceptions) vasoconstriction.

They are used in various techniques of local anesthesia such as:

- Topical anesthesia (surface)
- Topical administration of cream, gel, ointment, liquid, or spray of anaesthetic dissolved in DMSO or other solvents/carriers for deeper absorption
- Infiltration
- Brachial plexus block
- Epidural (extradural) block
- Spinal anesthesia (subarachnoid block)
- Iontophoresis

Medical Uses

Acute Pain

Acute pain may occur due to trauma, surgery, infection, disruption of blood circulation, or many other conditions in which tissue injury occurs. In a medical setting, pain alleviation is desired when its warning function is no longer needed. Besides improving patient comfort, pain therapy can also reduce harmful physiological consequences of untreated pain.

Acute pain can often be managed using analgesics. However, conduction anesthesia may be preferable because of superior pain control and fewer side effects. For purposes of pain therapy, LA drugs are often given by repeated injection or continuous infusion through a catheter. Low doses of LA drugs can be sufficient so that muscle weakness does not occur and patients may be mobilized.

Some typical uses of conduction anesthesia for acute pain are:

- Labor pain (epidural anesthesia, pudendal nerve blocks)
- Postoperative pain (peripheral nerve blocks, epidural anesthesia)
- Trauma (peripheral nerve blocks, intravenous regional anesthesia, epidural anesthesia)

Chronic Pain

Chronic pain is a complex and often serious condition that requires diagnosis and treatment by an expert in pain medicine. LAs can be applied repeatedly or continuously for prolonged periods to relieve chronic pain, usually in combination with medication such as opioids, NSAIDs, and anticonvulsants.

Surgery

Virtually every part of the body can be anesthetized using conduction anesthesia. However, only a limited number of techniques are in common clinical use. Sometimes, conduction anesthesia is combined with general anesthesia or sedation for the patient's comfort and ease of surgery. Typical operations performed under conduction anesthesia include:

- Dentistry (surface anesthesia, infiltration anesthesia or intraligamentary anesthesia during restorative operations or extractions, and regional nerve blocks during extractions and surgeries)
- Podiatry (cutaneous, nail avulsions, matricectomy, and various other podiatric procedures)
- Eye surgery (surface anesthesia with topical anesthetics or retrobulbar block)
- ENT operations, head and neck surgery (infiltration anesthesia, field blocks, or peripheral nerve blocks, plexus anesthesia)
- Shoulder and arm surgery (plexus anesthesia or intravenous regional anesthesia)
- Heart and lung surgery (epidural anesthesia combined with general anesthesia)
- Abdominal surgery (epidural anesthesia/spinal anesthesia, often combined with general anesthesia)

- Gynecological, obstetrical, and urological operations (spinal/epidural anesthesia)
- Bone and joint surgery of the pelvis, hip, and leg (spinal/epidural anesthesia, peripheral nerve blocks, or intravenous regional anesthesia)
- Surgery of skin and peripheral blood vessels (topical anesthesia, field blocks, peripheral nerve blocks, or spinal/epidural anesthesia)

Other Uses

Topical anesthesia, in the form of lidocaine/prilocaine (EMLA) is most commonly used to enable relatively painless venipuncture (blood collection) and placement of intravenous cannulae. It may also be suitable for other kinds of punctures such as ascites drainage and amniocentesis.

Surface anesthesia also facilitates some endoscopic procedures such as bronchoscopy (visualization of the lower airways) or cystoscopy (visualization of the inner surface of the bladder).

Side Effects

Localized Side Effects

The local adverse effects of anesthetic agents include neurovascular manifestations such as prolonged anesthesia (numbness) and paresthesia (tingling, feeling of "pins and needles", or strange sensations). These are symptoms of localized nerve impairment or nerve damage. Of particular note, the use of topical anesthetics for relief of eye pain can result in severe corneal damage.

Risks

The risk of temporary or permanent nerve damage varies between different locations and types of nerve blocks.

Recovery

Permanent nerve damage after a peripheral nerve block is rare. Symptoms are likely to resolve within a few weeks. The vast majority of those affected (92%–97%) recover within four to six weeks; 99% of these people have recovered within a year. An estimated one in 5,000 to 30,000 nerve blocks results in some degree of permanent persistent nerve damage.

Symptoms may continue to improve for up to 18 months following injury.

Causes

Causes of localized symptoms include:

1. neurotoxicity due to allergenic reaction
2. excessive fluid pressure in a confined space
3. severing of nerve fibers or support tissue with the needle/catheter
4. injection-site hematoma that puts pressure on the nerve
5. injection-site infection that produces inflammatory pressure on the nerve and/or necrosis

General Side Effects

General systemic adverse effects are due to the pharmacological effects of the anesthetic agents used. The conduction of electric impulses follows a similar mechanism in peripheral nerves, the central nervous system, and the heart. The effects of local anesthetics are, therefore, not specific for the signal conduction in peripheral nerves. Side effects on the central nervous system and the heart may be severe and potentially fatal. However, toxicity usually occurs only at plasma levels which are rarely reached if proper anesthetic techniques are adhered to. High plasma levels might arise, for example, when doses intended for epidural or intrasupport tissue administration are accidentally delivered as intravascular injection.

Central Nervous System

Depending on local tissue concentrations of local anesthetics, excitatory or depressant effects on the central nervous system may occur. Initial symptoms suggest some form of central nervous system excitation such as a ringing in the ears (tinnitus), a metallic taste in the mouth, or tingling or numbness of the mouth. As the concentration rises, a relatively selective depression of inhibitory neurons results in cerebral excitation, which may lead to more advanced symptoms include motor twitching in the periphery followed by grand mal seizures. A profound depression of brain functions occurs at higher concentrations which may lead to coma, respiratory arrest, and death. Such tissue concentrations may be due to very high plasma levels after intravenous injection of a large dose. Another possibility is direct exposure of the central nervous system through the cerebrospinal fluid, i.e., overdose in spinal anesthesia or accidental injection into the subarachnoid space in epidural anesthesia.

Cardiovascular System

Cardiac toxicity associated with overdose of intravascular injection of local anesthetic is characterized by hypotension, atrioventricular conduction delay, idioventricular rhythms, and eventual cardiovascular collapse. Although all local anesthetics potentially shorten the myocardial refractory period, bupivacaine avidly blocks the cardiac sodium channels, thereby making it most likely to precipitate malignant arrhythmias. Even levobupivacaine and ropivacaine (single-enantiomer derivatives), developed to ameliorate cardiovascular side effects, still harbor the potential to disrupt cardiac function.

Hypersensitivity/allergy

Adverse reactions to local anesthetics (especially the esters) are not uncommon, but true allergy is very rare. Allergic reactions to the esters is usually due to a sensitivity to their metabolite, para-aminobenzoic acid, and does not result in cross-allergy to amides. Therefore, amides can be used as alternatives in those patients. Nonallergic reactions may resemble allergy in their manifestations. In some cases, skin tests and provocative challenge may be necessary to establish a diagnosis of allergy. Also cases of allergy to paraben derivatives occur, which are often added as preservatives to local anesthetic solutions.

Methemoglobinemia

Methemoglobinemia is a process where iron in hemoglobin is altered, reducing its oxygen-carrying capability, which produces cyanosis and symptoms of hypoxia. Benzocaine, lidocaine, and prilocaine all produce this effect, especially benzocaine. The systemic toxicity of prilocaine is comparatively low, but its metabolite, o-toluidine, is known to cause methemoglobinemia.

Treatment of Overdose: "Lipid Rescue"

This method of toxicity treatment was invented by Dr. Guy Weinberg in 1998, and had not been widely used until after the first published successful rescue in 2006. Evidence indicates Intralipid, a commonly available intravenous lipid emulsion, can be effective in treating severe cardiotoxicity secondary to local anesthetic overdose, including human case reports of successful use in this way (lipid rescue). However, the evidence at this point is still limited.

Though most reports to date have used Intralipid, a commonly available intravenous lipid emulsion, other emulsions, such as Liposyn and Medialipid, have also been shown to be effective.

Ample supporting animal evidence and human case reports show successful use in this way. In the UK, efforts have been made to publicise this use more widely and lipid rescue has now been officially promoted as a treatment by the Association of Anaesthetists of Great Britain and Ireland. One published case has been reported of successful treatment of refractory cardiac arrest in bupropion and lamotrigine overdose using lipid emulsion.

The design of a 'homemade' lipid rescue kit has been described.

Although lipid rescue mechanism of action is not completely understood, the added lipid in the blood stream may act as a sink, allowing for the removal of lipophilic toxins from affected tissues. This theory is compatible with two studies on lipid rescue for clomipramine toxicity in rabbits and with a clinical report on the use of lipid rescue in veterinary medicine to treat a puppy with moxidectin toxicosis.

Mechanism of Action

All LAs are membrane-stabilizing drugs; they reversibly decrease the rate of depolarization and repolarization of excitable membranes (like nociceptors). Though many other drugs also have membrane-stabilizing properties, not all are used as LAs (propranolol, for example). LA drugs act mainly by inhibiting sodium influx through sodium-specific ion channels in the neuronal cell membrane, in particular the so-called voltage-gated sodium channels. When the influx of sodium is interrupted, an action potential cannot arise and signal conduction is inhibited. The receptor site is thought to be located at the cytoplasmic (inner) portion of the sodium channel. Local anesthetic drugs bind more readily to sodium channels in an activated state, thus onset of neuronal blockade is faster in rapidly firing neurons. This is referred to as state-dependent blockade.

LAs are weak bases and are usually formulated as the hydrochloride salt to render them water-soluble. At a pH equal to the protonated base's pKa, the protonated (ionized) and unprotonated (unionized) forms of the molecule exist in equimolar amounts, but only the unprotonated base diffuses readily across cell membranes. Once inside the cell, the local anesthetic will be in equilibrium, with the formation of the protonated (ionized form), which does not readily pass back out of the cell. This is referred to as "ion-trapping". In the protonated form, the molecule binds to the LA binding site on the inside of the ion channel near the cytoplasmic end. Most LAs work on the internal surface of the membrane - the drug has to penetrate the cell membrane, which is achieved best in the nonionised form.

Acidosis such as caused by inflammation at a wound partly reduces the action of LAs. This is partly because most of the anesthetic is ionized and therefore unable to cross the cell membrane to reach its cytoplasmic-facing site of action on the sodium channel.

All nerve fibers are sensitive to LAs, but due to a combination of diameter and myelination, fibers have different sensitivities to LA blockade, termed differential blockade. Type B fibers (sympathetic tone) are the most sensitive followed by type C (pain), type A delta (temperature), type A gamma (proprioception), type A beta (sensory touch and pressure), and type A alpha (motor). Although type B fibers are thicker than type C fibers, they are myelinated, thus are blocked before the unmyelinated, thin C fiber.

Techniques

Local anesthetics can block almost every nerve between the peripheral nerve endings and the central nervous system. The most peripheral technique is topical anesthesia to the skin or other body surface. Small and large peripheral nerves can be anesthetized individually (peripheral nerve block) or in anatomic nerve bundles (plexus anesthesia). Spinal anesthesia and epidural anesthesia merge into the central nervous system.

Injection of LAs is often painful. A number of methods can be used to decrease this pain, including buffering of the solution with bicarbonate and warming.

Clinical techniques include:

- Surface anesthesia is the application of an LA spray, solution, or cream to the skin or a mucous membrane; the effect is short lasting and is limited to the area of contact.
- Infiltration anesthesia is infiltration of LA into the tissue to be anesthetized; surface and infiltration anesthesia are collectively topical anesthesia
- Field block is subcutaneous injection of an LA in an area bordering on the field to be anesthetized.
- Peripheral nerve block is injection of LA in the vicinity of a peripheral nerve to anesthetize that nerve's area of innervation.
- Plexus anesthesia is injection of LA in the vicinity of a nerve plexus, often inside a tissue compartment that limits the diffusion of the drug away from the intended site of action. The anesthetic effect extends to the innervation areas of several or all nerves stemming from the plexus.
- Epidural anesthesia is an LA injected into the epidural space, where it acts primarily on the spinal nerve roots; depending on the site of injection and the volume injected, the anesthetized area varies from limited areas of the abdomen or chest to large regions of the body.
- Spinal anesthesia is an LA injected into the cerebrospinal fluid, usually at the lumbar spine (in the lower back), where it acts on spinal nerve roots and part of the spinal cord; the resulting anesthesia usually extends from the legs to the abdomen or chest.
- Intravenous regional anesthesia (Bier's block) is when blood circulation of a limb is interrupted using a tourniquet (a device similar to a blood-pressure cuff), then a large volume of LA is injected into a peripheral vein. The drug fills the limb's venous system and diffuses into tissues, where peripheral nerves and nerve endings are anesthetized. The anesthetic effect is limited to the area that is excluded from blood circulation and resolves quickly once circulation is restored.
- Local anesthesia of body cavities includes intrapleural anesthesia and intra-articular anesthesia.

- Transincision (or transwound) catheter anesthesia uses a multilumen catheter inserted through an insicion or wound and aligned across it on the inside as the incision or wound is closed, providing continuous administration of local anesthetic along the incision or wound.

Types

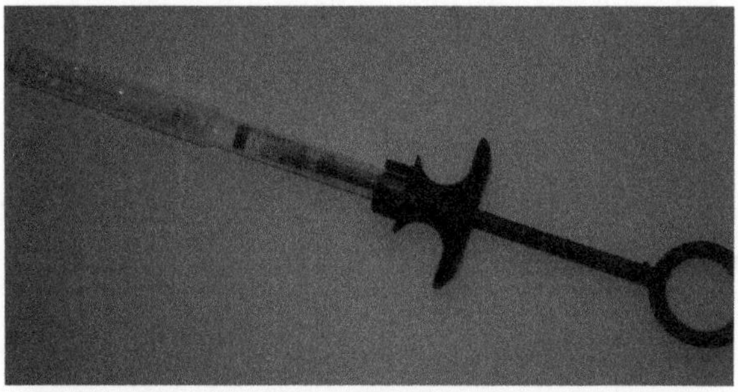

This LA system is designed to prevent needlestick injury. A cartridge of LA fits into the disposable needle, which can be locked when not in use and can be separated from the handle.

Local anesthetic solutions for injection typically consist of:

- The local anesthetic agent itself
- A vehicle, which is usually water-based or just sterile water
- Vasoconstrictor possibly
- Reducing agent (antioxidant), e.g. if epinephrine is used, then sodium metabisulfite is used as a reducing agent
- Preservative, e.g. methylparaben
- Buffer

Esters are prone to producing allergic reactions, which may necessitate the use of an amide. The names of each locally clinical anesthetic have the suffix "-caine". Most ester LAs are metabolized by pseudocholinesterase, while amide LAs are metabolized in the liver. This can be a factor in choosing an agent in patients with liver failure, although since cholinesterases are produced in the liver, physiologically (e.g. very young or very old individual) or pathologically (e.g. cirrhosis) impaired hepatic metabolism is also a consideration when using amides.

Sometimes, LAs are combined, e.g.:

- Lidocaine/prilocaine (EMLA, eutectic mixture of local anesthetic)
- Lidocaine/tetracaine (Rapydan)
- TAC

LA solutions for injection are sometimes mixed with vasoconstrictors (combination drug) to increase the duration of local anesthesia by constricting the blood vessels, thereby safely concentrating the anesthetic agent for an extended duration, as well as reducing hemorrhage. Because the vasoconstrictor temporarily reduces the rate at which the systemic circulation removes the local anesthetic from the area of the injection, the maximum doses of LAs when combined with a vasoconstrictor is higher compared to the same LA without any vasoconstrictor. Occasionally, cocaine is administered for this purpose. Examples include:

- Prilocaine hydrochloride and epinephrine (trade name Citanest Forte)
- Lidocaine, bupivacaine, and epinephrine (recommended final concentrations of 0.5, 0.25, and 0.5%, respectively)
- Iontocaine, consisting of lidocaine and epinephrine
- Septocaine (trade name Septodont), a combination of articaine and epinephrine

One combination product of this type is used topically for surface anaesthesia, TAC (5-12% tetracaine, $^1/_{2000}$ (0.05%, 500 ppm, ½ per mille) adrenaline, 4 or 10% cocaine).

Using LA with vasoconstrictor is safe in regions supplied by end arteries. The commonly held belief that LA with vasoconstrictor can cause necrosis in extremities such as the nose, ears, fingers, and toes due to constriction of end arteries], is invalidated, since no case of necrosis has been reported since the introduction of commercial lidocaine with epinephrine in 1948.

Ester Group

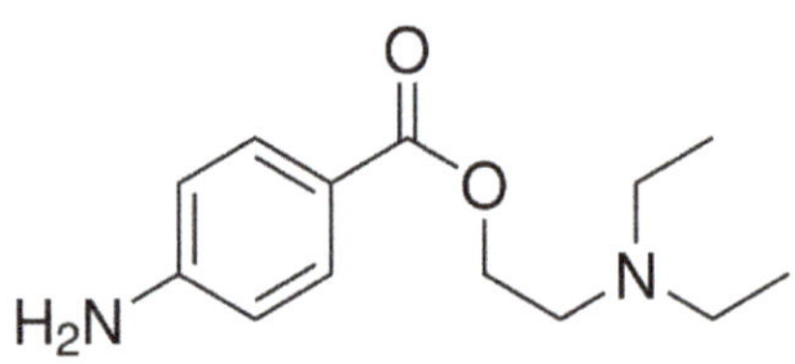

Procaine

- Benzocaine
- Chloroprocaine
- Cocaine
- Cyclomethycaine
- Dimethocaine/Larocaine
- Piperocaine

- Propoxycaine
- Procaine/Novocaine
- Proparacaine
- Tetracaine/Amethocaine

Amide Group

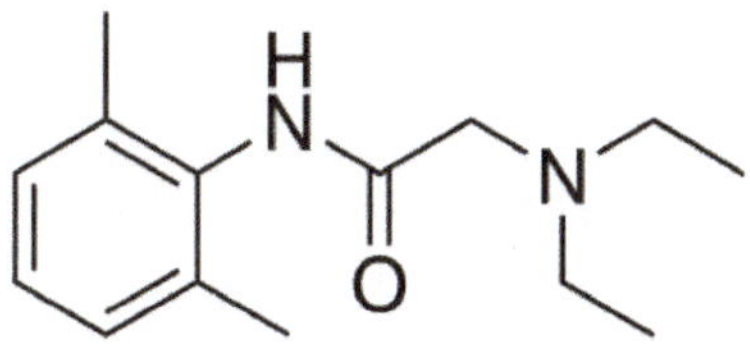

Lidocaine

- Articaine
- Bupivacaine
- Cinchocaine/Dibucaine
- Etidocaine
- Levobupivacaine
- Lidocaine/Lignocaine
- Mepivacaine
- Prilocaine
- Ropivacaine
- Trimecaine

Naturally Derived

- Saxitoxin
- Neosaxitoxin
- Tetrodotoxin
- Menthol
- Eugenol
- Cocaine

Naturally occurring local anesthetics not derived from cocaine are usually neurotoxins, and have the suffix -toxin in their names. Unlike cocaine produced local anesthetics which are intracellular in effect, saxitoxin, neosaxitoxin & tetrodotoxin bind to the extracellular side of sodium channels.

History

In Peru, the ancient Incas are believed to have used the leaves of the coca plant as a local anaesthetic in addition to its stimulant properties. It was also used for slave payment and is thought to play a role in the subsequent destruction of Incas culture when Spaniards realized the effects of chewing the coca leaves and took advantage of it. Cocaine was isolated in 1860 and first used as a local anesthetic in 1884. The search for a less toxic and less addictive substitute led to the development of the aminoester local anesthetics stovaine in 1903 and procaine in 1904. Since then, several synthetic local anesthetic drugs have been developed and put into clinical use, notably lidocaine in 1943, bupivacaine in 1957, and prilocaine in 1959.

Shortly after the first use of cocaine for topical anesthesia, blocks on peripheral nerves were described. Brachial plexus anesthesia by percutaneous injection through axillary and supraclavicular approaches was developed in the early 20th century. The search for the most effective and least traumatic approach for plexus anesthesia and peripheral nerve blocks continues to this day. In recent decades, continuous regional anesthesia using catheters and automatic pumps has evolved as a method of pain therapy.

Intravenous regional anesthesia was first described by August Bier in 1908. This technique is still in use and is remarkably safe when drugs of low systemic toxicity such as prilocaine are used.

Spinal anesthesia was first used in 1885, but not introduced into clinical practice until 1899, when August Bier subjected himself to a clinical experiment in which he observed the anesthetic effect, but also the typical side effect of postpunctural headache. Within a few years, spinal anesthesia became widely used for surgical anesthesia and was accepted as a safe and effective technique. Although atraumatic (noncutting-tip) cannulae and modern drugs are used today, the technique has otherwise changed very little over many decades.

Epidural anesthesia by a caudal approach had been known in the early 20th century, but a well-defined technique using lumbar injection was not developed until 1921, when Fidel Pagés published his article "Anestesia Metamérica". This technique was popularized in the 1930s and 1940s by Achile Mario Dogliotti. With the advent of thin, flexible catheters, continuous infusion and repeated injections have become possible, making epidural anesthesia still a highly successful technique. Beside its many uses for surgery, epidural anesthesia is particularly popular in obstetrics for the treatment of labor pain.

Spinal Anaesthesia

Spinal anaesthesia (or spinal anesthesia), also called spinal block, subarachnoid block, intradural block and intrathecal block, is a form of regional anaesthesia involving the injection of a local anaesthetic into the subarachnoid space, generally through a fine needle, usually 9 cm (3.5 in) long. For obese patients longer needles are available (12.7 cm / 5 inches). The tip of the spinal needle has a point or small bevel. Recently, pencil point needles have been made available (Whitacre, Sprotte, Gertie Marx and others).

Medical Uses

Spinal anaesthesia is a commonly used technique, either on its own or in combination with sedation or general anaesthesia. Examples of uses include:

- Orthopaedic surgery on the pelvis, hip, femur, knee, tibia, and ankle, including arthroplasty and joint replacement
- Vascular surgery on the legs
- Endovascular aortic aneurysm repair
- Hernia (inguinal or epigastric)
- Haemorrhoidectomy
- Nephrectomy and cystectomy in combination with general anaesthesia
- Transurethral resection of the prostate and transurethral resection of bladder tumours
- Hysterectomy in different techniques used
- Caesarean sections

Spinal anaesthesia is the technique of choice for Caesarean section as it avoids a general anaesthetic and the risk of failed intubation (which is approximately 1 in 250 in pregnant women). It also means the mother is conscious and the partner is able to be present at the birth of the child. The post operative analgesia from intrathecal opioids in addition to non-steroidal anti-inflammatory drugs is also good.

If surgery allows, spinal anaesthesia is very useful in patients with severe respiratory disease such as COPD as it avoids intubation and ventilation. It may also be useful in patients where anatomical abnormalities may make tracheal intubation very difficult.

Contraindications

- Non-availability of patient's consent

- Local infection or sepsis at the site of lumbar puncture
- Bleeding disorders, thrombocytopaenia, or systemic anticoagulation (secondary to an increased risk of a spinal epidural hematoma)
- Space occupying lesions of the brain
- Anatomical disorders of the spine
- Hypovolaemia e.g. following massive haemorrhage, including in obstetric patients

Risks/Complications

Can be broadly classified as immediate (on the operating table) or late (in the post-anaesthesia care unit or ward):

- Hypotension (Neurogenic shock) - Due to sympathetic nervous system blockade. Common but usually easily treated with intravenous fluid and sympathomimetic drugs such as Ephedrine, Phenylephrine or Metaraminol
- Post dural puncture head ache or post spinal head ache - Associated with the size and type of spinal needle used
- Cauda equina injury - very rare, due to the insertion site being too high
- Cardiac arrest - very rare, usually related to the underlying medical condition of the patient
- Spinal canal haematoma, with or without subsequent neurological sequelae due to compression of the spinal nerves. Urgent CT/MRI to confirm the diagnosis followed by urgent surgical decompression to avoid permanent neurological damage
- Epidural abscess, again with potential permanent neurological damage. May present as meningitis or and abscess with back pain, fever, lower limb neurological impairment and loss of bladder/bowel function. Urgent CT/MRI confirms the diagnosis followed by antibiotics and urgent surgical drainage

Technique

Regardless of the anaesthetic agent (drug) used, the desired effect is to block the transmission of afferent nerve signals from peripheral nociceptors. Sensory signals from the site are blocked, thereby eliminating pain. The degree of neuronal blockade depends on the amount and concentration of local anaesthetic used and the properties of the axon. Thin unmyelinated C-fibres associated with pain are blocked first, while thick, heavily myelinated A-alpha motor neurons are blocked moderately. Heavily myelinated, small preganglionic sympathetic fibers are blocked first. The desired result is total numbness of the area. A pressure sensation is permissible and often occurs due to incomplete blockade of the thicker A-beta mechanoreceptors. This allows surgical procedures to be performed with no painful sensation to the person undergoing the procedure.

Some sedation is sometimes provided to help the patient relax and pass the time during the procedure, but with a successful spinal anaesthetic the surgery can be performed with the patient wide awake.

Limitations

Spinal anaesthetics are typically limited to procedures involving most structures below the upper abdomen. To administer a spinal anaesthetic to higher levels may affect the ability to breathe by paralysing the intercostal respiratory muscles, or even the diaphragm in extreme cases (called a "high spinal", or a "total spinal", with which consciousness is lost), as well as the body's ability to control the heart rate via the cardiac accelerator fibres. Also, injection of spinal anaesthesia higher than the level of L1 can cause damage to the spinal cord, and is therefore usually not done.

Difference From Epidural Anesthesia

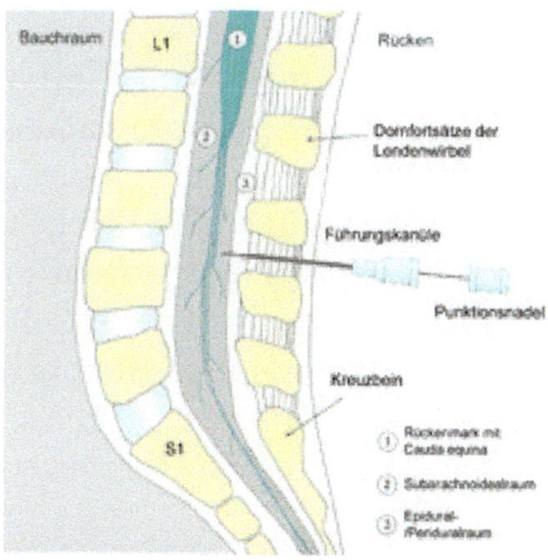

Schematic drawing showing the principles of spinal anesthesia.

Epidural anesthesia is a technique whereby a local anesthetic drug is injected through a catheter placed into the epidural space. This technique has some similarity to spinal anesthesia, both are neuraxial, and the two techniques may be easily confused with each other. Differences include:

- A spinal anaesthetic delivers drug to the intrathecal space (the CSF), and acts on the spinal cord directly. An epidural delivers drugs outside the dura (outside CSF), and has its main effect on nerve roots leaving the dura at the level of the epidural, rather than on the spinal cord itself.
- A spinal gives profound block of all motor and sensory function below the level of injection, whereas an epidural blocks a 'band' of nerve roots around the site

of injection, with normal function above, and close-to-normal function below the levels blocked.

- The injected dose for an epidural is larger, being about 10–20 mL compared to 1.5–3.5 mL in a spinal.
- In an epidural, an indwelling catheter may be placed that serves for additional injections, while a spinal is almost always a one-shot only.
- The onset of analgesia is approximately 25–30 minutes in an epidural, while it is approximately 5 minutes in a spinal.
- An epidural often does not cause as significant a neuromuscular block as a spinal, unless specific local anesthetics are also used which block motor fibres as readily as sensory nerve fibres.
- An epidural may be given at a cervical, thoracic, or lumbar site, while a spinal must be injected below L2 to avoid piercing the spinal cord.

Injected Substances

Bupivacaine (Marcaine) is the local anaesthetic most commonly used, although lidocaine (lignocaine), tetracaine, procaine, ropivacaine, levobupivicaine, prilocaine and cinchocaine may also be used. Commonly opioids are added to improve the block and provide post-operative pain relief, examples include morphine, fentanyl, diamorphine or buprenorphine. Non-opioids like clonidine may also be added to prolong the duration of analgesia (although Clonidine may cause hypotension). In the United Kingdom, since 2004 the National Institute for Health and Care Excellence recommends that spinal anaesthesia for Caesarean section is supplemented with intrathecal diamorphine and this combination is now the modal form of anaesthesia for this indication in that country. The peculiar legal status of diamorphine (heroin) means that this cannot easily occur elsewhere.

Baricity refers to the density of a substance compared to the density of human cerebrospinal fluid. Baricity is used in anaesthesia to determine the manner in which a particular drug will spread in the intrathecal space. Usually, the hyperbaric, (for example, hyperbaric bupivacaine) is chosen, as its spread can be effectively and predictably controlled by the Anaesthesiologist or Nurse Anesthetist, by tilting the patient. Hyperbaric solutions are made more dense by adding glucose to the mixture.

Baricity is one factor that determines the spread of a spinal anaesthetic but the effect of adding a solute to a solvent, i.e. solvation or dissolution, also has an effect on the spread of the spinal anaesthetic. In tetracaine spinal anaesthesia, it was discovered that the rate of onset of analgesia was faster and the maximum level of analgesia was higher with a 10% glucose solution than with a 5% glucose spinal anaesthetic solution. Also, the amount of ephedrine required was less in the patients who received the 5% glucose solution. In another study this time with 0.5% bupivacaine the mean maximum extent of sensory block was significantly higher with 8% glucose (T3.6) than with 0.83% glucose (T7.2) or 0.33% glucose (T9.5). Also the rate of onset of sensory block to T12 was fastest with solutions containing 8% glucose.

History

The first spinal analgesia was administered in 1885 by James Leonard Corning (1855–1923), a neurologist in New York. He was experimenting with cocaine on the spinal nerves of a dog when he accidentally pierced the dura mater.

The first planned spinal anaesthesia for surgery in man was administered by August Bier (1861–1949) on 16 August 1898, in Kiel, when he injected 3 ml of 0.5% cocaine solution into a 34-year-old labourer. After using it on 6 patients, he and his assistant each injected cocaine into the other's spine. They recommended it for surgeries of legs, but gave it up due to the toxicity of cocaine.

Society and Culture

Current usage of this technique is waning in the developed world, with epidural analgesia or combined spinal-epidural anaesthesia emerging as the techniques of choice where the cost of the disposable 'kit' is not an issue.

However spinal analgesia is the mainstay of anaesthesia in countries like India, Pakistan and parts of Africa, excluding the major centres. Thousands of spinal anaesthetics are administered daily in hospitals and nursing homes. At a low cost, a surgery of up to two hours duration can be performed below the umbilicus of the patient.

Anaesthetic Machine

The anaesthetic machine (UK English) or anesthesia machine (US English) or Boyle's machine is used by anaesthesiologists, nurse anaesthetists, and anaesthesiologist assistants to support the administration of anaesthesia. The most common type of anaesthetic machine in use in the developed world is the continuous-flow anaesthetic machine, which is designed to provide an accurate and continuous supply of medical gases (such as oxygen and nitrous oxide), mixed with an accurate concentration of anaesthetic vapour (such as isoflurane), and deliver this to the patient at a safe pressure and flow. Modern machines incorporate a ventilator, suction unit, and patient monitoring devices.

The original concept of Boyle's machine was invented by the British anaesthetist Henry Boyle (1875–1941) in 1917. Prior to this time, anaesthetists often carried all their equipment with them, but the development of heavy, bulky cylinder storage and increasingly elaborate airway equipment meant that this was no longer practical for most circumstances. The anaesthetic machine is usually mounted on anti-static wheels for convenient transportation.

Simpler anaesthetic apparatus may be used in special circumstances, such as the Tri-Service Apparatus, a simplified anaesthesia delivery system invented for the British armed forces, which is light and portable and may be used effectively even when no medical gases are available. This device has unidirectional valves which suck in ambient air which can be enriched with oxygen from a cylinder, with the help of a set of bellows. A large number of draw-over type of anaesthesia devices are still in use in India for administering an air-ether mixture to the patient, which can be enriched with oxygen.

Many of the early innovations in U.S. anaesthetic equipment, including the closed circuit carbon-dioxide absorber (a.k.a. the Guedel-Foregger Midget) and diffusion of such equipment to anaesthetists within the United States can be attributed to Richard von Foregger and The Foregger Company.

In dentistry a simplified version of the anaesthetic machine, without a ventilator or anaesthetic vaporiser, is referred to as a relative analgesia machine. By using this machine, the dentist can administer a mild inhalation sedation with nitrous oxide and oxygen, in order to keep his patient in a conscious state while depressing the feeling of pain.

Components of a Typical Machine

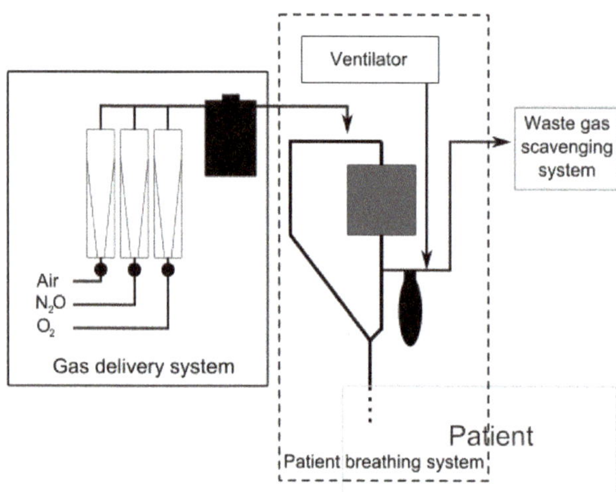

Simple schematic of an anaesthesia machine

A modern anaesthesia machine includes the following components:

- Connections to piped hospital oxygen, medical air, and nitrous oxide.

- Reserve gas cylinders of oxygen, air, and nitrous oxide attached via a specific yoke with a Bodok seal.
- A high-flow oxygen flush which provides pure oxygen at 30-75 litres/minute.
- Pressure gauges, regulators and 'pop-off' valves, to protect the machine components and patient from high-pressure gases.
- Flow meters (rotameters) for oxygen, air, and nitrous oxide, low Flow meters oxygen nitrous oxide.
- Updated vaporizers to provide accurate dosage control when using volatile anaesthetics such as isoflurane and sevoflurane.
- An integrated ventilator to properly ventilate the patient during administration of anaesthesia.
- A manual ventilation bag in combination with an Adjustable Pressure Limiting (APL) valve.
- Systems for monitoring the gases being administered to, and exhaled by the patient.
- Systems for monitoring the patient's heart rate, ECG, blood pressure and oxygen saturation, in some cases with additional options for monitoring end-tidal carbon dioxide and temperature.
- Breathing circuits, circle attachment, or a Bain's breathing system.

Safety Features of Modern Machines

Based on experience gained from analysis of mishaps, the modern anaesthetic machine incorporates several safety devices, including:

- An oxygen failure alarm (a.k.a. 'Oxygen Failure Warning Device' or OFWD). In older machines this was a pneumatic device called a Ritchie whistle which sounds when oxygen pressure is 38 psi descending. Newer machines have an electronic sensor.
- Nitrous cut-off or oxygen failure protection device, OFPD: the flow of medical nitrous-oxide is dependent on oxygen pressure. This is done at the regulator level. In essence, the nitrous-oxide regulator is a 'slave' of the oxygen regulator. i.e., if oxygen pressure is lost then the other gases can not flow past their regulator.
- Hypoxic-mixture alarms (hypoxy guards or ratio controllers) to prevent gas mixtures which contain less than 21-25% oxygen being delivered to the patient.

In modern machines it is impossible to deliver 100% nitrous oxide (or any hypoxic mixture) to the patient to breathe. Oxygen is automatically added to the fresh gas flow even if the anaesthetist should attempt to deliver 100% nitrous oxide. Ratio controllers usually operate on the pneumatic principle or are chain linked (link 25 system). Both are located on the rotameter assembly, unless electronically controlled.

- Ventilator alarms, which warn of low or high airway pressures.
- Interlocks between the vaporizers preventing inadvertent administration of more than one volatile agent concurrently.
- Alarms on all the above physiological monitors.
- The Pin Index Safety System prevents cylinders being accidentally connected to the wrong yoke.
- The NIST (Non-Interchangeable Screw Thread) or Diameter Index Safety System, DISS system for pipeline gases, which prevents piped gases from the wall being accidentally connected to the wrong inlet on the machine.
- Pipeline gas hoses have non-interchangeable Schrader valve connectors, which prevents hoses being accidentally plugged into the wrong wall socket.

The functions of the machine should be checked at the beginning of every operating list in a "cockpit-drill". Machines and associated equipment must be maintained and serviced regularly.

Older machines may lack some of the safety features and refinements present on newer machines. However, they were designed to be operated without mains electricity, using compressed gas power for the ventilator and suction apparatus. Modern machines often have battery backup, but may fail when this becomes depleted.

The modern anaesthetic machine still retains all the key working principles of the Boyle's machine (a British Oxygen Company trade name) in honour of the British anaesthetist Henry Boyle. In India, however, the trade name 'Boyle' is registered with Boyle HealthCare Pvt. Ltd., Indore MP.

A two-person pre-use check (consisting of an anaesthetist and an operating department practitioner) of the anaesthetic machine is recommended before every single case and has been shown to decrease the risk of 24-hour severe postoperative morbidity and mortality. Various regulatory and professional bodies have formulated checklists for different countries. A free transparent reality simulation of the checklist recommended by the United States Food & Drug Administration is available from the Virtual Anesthesia Machine web site after registration which is also free. Machines should be cleaned between cases as they are at considerable risk of contamination with pathogens.

Anesthesia Machine vs. Anesthesia Cart

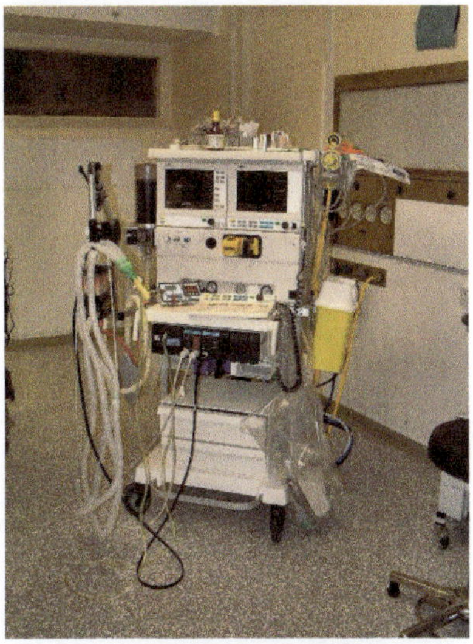

An anaesthetic machine

The Anesthesia machine contains mechanical respiratory support (ventilator) and O2 support as well as being a means for administering anesthetic gases which may be used for sedation as well as total anesthesia. An anesthesia cart holds extra IV push meds for anesthesia, sedation and reversal, extra equipment that the person giving anesthesia/ sedation might need, and the hardware for respiratory support and resuscitation.

References

- Subrahmanyam M, Mohan S (Sep 2013). "Safety Features in Anaesthesia Machine". Indian Journal of Anaesthesia. 57 (5): 472–480. doi:10.4103/0019-5049.120143. PMC 3821264. PMID 24249880
- Hademenos, George J.; Murphree, Shaun; Zahler, Kathy; Warner, Jennifer M. (2008-11-12). McGraw-Hill's PCAT. McGraw-Hill. p. 39. ISBN 978-0-07-160045-3. CS1 maint: Uses authors parameter (link)
- Ludwig Christian Stern (1889). Ebers G, ed. Papyrus Ebers (in German). 2 (1 ed.). Leipzig: Bei S. Hirzel. OCLC 14785083. Retrieved 2010-09-18
- Reddy S, Patt RB (Nov 1994). "The benzodiazepines as adjuvant analgesics". Journal of Pain and Symptom Management. 9 (8): 510–4. doi:10.1016/0885-3924(94)90112-0
- Fenster, JM (2001). "Power Struggle". Ether Day: The Strange Tale of America's Greatest Medical Discovery and the Haunted Men Who Made It. New York: HarperCollins. pp. 106–16. ISBN 978-0-06-019523-6
- McAuliffe, MS; Henry, B (2010). "Nurse anesthesia worldwide: practice, education and regulation" (PDF). Downloads. Silver Spring, Maryland: International Federation of Nurse Anesthetists. Retrieved 2012-06-13
- Chaloner EJ, Ham RJ (Aug 2001). "Amputations at the London Hospital 1852–1857". Journal of the Royal Society of Medicine. 94 (8): 409–412. PMC 1281639. PMID 11461989

- Rod Flower; Humphrey P. Rang; Maureen M. Dale; Ritter, James M. (2007). Rang & Dale's pharmacology (6th ed.). Edinburgh: Churchill Livingstone. ISBN 0-443-06911-5
- Fowler, B; Ackles, KN; Porlier, G (1985). "Effects of inert gas narcosis on behavior—a critical review.". Undersea Biomed. Res. 12 (4): 369–402. PMID 4082343. Retrieved 2008-09-21
- Deiner S, Silverstein JH (2009). "Postoperative delirium and cognitive dysfunction". British Journal of Anaesthesia. 103 (Suppl 1): i41–i46. doi:10.1093/bja/aep291
- Arnold Stern (2002). Pharmacology: PreTest self-assessment and review. New York: McGraw-Hill, Medical Pub. Division. ISBN 0-07-136704-7
- Guadagnino C (2000). "Improving anesthesia safety". Narberth, Pennsylvania: Physician's News Digest, Inc. Retrieved 8 September 2010. External link in |publisher= (help)
- Pahor, AL (1992). "Ear, nose and throat in ancient Egypt: Part I". Journal of Laryngology & Otology. 106 (8): 677–87. doi:10.1017/S0022215100120560. PMID 1402355. Retrieved 2010-09-16
- Bronwen Jean Bryant; Kathleen Mary Knights (2011). Pharmacology for Health Professionals. Elsevier Australia. pp. 273–. ISBN 978-0-7295-3929-6
- Cottrell, J.E. (2003). "Uncle Sam, Anesthesia-Related Mortality and New Directions: Uncle Sam Wants You!". ASA Newsletter. 67 (1). Retrieved 8 September 2010
- Sullivan, R (1996). "The identity and work of the ancient Egyptian surgeon". Journal of the Royal Society of Medicine. 89 (8): 467–73. PMC 1295891. PMID 8795503
- English W (2002). "Post-operative shivering, causes, prevention and treatment (letter)". Update in Anaesthesia (15). Archived from the original on 29 May 2011. Retrieved 8 September 2010
- Brill, S; Gurman, GM; Fisher, A (2003). "A history of neuraxial administration of local analgesics and opioids". European Journal of Anaesthesiology. 20 (9): 682–9. doi:10.1017/S026502150300111X. PMID 12974588

Permissions

All chapters in this book are published with permission under the Creative Commons Attribution Share Alike License or equivalent. Every chapter published in this book has been scrutinized by our experts. Their significance has been extensively debated. The topics covered herein carry significant information for a comprehensive understanding. They may even be implemented as practical applications or may be referred to as a beginning point for further studies.

We would like to thank the editorial team for lending their expertise to make the book truly unique. They have played a crucial role in the development of this book. Without their invaluable contributions this book wouldn't have been possible. They have made vital efforts to compile up to date information on the varied aspects of this subject to make this book a valuable addition to the collection of many professionals and students.

This book was conceptualized with the vision of imparting up-to-date and integrated information in this field. To ensure the same, a matchless editorial board was set up. Every individual on the board went through rigorous rounds of assessment to prove their worth. After which they invested a large part of their time researching and compiling the most relevant data for our readers.

The editorial board has been involved in producing this book since its inception. They have spent rigorous hours researching and exploring the diverse topics which have resulted in the successful publishing of this book. They have passed on their knowledge of decades through this book. To expedite this challenging task, the publisher supported the team at every step. A small team of assistant editors was also appointed to further simplify the editing procedure and attain best results for the readers.

Apart from the editorial board, the designing team has also invested a significant amount of their time in understanding the subject and creating the most relevant covers. They scrutinized every image to scout for the most suitable representation of the subject and create an appropriate cover for the book.

The publishing team has been an ardent support to the editorial, designing and production team. Their endless efforts to recruit the best for this project, has resulted in the accomplishment of this book. They are a veteran in the field of academics and their pool of knowledge is as vast as their experience in printing. Their expertise and guidance has proved useful at every step. Their uncompromising quality standards have made this book an exceptional effort. Their encouragement from time to time has been an inspiration for everyone.

The publisher and the editorial board hope that this book will prove to be a valuable piece of knowledge for students, practitioners and scholars across the globe.

Index